Your *Clinics* subscription just got better!

You can now access the FULL TEXT of this publication online at no additional cost! Activate your online subscription today and receive...

- Full text of all issues from 2002 to the present
- Photographs, tables, illustrations, and references
- Comprehensive search capabilities
- Links to MEDLINE and Elsevier journals

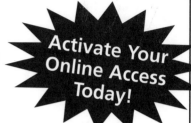

Activate Your Online Access Today!

Plus, you can also sign up for E-alerts of upcoming issues or articles that interest you, and take advantage of exclusive access to bonus features!

To activate your individual online subscription:

1. Visit our website at **www.TheClinics.com**.

2. Click on "Register" at the top of the page, and follow the instructions.

3. To activate your account, you will need your subscriber account number, which you can find on your mailing label (note: the number of digits in your subscriber account number varies from six to ten digits). See the sample below where the subscriber account number has been circled.

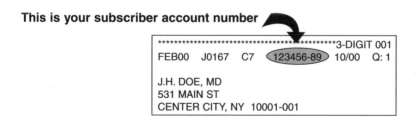

This is your subscriber account number

```
**********************************************3-DIGIT 001
FEB00  J0167  C7  ( 123456-89 )  10/00  Q: 1

J.H. DOE, MD
531 MAIN ST
CENTER CITY, NY  10001-001
```

4. That's it! Your online access to the most trusted source for clinical reviews is now available.

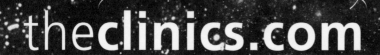

theclinics.com

ELSEVIER

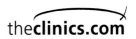

MAGNETIC RESONANCE IMAGING CLINICS
of North America

Body MR Angiography

VINCENT B. HO, MD
Guest Editor

February 2005 • Volume 13 • Number 1

SAUNDERS

An Imprint of Elsevier, Inc.
PHILADELPHIA   LONDON   TORONTO   MONTREAL   SYDNEY   TOKYO

W.B. SAUNDERS COMPANY
A Divison of Elsevier Inc.

The Curtis Center • Independence Square West • Philadelphia, Pennsylvania 19106

http://www.theclinics.com

MRI CLINICS OF NORTH AMERICA
February 2005
Editor: Barton Dudlick

Volume 13, Number 1
ISSN 1064-9689
ISBN 1-4160-2728-9

Reprints: For copies of 100 or more, of articles in this publication, please contact the Commercial Reprints Department, Elsevier Inc., 360 Park Avenue South, New York, New York 10010-1710. Tel. (212) 633-3813 Fax: (212) 462-1935 email: reprints@elsevier.com.

The ideas and opinions expressed in *Magnetic Resonance Imaging Clinics of North America* do not necessarily reflect those of the Publisher. The Publisher does not assume any responsibility for any injury and/or damage to persons or property arising out of or related to any use of the material contained in this periodical. The reader is advised to check the appropriate medical literature and the product information currently provided by the manufacturer of each drug to be administered to verify the dosage, the method and duration of administration, or contraindications. It is the responsibility of the treating physician or other health care professional, relying on independent experience and knowledge of the patient, to determine drug dosages and the best treatment for the patient. Mention of any product in this issue should not be construed as endorsement by the contributors, editors, or the Publisher of the product or manufacturers' claims.

Magnetic Resonance Imaging Clinics of North America (ISSN 1064-9689) is published quarterly by the W.B. Saunders Company. Corporate and editorial offices: The Curtis Center, Independence Square West, Philadelphia, PA 19106-3399. Accounting and circulation offices: 6277 Sea Harbor Drive, Orlando, FL 32887-4800. Periodicals postage paid at Orlando, FL 32862, and additional mailing offices. Subscription prices are $190.00 per year (US individuals), $290.00 per year (US institutions), $95.00 (US students and residents), $214.00 per year (Canadian individuals), $352.00 per year (Canadian institutions), $255.00 per year (foreign individuals), and $352.00 per year (foreign institutions). To receive student and resident rate, orders must be accompanied by name of affiliated institution, date of term, and the *signature* of program/residency coordinator on institution letter-head. Orders will be billed at individual rate until proof of status is received. Foreign air speed delivery is included in all *Clinics* subscription prices. All prices are subject to change without notice. POSTMASTER: Send address changes to *Magnetic Resonance Imaging Clinics of North America*, W.B. Saunders Company, Periodicals Fulfillment, Orlando, FL 32887-4800. **Customer Service: 1-800-654-2452 (US). From outside of the US, call 1-407-345-4000. E-mail: hhspcs@harcourt.com.**

Magnetic Resonance Imaging Clinics of North America is covered in the *RSNA Index of Imaging Literature, Index Medicus, MEDLINE*, and *EMBASE/Excerpta Medica*.

Printed in the United States of America.

GUEST EDITOR

VINCENT B. HO, MD, Vice Chair and Professor, Department of Radiology and Radiological Sciences, Uniformed Services University of the Health Sciences, Bethesda, Maryland

CONTRIBUTORS

DAVID A. BLUEMKE, MD, PhD, Associate Professor of Radiology and Medicine, Russell H. Morgan Department of Radiology and Radiologic Sciences, Johns Hopkins University, Baltimore, Maryland

TAYLOR CHUNG, MD, Associate Professor, Departments of Radiology and Pediatrics, Baylor College of Medicine; and Head, Edward B. Singleton Department of Diagnostic Imaging, Texas Children's Hospital, Houston, Texas

WILLIAM R. CORSE, DO, Director of MR Imaging, Department of Radiology, Doylestown Hospital, Doylestown, Pennsylvania; and Assistant Professor, Department of Radiology and Radiological Sciences, Uniformed Services University of the Health Sciences, Bethesda, Maryland

JULIANNA M. CZUM, MD, Assistant Professor of Radiology, Department of Radiology, Weill Medical College of Cornell University, New York, New York

MILIND Y. DESAI, MD, Clinical Fellow, National Institute of Biomedical Imaging and Bioengineering, National Institutes of Health, Bethesda; and Russell H. Morgan Department of Radiology and Radiologic Sciences, Johns Hopkins University, Baltimore, Maryland

THOMAS K.F. FOO, PhD, Chief Scientist/Manager, General Electric Healthcare Technologies, Applied Science Laboratory - East, Baltimore, Maryland

JAMES F. GLOCKNER, MD, PhD, Assistant Professor, Department of Radiology, Mayo Clinic, Rochester, Minnesota

MATHIAS GOYEN, MD, Department of Diagnostic and Interventional Radiology, University Hospital Essen, Essen, Germany

CHRISTOPH U. HERBORN, MD, Department of Diagnostic and Interventional Radiology, University Hospital Essen, Essen, Germany

VINCENT B. HO, MD, Vice Chair and Professor, Department of Radiology and Radiological Sciences, Uniformed Services University of the Health Sciences, Bethesda, Maryland

MAUREEN N. HOOD, MS, RN, RT-R, MR, Assistant Professor, Department of Radiology and Radiological Sciences, Uniformed Services University of the Health Sciences, Bethesda, Maryland

SCOTT A. KOSS, MD, Division of Cardiovascular Imaging, Department of Radiology, Brigham and Women's Hospital, Harvard Medical School, Boston, Massachusetts

RAJESH KRISHNAMURTHY, MD, Assistant Professor, Department of Radiology, Baylor College of Medicine; and Staff Radiologist, Edward B. Singleton Department of Diagnostic Imaging, Texas Children's Hospital, Houston, Texas

ELIZABETH A. McGUIGAN, MD, Assistant Professor, Department of Radiology and Radiological Sciences, Uniformed Services University of the Health Sciences; and Head, Cross-Sectional Imaging, Department of Radiology, National Naval Medical Center, Bethesda, Maryland

JAMES F.M. MEANEY, FRCR, Consultant Radiologist, Department of Diagnostic Imaging, St. James's Hospital, Dublin, Ireland

HENRIK J. MICHAELY, MD, Department of Clinical Radiology, University Hospitals, Ludwig Maximilians University-Munich, Munich, Germany

JASON A. POLZIN, PhD, Chief Engineer, MR Engineering, General Electric Healthcare Technologies, Waukesha, Wisconsin

MARTIN R. PRINCE, MD, PhD, Weill Medical College of Cornell University; and Columbia College of Physicians and Surgeons, New York, New York

MAXIMILIAN F. REISER, MD, Department of Clinical Radiology, University Hospitals, Ludwig Maximilians University-Munich, Munich, Germany

JOHANNES R. RIEGER, MD, Department of Clinical Radiology, University Hospitals, Ludwig Maximilians University-Munich, Munich, Germany

STEFAN O. SCHOENBERG, MD, Department of Clinical Radiology, University Hospitals, Ludwig Maximilians University-Munich, Munich, Germany

STEPHEN T. SEARS, MD, Staff Radiologist, Department of Radiology, National Naval Medical Center, Bethesda, Maryland

NIALL SHEEHY, MRCPI, Registrar in Radiology, Department of Diagnostic Imaging, St. James's Hospital, Dublin, Ireland

DAVID M. THOMASSON, PhD, Senior Scientist, Diagnostic Radiology Department, Clinical Center, National Institutes of Health, Bethesda, Maryland

FLORIAN M. VOGT, MD, Department of Diagnostic and Interventional Radiology, University Hospital Essen, Essen, Germany

E. KENT YUCEL, MD, Associate Professor of Radiology, Director, Division of Cardiovascular Imaging, Department of Radiology, Brigham and Women's Hospital, Harvard Medical School, Boston, Massachusetts

HONGLEI ZHANG, MD, Weill Medical College of Cornell University, New York, New York

CONTENTS

Preface   xi
Vincent B. Ho

MR Angiography Physics: an Update   1
Thomas K.F. Foo, Jason A. Polzin, and David M. Thomasson

> This article reviews the most common MR angiography techniques in clinical use and
> highlights some of the more promising emerging methods for vascular imaging.

MR Angiography Interpretation: Techniques and Pitfalls   23
James F. Glockner

> Although three-dimensional contrast-enhanced (3-D CE) MR angiography reliably pro-
> duces images of outstanding quality, there are a number of common pitfalls and artifacts
> to avoid. In addition, the widespread application of 3-D CE MR angiography has led to
> the generation of enormous amounts of data. Efficient reconstruction, display, and inter-
> pretation of MR angiography data are important, especially as the number of source
> images becomes increasingly unwieldy. This article examines the variety of reconstruc-
> tion techniques available, discusses their strengths and weaknesses, and describes com-
> mon pitfalls and artifacts in 3-D CE MR angiography.

MR Angiography of the Thoracic Aorta   41
Julianna M. Czum, William R. Corse, and Vincent B. Ho

> This article reviews MR and MR angiographic techniques for evaluation of the thoracic
> aorta and the practical issues for their implementation. Common diseases of the thoracic
> aorta will be discussed focusing of their anticipated locations, and unique morphologic
> and functional features. An understanding of both the MR techniques and pathologic
> considerations will enable the formulation of tailored imaging strategies for a thorough,
> accurate and time-efficient aortic MR evaluation.

MR Angiography of the Abdominal Aorta   65
Elizabeth A. McGuigan, Stephen T. Sears, William R. Corse, and Vincent B. Ho

> MR angiography has evolved rapidly into a robust diagnostic tool with ever-increasing
> flexibility for tailored applications for illustration of the abdominal aorta and its

branches. The abdominal indications for MR angiography continue to expand as technical advances overcome old barriers, such as motion and the time required for a high-quality diagnostic study. Three-dimensional contrast-enhanced MR angiography is now standard practice in the noninvasive evaluation of a wide range of clinical situations and is particularly well suited for imaging patients who are not able to tolerate invasive procedures or iodinated contrast material.

MR Angiography of the Peripheral Arteries   91
James F.M. Meaney and Niall Sheehy

> This article discusses the use of MR angiography in the evaluation of patients with peripheral vascular disease. A carefully tailored three-station moving table study performed on a scanner equipped with fast gradient technology in association with parallel imaging at the first two (and preferably all three) locations with bolus detection, optimized k-space filling strategies, and thigh compression to delay the onset of venous enhancement will deliver high spatial resolution images free from venous contamination in virtually all patients.

MR Venography   113
Florian M. Vogt, Christoph U. Herborn, and Mathias Goyen

> This article describes existing MR techniques for the assessment of the venous system and summarizes the clinical experience. It also discusses new applications that are likely to increase the use of MR venography in clinical practice.

MR Angiography in Patients with Renal Disease   131
Henrik J. Michaely, Stefan O. Schoenberg, Johannes R. Rieger, and
Maximilian F. Reiser

> This article discusses the advantages and applications of MR angiography in patients with renal disease.

Role of MR Angiography in Vascular Interventional Planning   153
Scott A. Koss and E. Kent Yucel

> Peripheral vascular disease is a common problem in the United States. MR angiography is a high-quality noninvasive imaging tool for planning vascular intervention. This technique has supplanted conventional angiography as the tool of choice for planning surgery and percutaneous intervention. The evolution from two-dimensional time-of-flight MR angiography to three-dimensional contrast-enhanced MR angiography has provided improved imaging quality and reduced examination times. Further advancements in the field will continue to improve this technique.

Contrast-Enhanced MR Angiography in Infants and Children   161
Taylor Chung and Rajesh Krishnamurthy

> There are challenges to performing contrast-enhanced MR angiography in infants and children because of the more rapid circulation times, higher respiratory rates, and the inability to suspend respiration. With the advances in MR techniques and stronger gradients, however, diagnostic-quality MR angiographic studies can be obtained. One

approach is to incorporate parallel-imaging techniques to achieve a time-resolved method to perform the MR angiography without the need for bolus timing. This article describes one implementation of time-resolved MR angiography with sensitivity encoding and provides clinical examples.

Atherosclerosis Imaging Using MR Imaging: Current and Emerging Applications 171
Milind Y. Desai and David A. Bluemke

Because of its high resolution, 3-D capabilities, noninvasive nature, and capacity for soft tissue characterization, MR imaging has emerged as a powerful modality to assess the process of atherosclerosis comprehensively in different arterial beds, including the coronary arteries. It holds great promise in studies involving longitudinal follow-up of plaque progression and for detection of therapeutic intervention-related changes. With the development of newer, target-specific contrast agents and molecular imaging applications, an exponential growth in its current applications is anticipated. This article reviews the technical principles and current status of in vivo MR imaging of atherosclerosis in various arterial beds and briefly discusses ongoing research in this field.

Emerging Functional MR Angiographic Techniques 181
Honglei Zhang, Julianna M. Czum, and Martin R. Prince

As the accuracy of MR angiography approaches that of conventional digital subtraction angiography, further refinements will focus on providing functional information about the normal and pathologic vasculature. In particular, PC flow measurement, time-resolved contrast-enhanced MR angiography, and detection of turbulent flow jets help to establish the functional significance of stenoses. This article discusses these emerging functional MR angiographic techniques.

Contrast Agents: Innovations and Potential Applications for Body MR Angiography 189
Maureen N. Hood and Vincent B. Ho

This article reviews some promising contrast agents and potential benefits for vascular imaging. The future of contrast-enhanced (CE) MR angiography is full of a wide variety of imaging options, from time-resolved CE MR angiography, to steady-state high-resolution imaging, to tissue-specific imaging. The growth in the complexity of contrast agent formulation for CE MR angiography and improvements in pulse sequence design are providing countless opportunities for improved applications of MR and MR angiography for the evaluation of cardiovascular disease.

Index 205

FORTHCOMING ISSUES

May 2005
MR-Guided Interventions
Jonathan S. Lewin, MD, *Guest Editor*

August 2005
Abdominal MR Imaging
Diego R. Martin, MD, PhD, *Guest Editor*

RECENT ISSUES

November 2004
Selected Topics

August 2004
Genitourinary MR Imaging
Vivian S. Lee, MD, PhD, *Guest Editor*

May 2004
MR Imaging of the Upper Extremity
Javier Beltran, MD, *Guest Editor*

GOAL STATEMENT

The goal of *Magnetic Resonance Imaging Clinics of North America* is to keep practicing radiologists and radiology residents up to date with current clinical practice in radiology by providing timely articles reviewing the state of the art in patient care.

ACCREDITATION

The *Magnetic Resonance Imaging Clinics of North America* is planned and implemented in accordance with the Essential Areas and Policies of the Accreditation Council for Continuing Medical Education (ACCME) through the joint sponsorship of the University of Virginia School of Medicine and Elsevier. The University of Virginia School of Medicine is accredited by the ACCME to provide continuing medical education for physicians.

The University of Virginia School of Medicine designates this educational activity for a maximum of 60 category 1 credits per year, 15 category 1 credits per issue, toward the AMA Physician's Recognition Award. Each physician should claim only those credits that he/she actually spent in the activity.

The American Medical Association has determined that physicians not licensed in the US who participate in this CME activity are eligible for AMA PRA category 1 credit.

Category 1 credit can be earned by reading the text material, taking the CME examination online at http://www.theclinics.com/home/cme, and completing the evaluation. After taking the test, you will be required to review any and all incorrect answers. Following completion of the test and evaluation, your credit will be awarded and you may print your certificate.

FACULTY DISCLOSURE

As a provider accredited by the Accreditation Council for Continuing Medical Education (ACCME), the Office of Continuing Medical Education of the University of Virginia School of Medicine must ensure balance, independence, objectivity, and scientific rigor in all its individually sponsored or jointly sponsored educational activities. All authors/editors participating in a sponsored activity are expected to disclose to the readers any significant financial interest or other relationship (1) with the manufacturer(s) of any commercial product(s) and/or provider(s) of commercial services discussed in an educational presentation and (2) with any commercial supporters of the activity (significant financial interest or other relationship can include such things as grants or research support, employee, consultant, stock holder, member of speakers bureau, etc.). The intent of this disclosure is not to prevent authors/editors with a significant financial or other relationship from writing an article, but rather to provide readers with information on which they can make their own judgments. It remains for the readers to determine whether the author's/editor's interest or relationships may influence the article with regard to exposition or conclusion.

The authors/editors listed below have identified no professional or financial affiliations related to their presentation:
David A. Bluemke, MD, PhD; William R. Corse, DO; Taylor Chung, MD; Julianna M. Czum, MD; Barton Dudlick, Acquisitions Editor; Mathias Goyen, MD; Christoph U. Herborn, MD; Maureen N. Hood, MS, RN, RT-R, MR; Scott A. Koss, MD; Rajesh Krishnamurthy, MD; Elizabeth A. McGuigan, MD; Henrik J. Michaely, MD; Maximilian F. Reiser, MD; Johannes R. Rieger, MD; Stefan O. Schoenberg, MD; Stephen T. Sears, MD; Niall Sheehy, MRCPI; David M. Thomasson, PhD; Florian M. Vogt, MD; and HongLei Zhang, MD.

The author listed below has identified the following professional or financial affiliation related to his presentation:
Vincent B. Ho, MD receives research support from GE Medical Systems and is on the speakers' bureau for Bracco Diagnostics.

Disclosure of Discussion of non-FDA approved uses for pharmaceutical products and/or medical devices: The University of Virginia School of Medicine, as an ACCME provider, requires that all authors identify and disclose any "off label" uses for pharmaceutical and medical device products. The University of Virginia School of Medicine recommends that each physician fully review all the available data on new products or procedures prior to instituting them with patients.

All authors who provided disclosures will not be discussing off-label uses except the following:
William R. Corse, DO will discuss the use of gadolinium for MRA.
Mathias Goyen, MD, Christoph U. Herborn, MD, and Florian M. Vogt, MD will discuss the use of paramagnetic contrast agents for MR Venography.
Vincent B. Ho, MD will discuss the use of contrast agents from MR angiography in all 3 articles. The article "Contrast Agents: Innovations and Potential Applications for Body MR Angiography" also discussed investigational contrast agents.
Maureen N. Hood, MS, RN, RT-R, MR will discuss contrast enhanced MRA.
Rajesh Krishnamurthy, MD will discuss the use of gadolinium as an intravascular contrast agent in MR angiography in pediatric patients.
Elizabeth A. McGuigan, MD will discuss the use of gadolinium agents for MRA.
Henrik J. Michaely, MD, Johannes R. Rieger, MD, Maximilian F. Reiser, MD, and Stefan O. Schoenberg, MD will discuss the measurement of renal perfusion and MRA using all contrast agents including investigational drugs.
Stephen T. Sears, MD will discuss the use of gadolinium chelates for magnetic resonance angiography.
Niall Sheehy, MRCPI will discuss the use of gadolinium contrast agents for contrast enhanced MRA not approved for use in this context by the FDA.

The authors listed below have not provided disclosure or off-label information:
Milind Y. Desai, MD; Thomas K.F. Foo, PhD; James F. Glockner, MD, PhD; James F.M. Meaney, FRCR; Jason A. Polzin, PhD; Martin R. Prince, MD, PhD; and E. Kent Yucel, MD.

TO ENROLL

To enroll in the Magnetic Resonance Imaging Clinics of North America Continuing Medical Education program, call customer service at 1-800-654-2452 or visit us online at www.theclinics.com/home/cme. The CME program is available to subscribers for an additional fee of $165.00.

ELSEVIER
SAUNDERS

Magn Reson Imaging Clin N Am
13 (2005) xi–xii

MAGNETIC
RESONANCE
IMAGING CLINICS
of North America

Preface

Body MR Angiography

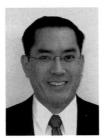

Vincent B. Ho, MD
Guest Editor

This issue of the *Magnetic Resonance Imaging Clinics of North America* is the latest of three on body MR angiography. Each issue represents a snapshot of state-of-the-art body MR angiography by recognized experts. The initial issue (December 1993) highlighted the ability of MR to illustrate vessels based on their blood flow characteristics, namely using time-of-flight and phase contrast pulse sequences. In practice, these techniques were often time-consuming and fraught with flow-related artifacts, which greatly hampered their wide clinical appeal. However, in the mid-1990s, with the introduction of contrast-enhanced (CE) MR angiography, high-performance gradient subsystems, and improved three-dimensional image processing workstations, MR angiography made a monumental leap into clinical radiology. By the second issue (May 1998), body MR angiography was well on its way into mainstream clinical radiology.

Today body MR angiography has become routine in most practices. CE MR angiography continues to be the centerpiece of most protocols but has greatly improved in its reliability and speed with further improvements in gradient performance, innovations in pulse sequence design, and the invention of specialized software/hardware combinations such as parallel imaging. These advances have dramatically improved the speed of MR data acquisition and have enabled the performance of time-resolved CE MR angiography and multistation bolus chasing.

This issue provides an update of the current state-of-the-art in body MR angiography by many of the leading experts in the field. It begins with reviews of MR angiography physics and image interpretation. This is followed by four articles that detail the techniques and common clinical applications for MR angiography within the body, namely illustration of the thoracic aorta, abdominal aorta, peripheral arteries, and venous system. In the third section, pertinent considerations for MR angiography in special populations (patients with renal disease, patients undergoing vascular intervention and pediatric patients) are addressed. The final section is comprised of several articles that describe the "new frontiers" of body MR angiography, notably atherosclerotic plaque imaging, functional MR angiography, and new contrast agents for MR angiography. This issue and the field of body MR angiography is far from complete, and it is hoped that readers may themselves invent novel methods or new applications.

I would like to take this opportunity to thank Barton Dudlick and Elsevier for the privilege of editing this special issue, their staff for the professional and efficient production of this issue, and, of course, all the contributors for not only sharing their expertise but also for expending the

1064-9689/05/$ - see front matter © 2005 Elsevier Inc. All rights reserved.
doi:10.1016/j.mric.2005.01.001

mri.theclinics.com

extra time and energy to prepare such exceptional manuscripts. I would be remiss if I did not also thank the many technologists, residents, and fellows who no doubt were responsible for generating many if not most of the images shown in this issue and the families of all involved for their understanding and patience with us during the preparation of this issue.

Vincent B. Ho, MD
Department of Radiology and Radiological Sciences
Uniformed Services University of the Health Sciences
4301 Jones Bridge Road
Bethesda, MD 20814-4799, USA

E-mail address: vho@usuhs.mil

ELSEVIER
SAUNDERS

Magn Reson Imaging Clin N Am
13 (2005) 1–22

MAGNETIC
RESONANCE
IMAGING CLINICS
of North America

MR Angiography Physics: An Update

Thomas K.F. Foo, PhD[a], Jason A. Polzin, PhD[b],
David M. Thomasson, PhD[c,*]

[a]Applied Science Laboratory - East, General Electric Healthcare Technologies,
600 N Wolfe Street, Baltimore, MD 21287, USA
[b]MR Engineering, General Electric Healthcare, 3200 N Grandview Boulevard, Waukesha, WI 53188, USA
[c]Diagnostic Radiology Department, Clinical Center, National Institutes of Health, 10 Center Drive,
Building 10-IC660, Room IC660, Bethesda, MD 20892, USA

MR imaging of blood vessels has improved significantly during the past 2 decades. The goal of MR angiography has been the accurate and reliable imaging of blood vessels. Technically, preferential vascular illustration is determined by a technique's ability to generate differences in signal intensity sufficient to distinguish blood vessels from their adjacent surrounding tissues (ie, high vessel-to-background image contrast-to-noise ratio). A wide variety of techniques is used to create such contrast. This article reviews the most common MR angiography techniques in clinical use and highlights some of the more promising emerging methods for vascular imaging.

One of the earliest methods for MR angiography is time-of-flight (TOF), which uses the signal differences between flowing blood and stationary tissues to generate vascular illustration [1–4]. With this method, stationary spins within the imaged slice are subjected to a series of radiofrequency (rf) excitation pulses with a short repetition time (TR) and high flip angle. The use of repetitive rf pulses has the effect of saturating spins in the imaged slice (ie, diminishing the signal intensity of stationary tissue resulting from a low value of the steady-state longitudinal magnetization). Stationary tissue and blood remain in a saturated or nearly saturated state. Because of the relatively long time required for recovery of their longitudinal magnetization (ie, long longitudinal relaxation [T1] times), there is insufficient time between successive rf excitation

pulses for full recovery. As shown in Fig. 1, signal intensity decreases as the number of rf excitation pulses increases. In addition, the longer the T1 relaxation time, the lower the resulting signal intensity. Tissues with shorter T1 relaxation times exhibit greater recovery of magnetization during the TR period of the sequence, yielding an overall greater signal intensity (transverse magnetization).

In the presence of through-plane flow, fresh, unsaturated spins transit through the imaged slice replacing the saturated spins and producing, on the average, a greater amount of available longitudinal magnetization between successive rf excitation pulses than for stationary tissue. This effect, known as TOF effect, is greatest if flow is traveling primarily through the imaging plane (ie, through-plane) and is equivalent to decreasing the effective T1 time in regions where there is substantial through-plane flow. The greater the flow, the greater the fraction of replenished fresh, unsaturated spins until an upper limit is reached in which all the saturated spins within the slice are replaced between rf excitation pulses. The difference in signal intensity then provides the necessary contrast mechanism to differentiate the vascular structures from the stationary background.

The TOF effect, however, depends on several factors that include TR, flow rate, slice thickness, and flip angle. TOF techniques produce the best results in vessels with fast flow and do not perform well in regions of slow flow such as aneurysms. To overcome this deficiency, longer TR times can be used but this will increase the overall scan time and introduce additional image artifacts from respiratory motion and pulsatile flow. Because of

---

* Corresponding author.
E-mail address: dt187i@nih.gov (D.M. Thomasson).

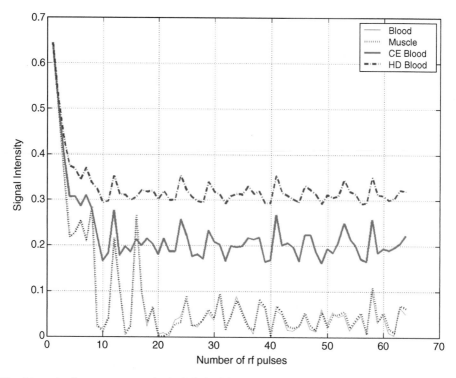

Fig. 1. Signal intensity (transverse magnetization) derived from Bloch equation simulations illustrating the differential saturation of different tissues as a function of the number of rf excitation pulses applied. Note that in the steady state, blood (T1 = 1200 milliseconds) and muscle (T1 = 800 milliseconds) are equally suppressed by a TR = 6 milliseconds, 40° flip angle, rf phase-spoiled gradient echo (SPGR) pulse sequence. CE blood at moderate (CE blood, T1 = 60 milliseconds) and high (HD blood, T1 = 30 milliseconds) concentration of contrast medium shows substantial signal difference over stationary tissues with longer T1 relaxation times.

inherently long scan times, TOF techniques do not provide satisfactory results in the abdomen (eg, in imaging the renal arteries), where respiratory motion is a persistent issue. Furthermore, in volume acquisitions in which the excitation volume is a thick slab, spins exiting the volume will have differential saturation (and lower signal intensity) than spins entering the volume, thus placing limitations on the acquisition parameters and spatial coverage for a single acquisition. Furthermore, for vessels or vascular lesions (eg, an arteriovenous malformation) with tortuous orientations within the imaging slab, there is minimal inflow refreshment, leading to poor visualization and contrast against the stationary background. Some of these volumetric limitations can be addressed by using multiple overlapping-slab techniques, also known as multiple overlapping thin slab acquisition (MOTSA) [5,6].

Contrast-enhanced (CE) MR angiography was developed to address the deficiencies in TOF MR angiography and to improve the reliability and reproducibility of MR angiographic examinations. To generate contrast between the vasculature and stationary tissue, contrast media (eg, gadolinium chelate) can be used as an intravenous bolus injection. At 1.5 T, the use of gadolinium chelate can substantially reduce the T1 time of blood from 1200 milliseconds to between 30 and 150 milliseconds, depending on the intravascular concentration of the contrast media. Because of the extracellular nature of contrast media in current use, however, normal physiologic extravascular leakage and renal extraction substantially reduce the concentration of the contrast media in blood subsequent to the first pass of the contrast bolus. Thus, to maximize the differences in signal between vessels and surrounding tissue, the MR angiography data acquisition must be timed accurately. It is critical that MR angiography imaging, specifically the acquisition of the central low-spatial-frequency k-space encoding views, coincide with the arrival of the contrast bolus in the vessel of interest [7–10].

Accurate timing of the data acquisition can also facilitate the discrimination between arteries and veins if imaging is sufficiently fast. By acquiring data during the first-pass arterial phase of the contrast bolus passage, before significant venous enhancement, the higher concentration of contrast media within the arteries will provide preferential arterial illustration. If the peak arterial phase is missed, the equivalent concentration of contrast media in the vasculature on recirculation results in arteries and veins being isointense, making differentiation between the two difficult. Spatial-saturation rf pulses to preferentially suppress arterial or venous flow are ineffective in CE MR angiography: the T1 of blood is substantially shortened because of the presence of contrast media. The shortened T1 relaxation time implies a greater recovery of magnetization after application of saturation rf pulses, making arterial–venous discrimination and background tissue suppression quite difficult.

Although there are different approaches to CE MR angiography, they involve the same basic salient features—synchronization of data acquisition to coincide with the arrival of the contrast bolus, speed of acquisition, and suppression of background tissue. Variations in the different acquisition techniques used in specific applications include single-station/location MR angiography or multistation MR angiography and the use of a single, large bolus or several smaller bolus injections of contrast agent.

Contrast-enhanced MR angiography examination

Single-scan location studies

Because the timing of the start of data acquisition is critical in CE MR angiography imaging, three basic options are available for a single-station study. If only a single scan location is required (eg, in the assessment of the renal arteries) arterial-only images with CE can be obtained using either time-resolved three-dimensional (3-D) volume acquisitions (as discussed in the next section) [11–13], automated bolus detection [14,15] or fluoroscopic triggering [16–18]. Alternately the data acquisition can be started at a time determined from an additional test-bolus study conducted before imaging [19–21]. Only the last technique requires a separate test bolus to be administered before imaging; the others can be used with the primary contrast administered as a single injection.

Timing bolus studies require the acquisition of a series of images with a temporal resolution of about 1 to 2 seconds per image or better, with magnetization preparation or saturation pulses to suppress signal from stationary tissue and non-enhanced blood. A small bolus (eg, 1–2 mL) of contrast medium is usually sufficient to evaluate the time between the start of the contrast injection and the arrival of the bolus in the imaging field-of-view (FOV). This technique can be performed on almost every MR imaging system. The operator inspects the resulting sequence of images, as shown in Fig. 2, to identify the image frame that shows the arrival of the contrast bolus. Blood without contrast is suppressed because of its long T1 relaxation time. CE blood, with a shortened T1 relaxation time, shows up distinctly as bright vascular signals over a suppressed background. Hence, the bright vascular signal indicates the arrival of the contrast bolus.

With knowledge of the image acquisition time per image, the bolus transit time can be computed and used to determine the start of data acquisition for the CE MR angiography. A standard formula can be used to calculate scan delay time but should be specific to the type of imaging sequence used. For example, a volume (3-D) imaging sequence with a sequential view acquisition order will have a different timing bolus formula than one that uses an elliptical centric view acquisition order. The difference arises from when the low-spatial-frequency data (center of k-space) are acquired with different acquisition schemes. Ideally, the central k-space views should be acquired during the peak transit of the contrast bolus. During sequential view acquisitions, the center of k-space is obtained during the middle of the acquisition. With elliptical centric (and centric) phase-ordered acquisitions, the acquisition of the center of k-space occurs at the beginning of the imaging period. The formula must be changed if the image acquisition and view acquisition order are changed.

The use of a test bolus, although straightforward, imposes the penalty of additional scan time and increases the complexity of set-up. Moreover, if the contrast dynamics change between the test bolus sequence and the imaging segment (eg, with breath-holding or with changes in the flush volume or heart rate), timing errors are introduced that lead to inaccurate synchronization of the acquisition with the arrival of the contrast bolus and suboptimal vascular image quality.

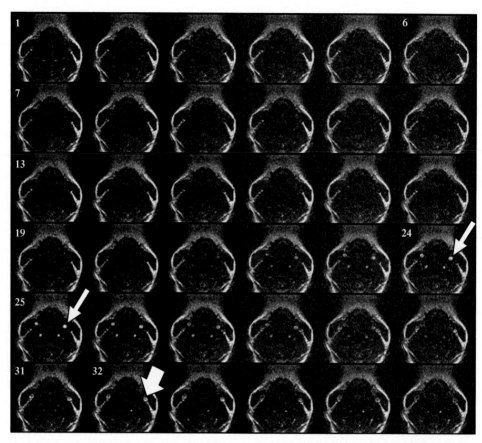

Fig. 2. Multiple image frames from a timing bolus sequence showing the arrival of a 1-mL contrast bolus. Images are from an rf phase spoiled gradient echo pulse sequence (SPGR) with saturation pulses to suppress the stationary background (including noncontrast blood). Images are acquired every 800 milliseconds. To obtain the arrival times of the contrast bolus, the operator reviews the images and selects the frame in which the contrast sufficiently fills the vessel of interest (here the carotid arteries) (*thin longer white arrow in frames 24 and 25*) and before the veins enhance (*wide shorter arrow in frame 32*). With knowledge of the scan time per image, this information is entered into a formula that determines when the operator should start scanning relative to the start of the primary bolus injection. Note that with advances in MR technology, the identical images, if displayed in real time, can be used for MR fluoroscopic triggering. When the operator observes the contrast filling the arteries, he or she can start the primary image acquisition segment. Fluoroscopic MR triggering or automated bolus detection obviates the need for a separate test bolus acquisition.

The alternative is to avoid using a test bolus altogether. The arrival of the primary contrast bolus can be monitored in real time, with data acquisition initiated in a single step. Real-time monitoring requires either operator intervention or an automated algorithm to initiate imaging. In the automated bolus arrival detection technique (SMARTPREP), real-time signal changes in a small (eg, 2 cm × 2 cm × 2 cm) voxel positioned in the descending aorta are monitored every 400 to 800 milliseconds for a rapid rise in signal intensity indicating the arrival of the contrast bolus [14,15]. As the signal intensity increases

beyond specified thresholds (determined from a baseline period to avoid false triggering from respiratory motion, Fig. 3) from the passage of the leading edge of the contrast bolus, a valid trigger is registered, and the MR imaging system automatically switches from the monitoring segment to the 3-D volume acquisition (imaging) sequence. Minimal operator intervention is needed other than positioning the monitoring volume on a scout image.

Fluoroscopic triggering involves the real-time acquisition and display of a rapid series of images with appropriate saturation rf pulses to suppress

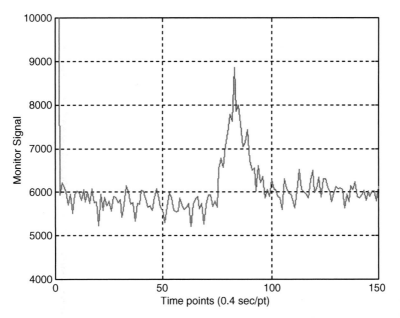

Fig. 3. Plot from a SMARTPREP monitoring sequence in response to a 1-mL test bolus similar to that in Fig. 2. The fluctuation in the baseline signal is caused by respiratory motion. In this example, the volume of interest was placed in the descending aorta. With a threshold level set at 20% of the mean baseline signal, a valid contrast arrival trigger registers as the signal intensity exceeds the 6800 level.

the stationary background and nonenhancing blood signal [16–18]. The operator watches for the arrival of the contrast test bolus by acquiring and displaying the monitored images every second (or faster). Fluoroscopic triggering requires that the operator switch manually between the monitoring and image acquisition segments, using a computer command.

The progression from a test bolus acquisition to fluoroscopic triggering has been made possible by technologic advances that allow fast image acquisition, real-time reconstruction and display, and the ability to interact with the MR imaging system in real-time with minimal lag between command and effect. Fluoroscopic MR images, similar in quality to that shown in Fig. 2 but acquired and displayed in real time, facilitate easy identification of the contrast bolus arrival. The tasks that remain for the operator are to recognize contrast arrival and to trigger manually the start of the MR angiography image acquisition.

Time-resolved MR angiography

An alternative method for timed or triggered CE MR angiography is to use a time-resolved imaging approach in which data are acquired continuously at multiple time-points during the passage of the contrast agent [12]. This approach does not require detection of the bolus either through timing or triggering and hence removes bolus detection as a source of error in the CE MR angiography scan. The time-resolved approach also provides information on bolus transit time, including differences in filling rates and retrograde flow.

The temporal resolution required to visualize the contrast bolus passage depends on the vascular bed being imaged. The carotids require an extremely high temporal resolution, approximately 1 to 2 seconds, whereas the popliteal arteries require a much lower temporal resolution, approximately 10 seconds. Before the introduction of high-speed imaging gradients in the late 1990s, it was not possible to acquire an entire 3-D dataset with adequate temporal resolution to visualize the passage of the contrast bolus.

Dynamic two-dimensional (2-D) thick-slice projection imaging can be used along with complex mask subtraction to remove the background signal [22,23]. This approach has adequate temporal resolution but provides only in-plane 2-D projectional viewing of vessels. Early investigators realized that the image contrast is principally determined by the low spatial frequency (central k-space lines) and applied techniques that sampled the central k-space lines more frequently than the outer k-space lines, thereby improving the effective temporal resolution.

The first such approach, by van Vaals et al [24], was termed "keyhole" imaging and was applied to 2-D imaging. This method acquires a full set of k-space data before the bolus injection. Then, after injection, a predetermined number of central k-space lines are repeatedly acquired. For each time-point the central k-space data are combined with the outer k-space data from the precontrast acquisition, and the result is reconstructed. The combined data set has the temporal characteristics of the low spatial frequency but preserves most of the edge detail seen in the precontrast images. This approach works well for showing uptake of contrast media into a specific organs such as the kidney but does not work as well for angiography. For angiographic applications, in which the vessels are quite small and are not well depicted on the precontrast images, significant high-spatial-frequency content is missing in the CE images. To visualize small vessels, a greater fraction of the center of k-space must be acquired (repeatedly). Furthermore, the image quality can be improved by acquiring the high-spatial-frequency data at the end of the acquisition series. This technique ensures that the resulting images have some signal enhancement of the vascular high-spatial-frequency (edge detail) data.

The TRICKS method is a 3-D–based approach that employs the following techniques to improve spatial and temporal resolution:

1. Variable rate k-space sampling. (The low spatial frequencies are sampled more often then high spatial frequencies, but, unlike the keyhole approach, all spatial frequencies are updated at some rate.)
2. Interpolation of data to improve the effective temporal resolution.
3. Zero-filling in the slice direction.

In the original TRICKS approach, k-space was divided into four equal-sized blocks along the phase-encoding (k_y) direction. When the total number of k-space lines is 128, the phase-encoding lines are divided as follows:

- A: 40–64, 65–80
- B: 33–48, 81–96
- C: 17–32, 97–112
- D: 1–16,113–128

where the center of k-space is between lines 64 and 65. For each phase encoding within the block, all slice encodings are also included. In other words, this scheme divides the data only along the phase-encoding direction.

In a conventional multiphase 3-D acquisition, the blocks would be acquired as follows:

D-C-B-A-D-C-B-A-D-C-B-A-D-C-B-A-D-C-B-A-D-C-B-A-D-C-B-A
—1   —-2   —-3   —-4   —-5   —-6   —-7

Improvements in time-resolved imaging: time-resolved imaging of contrast kinetics

Time-resolved imaging of contrast kinetics (TRICKS) was introduced in 1996 and addresses

The first row is the order in which the blocks are acquired, and the second row corresponds to the relative time-points for the reconstructed phases from 1 to 7. The corresponding TRICKS acquisition would be

D-C-B-A-D-A-C-A-B-A-D-A-C-A-B-A-D-A-C-A-B-A-D-A-C-A-B-A
—1 -2 -3 -4 -5 -6 -7 -8 -9 -0 -1 -2 -3 -4 -5 -6 -7 -8 -9 -0 -1 -2 -3 -4 -5

some of the shortcomings of the keyhole approach [25]. It is based on an earlier generalized keyhole approach called block regional interpolation scheme for k-space (BRISK) developed primarily for cardiac imaging [26]. In BRISK, the k-space acquisition is determined by the spatial and temporal characteristics of the object being imaged, so dynamic changes in small objects containing primarily high spatial frequencies are also visualized.

The first row is the order in which the blocks are acquired. Note that a complete 3-D acquisition is acquired first, followed by the TRICKS sampling scheme in which the A block is sampled every other block. The second row corresponds to the reconstructed phases in which a new phase is reconstructed for every block. This scheme includes a new reconstructed phase every time the A block is acquired as well as an intermediate phase between the acquisition of each A block. This scheme is made possible by linear interpolation of each block from the nearest two blocks of the same type (ie, A, B, C, or D). If data are acquired in the following order:

fact sampled less frequently than in a conventional acquisition. The time between samples of the non-A regions is, in fact, 50% longer than in a conventional 3-D acquisition.

$$\ldots D1\text{-}A1\text{-}C1\text{-}A2\text{-}B1\text{-}A3\text{-}D2\text{-}A4\text{-}C2\text{-}A5\text{-}B2 \ldots X$$

A1 would be the first acquisition of block A, and B2 would be the second acquisition of block B. If reconstruction data for time-point X are desired, the blocks AX, BX, CX, and DX can be calculated as follows:

$$AX = A3$$

$$BX = (5'B1 + 1'B2)/6$$

$$CX = (3'C1 + 3'C2)/6$$

$$DX = (1'D1 + 5'D2)/6$$

This scheme shows that the A region is sampled twice as often in TRICKS as it is in a conventional 3-D acquisition. The use of linear interpolation results in an additional increase by a factor of two in the reconstructed (or effective) temporal resolution, resulting in a fourfold total increase. Note that the increased temporal sampling rate of the A region means that the B, C, and D regions are in

The original TRICKS method divided the blocks along the phase-encoding direction. Along the slice-encoding direction, both central and outer k-space values were acquired in each block. Therefore the A region, which is supposed to contain only the central k-space values, also contains the outer slice-encoding values. An important improvement combined the benefits of elliptical centric view ordering [27,28] with TRICKS [29]. In elliptical centric view ordering, each encoding step (phase and slice) is sorted based on the distance from the center of k-space. The sorted k-space values are acquired in order, from closest to the center to the farthest from the center. This method provides a true centric weighting for 3-D acquisitions and is used commonly in single-phase CE imaging to provide optimal arterial vessel contrast without venous contamination.

In elliptical centric (EC)-TRICKS, the sorted encoding steps are divided evenly into blocks, as

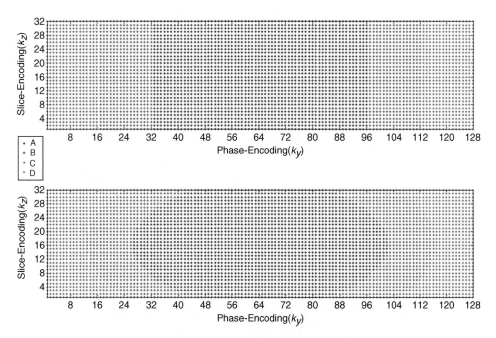

Fig. 4. Comparison of the k-space partitioning for a conventional TRICKS acquisition (*top*) and an EC-TRICKS acquisition (*bottom*) with four blocks (A-B-C-D) using 128 phase-encoding steps, 32 slice-encoding steps, a 42-cm FOV, and a 5-mm slice thickness.

in the original TRICKS approach. Fig. 4 shows the k-space partitioning for a conventional TRICKS acquisition and an EC-TRICKS acquisition with four blocks (A-B-C-D) using 128 phase-encoding steps, 32 slice-encoding steps, a 42-cm FOV, and a 5-mm slice thickness. The top plot shows the k-space partitioning for the original TRICKS approach in which the central A region is shown in blue. In this case, all slice encodings for phase-encoding steps 49 through 80 are acquired in the block A. The second plot shows the phase-encoding and slice-encoding steps for slice EC-TRICKS. Here, the central A region contains an ellipse of k-space values containing a wider range of phase-encoding values and a smaller range of slice-encoding values. Fig. 5 shows four temporal phases from an EC-TRICKS study of the pedal arch. The high temporal resolution and good in-plane resolution provide good visualization of the arterial phase. Some interpolation artifacts are seen on the second phase before the contrast bolus has fully arrived. These artifacts are a result of k-space interpolation from time-frames where the contrast bolus has not yet arrived.

Improvements in time-resolved imaging: fast three-dimensional imaging

Schoenberg et al [12] demonstrated that high-performance imaging gradients along with high bandwidth receivers are capable of acquiring time-resolved 3-D acquisitions without any k-space interpolation or keyhole approaches. In this work, a gradient system capable of reaching 25 mT/m in 300 microseconds along with a partially self-refocusing rf pulse, asymmetric (5/8) readout with 160 points, and a receiver bandwidth of 650 Hz/pixel were used to reduce the repetition time to 3.2 milliseconds. In addition, by using an asymmetric sampling factor of 5/8 along the phase- and slice-encoding direction and acquiring 90 and 22 encodings, respectively, the total acquisition time per phase was only 6.4 seconds. Zero-filling was used to interpolate the acquisition to a matrix size of $256 \times 135 \times 44$. This approach is advantageous for abdominal imaging where the breath-hold duration becomes a concern.

This approach has continued to evolve as the gradient and data acquisition platforms have continued to improve. In recent work by Goyen

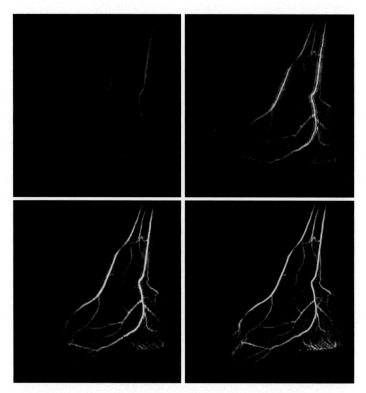

Fig. 5. Four temporal phases from an EC-TRICKS (time-resolved) study of the pedal arch. These results are the MIP images after mask subtraction. (Courtesy of J Glockner, MD, Mayo Clinic, Rochester, MN.)

et al [30], the TR was further reduced to 1.64 milliseconds using a receiver bandwidth of 1295 Hz/pixel and gradients capable of achieving a maximum amplitude of 40 mT/m in 200 microseconds. The acquired matrix size was 160 readout points × 88 phase encodings × 25 slice encodings. Zero-filling was used to interpolate the reconstruction to 256 × 140 × 40. The total scan time per phase was 3.74 seconds. (Note that zero-filling produces images with notable blurring because a high spatial frequency data component is missing.)

In this study, patients with suspected pulmonary embolism were injected with 20 mL of contrast agent. After a delay of 8 seconds, they were asked to hold their breath and were scanned for a total of 20 seconds (five phases). The researchers found that all eight patients were able to maintain the breath-hold for at least the first 8 seconds of the scan, but only two were able to hold their breath for the entire duration of the scan. Although the spatial resolution of this approach may not be as good as with the TRICKS approach, the short scan time per volume is preferred for acquisitions in which a breath-hold is required.

Projection reconstruction

In projection reconstruction (PR), data are sampled along radial lines through the center of k-space at different azimuthal angles. These lines are equivalent to the Fourier transform of a projection through the object at the same angle. A fully sampled PR acquisition requires approximately 57% more projections than the corresponding spin warp methods. Reducing the number of projections does not result in spatial aliasing or a loss of resolution but instead produces streak artifacts from undersampling in the azimuthal direction. For MR angiography when the vessels of interest are sparsely located throughout the FOV, these streak artifacts do not degrade the image quality as severely as in anatomic imaging where the structures are more closely spaced.

The original method by Peters et al [31] used a 3-D acquisition with PR in two directions (in-plane) and conventional Fourier encoding along the slice direction. Data could be acquired with the slice encodings as the inner loop Z-encoding inside projections (ZIPR) or as the outer loop, projections inside Z-encoding (PRIZE). In PRIZE only a single time-frame is acquired, with the central slice encoding timed to the peak arterial contrast. In ZIPR, by rotating the projections through several

revolutions and using sliding window reconstruction, multiple time-frames can be reconstructed.

One application for ZPIR is in fast pulmonary imaging when short breath-hold durations are desired (eg, to rule out pulmonary embolism). Fig. 6 compares a PRIZE acquisition with 170 projections and a conventional 3-D acquisition with 128 phase encodings. Both acquisitions had 16 slice encodings, a 17-second scan time, and were interpolated to a 512 × 512 × 32 reconstruction matrix. In this example, the PR acquisition has better resolution but exhibits a loss in signal-to-noise ratio (S/N).

Vigen et al [32] later extended this work to use a TRICKS acquisition along the slice-encoding

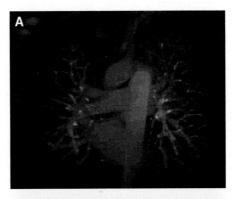

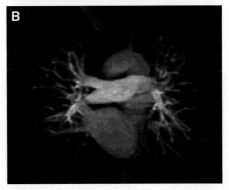

Fig. 6. Comparison of (*A*) PRIZE acquisition with 170 projections and (*B*) a conventional 3-D acquisition with 128 phase encodings. Both acquisitions had 16 slice encodings, a 17-second scan time, and were interpolated to a 512 × 512 × 32 reconstruction matrix. Note that in A the spatial resolution is improved with the PR acquisition, but a loss in S/N is noted with the PR acquisition. (*From* Peters DC, Korosec FR, Grist TM, et al. Undersampled projection reconstruction applied to MR angiography. Magn Reson Med 2000;43:91–101; with permission.)

direction. By combining this acquisition with a PRIZE acquisition and dividing the slice direction into three segments, imaging volumes could be reconstructed with a threefold improvement in temporal resolution. There is a slight increase in the time needed to acquire each volume, ranging from 1 to 1.33 times the time needed for the non-TRICKS scan.

PR-HyperTRICKS further improves the PR-TRICKS method by collecting additional high-spatial-frequency data during the contrast steady-state phase (eg, after the first pass) along with an improved sliding-window temporal filter for the in-plane (radial) spatial frequencies [33,34]. For CE MR angiography the PR method was extended to 3-D using a method called "vastly undersampled isotropic projection reconstruction" (VIPR) [35]. In this approach, data are symmetrically undersampled in all three dimensions. The resulting streak artifacts are distributed uniformly through the entire volume rather than in a single plane, so a larger degree of undersampling can be used. Furthermore, by interleaving the projections so that all spatial-frequency directions are at least coarsely sampled every few seconds, a sliding-window reconstruction can be used that reconstructs an entire imaging volume every few seconds. The isotropic nature of VIPR makes it ideal for large-FOV pulmonary imaging.

Fig. 7 shows the peak arterial phase (10 seconds) for three different orientations. The total acquisition time was 40 seconds for a 40 × 40 × 40 cm volume with a 256 × 256 × 256 matrix. This example demonstrates the isotropic nature,

large FOV, and good venous suppression of this technique.

Improvements in time-resolved imaging: parallel imaging

Recent work has demonstrated that parallel imaging is another promising technology that can be used to improve time-resolved CE MR angiography [36–40]. Both simultaneous acquisition of spatial harmonics (SMASH) and sensitivity encoding (SENSE) have been used, with the SENSE-based approaches being more common. In parallel imaging, the spatially varying sensitivity of receiver coils is used to encode the data and allow an increase in the phase-encoding step size. This increase in step size allows the scan time to be reduced by reducing the number of k-space views that need to be acquired. Alternately, the scan time can remain the same, and the resolution can be increased by acquiring a higher maximum spatial frequency view. The spatial decoding can be performed in either k-space (SMASH) or in image space (SENSE).

In early work, Sodickson et al [36] used a SMASH-based approach to reduce the encoding FOV along the phase direction. The total number of encodings was kept the same, doubling the resolution along the phase direction. In healthy subjects this improvement in resolution was easily seen. Similarly, Weiger et al [37] used a SENSE-based approach but instead increased the number of slice encodings and the resolution along the slice direction. This improvement in resolution was

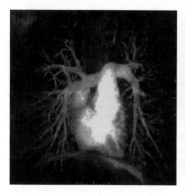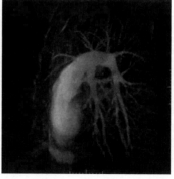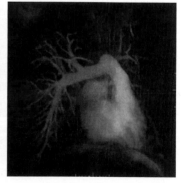

Fig. 7. MIP images from a VIPR acquisition of the pulmonary vessels at the peak arterial phase (10-second temporal resolution) for three different reformation orientations. The acquisition time was over a 40 × 40 × 40 cm³ volume with a 256 × 256 × 256 matrix, providing isotropic spatial resolution of 1.56 mm/pixel. This example demonstrates the isotropic nature, large FOV, and good venous suppression from a 40-mL contrast medium bolus. (*From* Barger AV, Block WF, Toropov Y, et al. Time-resolved contrast-enhanced imaging with isotropic resolution and broad coverage using an undersampled 3D projection trajectory. Magn Reson Med 2002;48:297–305; with permission.)

apparent when the coronal source images were reformatted along the axial direction. In one particular case, a right renal artery stenosis was depicted better on the higher-resolution axial reformat of the SENSE data.

Both Sodickson and Weiger also applied parallel imaging to reduce the acquisition time for time-resolved imaging, from 24 seconds to 8 seconds and from 12 seconds to 4 seconds, respectively. Both authors noted that although the reduction in scan time results in a reduction in the S/N, much of this reduction in S/N can be restored by using tighter bolus injections.

More recently Muthupillai et al [40] demonstrated the use of SENSE in imaging pediatric patients with congenital abnormalities. CE MR angiography is not commonly used in pediatrics because of difficulties in breath-holds, restrictions on contrast dosage, and shorter arterial–venous transit times. By employing SENSE, the acquisition can be done in a time-resolved fashion without requiring a test bolus or a breath-hold. This approach works well, specifically for imaging large thoracic and abdominal vessels.

The top row of Fig. 8 shows the full-volume maximum intensity projection (MIP) for four time-frames of a sedated, free-breathing 8-year-old boy with Kawasaki's disease. The temporal resolution of each phase was 6 seconds. The second row shows the same four time-frames with precontrast mask subtraction to remove the background signal. The second image clearly shows the arterial phase; the third and fourth show predominantly the venous phase.

Multiple-scanning-location MR angiography—peripheral run-off examinations

Patients with peripheral vascular occlusive disease often require studies that include assessment of the descending aorta and renal arteries through the tibial and pedal arteries. The vascular territory to be assessed is vast, and the total dose of contrast media administered and the overall examination time are important considerations for an efficacious MR angiography study.

There are several approaches to a multistation peripheral run-off MR angiography study. The peripheral vasculature can be divided into three or more stations with time-resolved MR angiography imaging performed at each station using 3-D EC-TRICKS [11] or similar fast 3-D time-resolved pulse sequences [12,13] with separate injections of contrast medium at each stage.

With each injection of contrast, however, precise registration of the contrast and mask images (for efficient background subtraction) becomes increasingly important. Each contrast injection increases the intensity of the background and residual vascular signal, making stationary spin suppression using rf excitation pulses alone rather difficult for subsequent MR angiography studies. Multistation, multiple-injection, peripheral MR angiography studies usually start by imaging the tibial or pedal arteries, with the abdominal station as the final imaging stage. Respiratory motion or peristalsis increases the difficulty of background mask suppression in the abdomen, especially with the cumulative dose of contrast media that increases with each injection. Additional delay time (approximately 15–20 minutes) can be imposed between image acquisitions to allow normal extravascular leakage or renal extraction of contrast media and a reduction in residual background signal enhancement. Such a delay is impractical in a clinical situation because of limited patient examination time. Hence, waiting for the contrast medium to dissipate is not a viable option when imaging many vascular territories.

In cases of multiple contiguous anatomic locations, the use of a single contrast injection is advantageous, because it greatly simplifies the scan set-up and data acquisition in addition to minimizing the sensitivity to misregistration artifacts. As in single-station acquisitions, multiple-station, single-bolus, peripheral MR angiography requires that the data acquisition be synchronized with the arrival of the contrast bolus, at each station or scan location. This technique is, in essence, a true bolus chase. Fluoroscopic triggering or automated bolus-detection techniques can easily be incorporated into a multiple-station MR angiography study, but currently available commercial software offers this feature only at the initial or proximal station.

Multistation bolus-chase studies can be performed in several ways. The simplest to implement is the incorporation of automated or manual table motion into the routine CE MR angiography technique [41–43]. In this example, the detection of contrast arrival and the acquisition of MR angiography data for the initial station (eg, abdominal aorta for a peripheral MR angiography) proceed as in a single-station study. Upon completion of scanning for station one (the abdominal station), the table automatically or manually translates to the next station (the iliac-femoral artery stage), repeating the process until data for the

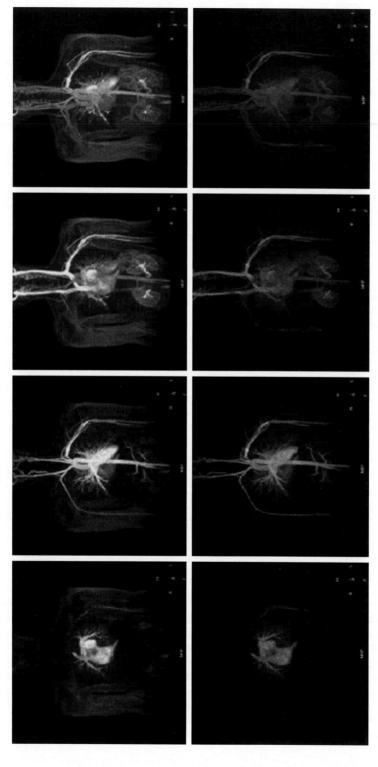

Fig. 8. MIP images for four time-frames of a time-resolved CE MR angiography acquisition with SENSE acceleration in a sedated, free-breathing 8-year-old boy with Kawasaki's disease. The top row shows the unsubtracted MIPs. The subtracted precontrast mask data for the same time-frames are shown in the bottom row. (*From* Muthupillai R, Vick GW III, Flamm SD, et al. Time-resolved contrast-enhanced magnetic resonance angiography in pediatric patients using sensitivity encoding. J Magn Reson Imaging 2003;17:559–64; with permission.)

tibial-pedal artery stage are completed. A premium is placed on the table translation speed to minimize dead time between image acquisitions. Using current techniques, overall scan times from the start of imaging at the abdominal station to the calves or feet are of the order of 70 to 90 seconds. Unfortunately, this relatively long scan time is associated with increased likelihood of venous contamination in the tibial-pedal vascular station, the last location of the bolus chase (Fig. 9). To optimize distal tibial and pedal arterial visualization, several researchers have suggested the use of a dual-rate (biphasic) bolus injection scheme] or venous compression [44,45].

Optimization of arterial visualization on multistation CE MR angiography is similar to that of single-station CE MR angiography and relies on proper synchronization of central k-space views for each station with arterial enhancement. Station-specific adjustment of the view acquisition order at each station may attempt to minimize the effects of venous contamination, but the problem of a long interval between the initiation of the contrast medium injection and the acquisition of data at the distal station remains [46].

Because the primary problem is venous contamination in the tibial-pedal station, an alternative solution is to segment the run-off study into a vascular-specific tibial-pedal study with 0.1 mmol/kg of gadolinium chelate contrast agent, followed by a two- or three-station moving-table multistation examination using a further 0.1 to 0.2 mmol/kg contrast bolus. The first part of the study can either be a time-resolved study [47] or a CE MR angiography study using a test bolus to determine the time of arrival of the contrast agent at the distal station. In the second part of this two-staged run-off study, the moving-table translation is only from the abdominal stage to the vascular segments at or about the level of the popliteal trifurcation.

Multistation peripheral run-off studies can be simplified greatly using a single injection of contrast agent if the scan time at each station can be substantially reduced while maintaining adequate spatial resolution. Such an approach would allow imaging at the distal station to begin before significant venous recirculation occurs. This goal can be accomplished using either parallel-imaging techniques [48,49] or a segmented volume-type acquisition (SNS) [50]. Parallel-imaging techniques have hitherto been limited by the availability of rf phased-array (receiver) coils: coils specifically optimized for parallel imaging

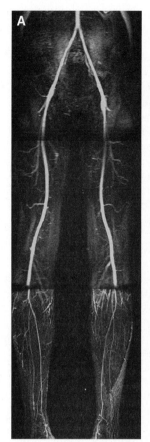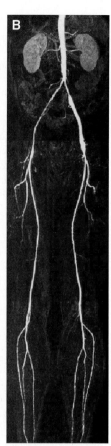

Fig. 9. Examples of a single-injection, multistation peripheral run-off examination. (*A*) With an acquisition time of 45 seconds at each station, the calf station was reached 100 seconds after the contrast was detected arriving in the abdominal aorta. With a 31-second contrast medium bolus (0.2 mmol/kg), it is clear that by the time data acquisition started at the tibial vascular stage, the arterial (and even the venous) phase was missed, resulting in poor depiction of the tibial and peroneal arteries. (*B*) A second example illustrating excellent depiction of the tibial and peroneal arteries using a 0.2 mmol/kg contrast bolus of 37-seconds duration. Minimal venous contamination and visualization of the arterial phase were accomplished in this example by reducing the scan time per station to 14 seconds. With a 5-second table translation time between stations, the data acquisition at the distal station started only 38 seconds after the contrast bolus was detected in the descending aorta. The reduction in scan time was achieved by compromising on the image spatial resolution. (Courtesy of Prof. D. Regent, CHU-Nancy, France.)

must be placed at each station. The initial work of Maki et al [48] (using a technique called wide apart kinematic table isotropic imaging or "WAKI-TRAK") involved the use of parallel imaging in the abdominal station followed by reduced spatial resolution in the iliac-femoral stage. This limitation was imposed by the lack of available coils to span all three vascular imaging stages. With improvements in rf coil technology and an increased number of receiver channels available, further acceleration can be realized.

The acceleration factors, however, cannot be increased without bound. All current parallel-imaging methods incur increasing image S/N penalties with greater acceleration factors in a single encoding direction [36,51,52]. To achieve higher acceleration factors but maintain image S/N, a 2-D rather than a single-dimension acceleration strategy can be used. This method is ideal for 3-D volume acquisitions in which, for example, an acceleration factor of two can be used for both the phase- and slice-encoding directions, leading to an overall acceleration factor of four. This $n \times m$ acceleration scheme (where n and m denote the acceleration factors in the phase- and slice-encoding directions, respectively) has been demonstrated to provide improved S/N over a single-dimensional acceleration of equal ($n \times m$) acceleration. The potential for acceleration has already been demonstrated in large (32-channel) receiver systems with which 3-D vascular images with high spatial resolution can be acquired in a single breath-hold. With acceleration factors of between 9 and 12, 3-D volume acquisitions that would normally take 4 minutes or more can be acquired in a 22-second scan [53]. Massively parallel acceleration would allow the acquisition to proceed from the abdomen to the feet in a substantially shorter time than in current clinical practice.

A similar technique for a multistation, single-injection, peripheral run-off study uses segmented volume acquisition [50]. By acquiring only the central k-space views (in an elliptical centric view acquisition order) at the uppermost stations, data acquisition at the most distal station can be started between 30 and 40 seconds after the start of imaging at the abdominal vascular stage. This method ensures that the image contrast in the uppermost stations is heavily weighted to the arterial passage of the contrast agent. Because the remaining high-spatial-frequency data views are collected subsequent to the complete data acquisition at the distal station, arterial phase–only images can be reconstructed with relatively high spatial resolution (Fig. 10).

Both methods of single-injection, multistation CE MR angiography seek to minimize the imaging time in the uppermost stations. Because the arrival of the contrast agent at each station can

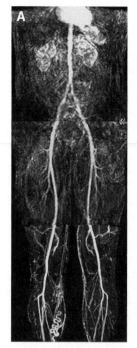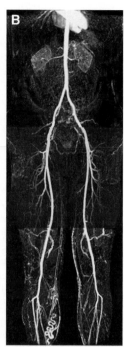

Fig. 10. MIP images showing a 3-D segmented multi-station, single-injection peripheral MR angiography study (SNS). (*A*) Images reconstructed from the first pass at the abdominal and iliac-femoral stations acquired using 40% of the central k-space data with an elliptical centric view acquisition order at the abdominal and thigh stations. At the distal (calf) station, minimal venous contamination is observed because the image acquisition started 40 seconds after the contrast bolus was detected in the abdominal aorta. (*B*) Images reconstructed after acquiring the remaining outer k-space data for the uppermost stations after completing data acquisition for the distal station. Note the improvement in the vascular definition in the renal arteries, abdominal aorta, iliac, and femoral arteries after the addition of the remaining high-spatial-frequency data views.

vary from patient to patient, however, the time available for data acquisition at each peripheral station must be adjusted to match the passage of contrast in the abdominal-iliac, femoral, and tibial-pedal stages. To time a multistation CE MR angiography, it often is sufficient to obtain information about the arrival of contrast only at the uppermost and distal stations. The timing of contrast arrival for the intermediate station can be interpolated from the two measurements.

The arrival of the contrast bolus for multiple scanning locations can be determined using two basic techniques, both of which use a small (2–5 mL) test bolus of contrast agent followed by a large (20–30 mL) normal saline flush. For a multiple-station timing bolus, arrival of the contrast medium at the abdominal station is first detected using either the automated SMART-PREP or a manual fluoroscopic trigger. This trigger initiates table motion to the final station. At the distal station, however, the small size of the vessels reduces the ability to detect an appreciable increase in signal intensity from a small test bolus, so real-time MR fluoroscopic imaging, rather than an automated technique such as SMARTPREP, is the preferred method to assess the arrival of the contrast bolus [54]. Maki et al [55,56] have described a similar technique using manual table motion. The arrival times at the uppermost and distal stations can then be measured from the saved fluoroscopic images or by automatic determination of the time between the trigger selections by the operator. An alternative to merely acquiring the arrival images of the test bolus is to use a slightly larger amount of contrast agent (eg, 5 mL) and, when the table reaches the distal station, switching to a multiphase, time-resolved volume acquisition that can determine the arrival of the contrast bolus and also provide preliminary diagnostic information as to the arterial filling of the distal vessels in the calves and feet [54].

With a priori knowledge (from the timing-bolus run) of the contrast dynamics, the multi-station acquisition can be tailored to match the available imaging time at each station before the onset of venous (enhancement) contamination. The tailored multistation run-off examination can be optimized by adjusting the acquisition time at each station (to maintain spatial resolution), by using parallel imaging, or by using a SNS-type image acquisition [48–50]. Ideally, the acquisition parameters for each vascular station should be adjusted to optimize the spatial resolution for the available imaging window (ie, period of preferential arterial enhancement before the onset of significant venous contamination).

Phase-contrast imaging improvements

Phase-contrast imaging remains an important tool for visualizing both the magnitude and direction of flow. Phase-contrast imaging relies on the inherent phase shifts that moving spins (blood) experience along a gradient field. Flowing blood thus is well differentiated from stationary background tissue. Improvements in phase-contrast imaging have focused on reducing the long scan times. Short scan times are essential in MR angiography applications, especially in the abdomen. Because of the long acquisition times for phase-contrast imaging, respiratory motion often degrades the ability to assess accurately velocity-directional information in the abdominal vessels (eg, the renal arteries). Breath-hold imaging adequately addresses the problems arising from respiratory motion, but reduction of scan time is necessary to ensure reasonable durations for patient compliance with breath-holding requirements. Scan time is usually shortened by degrading temporal resolution or spatial resolution or both.

Adequate visualization of peak flow velocities requires sufficient temporal resolution. In fast-segmented (gated) phase-contrast imaging, the temporal resolution can be controlled by the selection of the number of views acquired per R-R interval (views per segment, vps). For through-plane flow measurements, the temporal imaging window is given as

$$\text{Temporal resolution} = \text{vps} \times 2 \times \text{TR}$$

Similarly, for measurements of flow for three directions, the temporal resolution is

$$\text{Temporal resolution} = \text{vps} \times 4 \times \text{TR}$$

As demonstrated by Polzin et al [57], the temporal resolution in a phase-contrast acquisition has an effect similar to that of a low-pass filter on the time-varying flow velocities, blunting the flow-velocity response of the imaging sequence. The result is an underestimation of the overall flow and peak flow velocities.

Degradation in spatial resolution can also result in problems for phase-contrast imaging. An increase in voxel sizes increases the likelihood of intravoxel dephasing, especially in regions of high flow or complex flow patterns. In addition, with too large a voxel, the partial-volume effect of having both stationary and flowing spins in the same voxel reduces the measured velocities. This reduction results in a diminution of the signal intensity and decreases the overall image S/N in addition to decreasing the mean flow velocity in a voxel. Another potential issue is a reduction in spatial resolution that results in edge blurring of the vessel in the magnitude image. Because vessel boundaries are drawn in the magnitude images, imprecise vessel boundary delineation would overestimate the cross-sectional area of the vessel, leading to an overestimation of the overall flow.

To maintain images with high temporal and high spatial contrast in the resolution phase, several options are viable. The first is to use parallel imaging to reduce the overall scan time by reducing the number of k-space lines that need to be acquired [58–60]. The second technique is to use partial Fourier acquisition techniques (0.5 or 0.75 number of excitations or signal averages [NEX]) [61,62]. As shown in Fig. 11, breath-held 0.5 NEX phase-contrast measurements of renal artery flow with a temporal resolution of 58 milliseconds (4 vps, one flow direction) were completed in as little as 26 seconds. This time compared well with a full NEX (NSA) acquisition of 40 seconds' duration. Note that the flow measurements between the 0.5 NEX and the full NEX are within 2% of each other.

Phase-contrast angiography also benefits from the use of contrast media. In addition to improving the overall image S/N, the increase in vascular signal with contrast enhancement reduces the partial-volume effect from larger voxel sizes [63], leading to more accurate and improved phase-contrast images. Furthermore, by reducing the partial-volume effect, slightly thicker slices can be used to improve spatial coverage without a substantial increase in overall scan times.

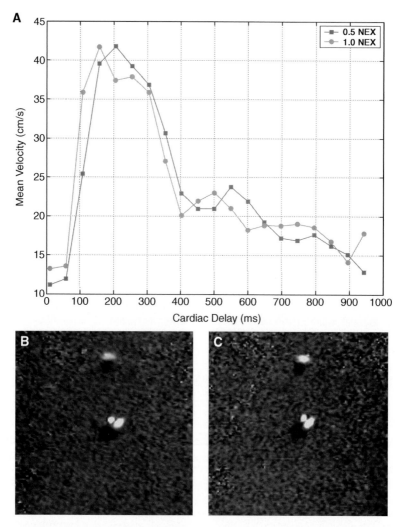

Fig. 11. (A) Comparison between phase-contrast flow measurements in the renal artery using (B) a partial (0.5) NEX acquisition technique and (C) the more conventional full (1.0) NEX (also known as NSA) approach. The phase-contrast acquisition was completed in 26 seconds with the partial NEX approach and in 40 seconds with the full NEX scan. The flow measurements obtained were within 2% of each other (401 mL/min and 409 mL/min, respectively). The temporal resolution attained was 58 milliseconds (TR = 7.3 milliseconds, 4 vps, VENC = 80 cm/s, 1 flow-encoding direction).

Cardiac MR angiography: coronary artery imaging

MR angiography of the coronary artery has been the focus of substantial development activity over the past few years but remains one of the most technically challenging areas for MR angiography [64–66]. Coronary MR angiography is challenged by the constraints imposed on the acquisition-sequence design by both respiratory and cardiac motion, by the inherent S/N and spatial-resolution requirements necessary for confident diagnosis, and by the tortuous anatomic arrangement of the coronary arterial tree. Historically, MR angiography has evolved along several acquisition pathways in which the basic imaging constraints of the S/N ratio and spatial resolution are continuously addressed. The physiologic constraints of cardiac and breathing motion have made traditional, time-consuming spin-echo techniques for black-blood vessel contrast far too problematic. This approach has been superceded by fast spin echo techniques in which the spin echo signal is refocused multiple times, with each echo representing a k-space acquisition view. In this manner, the scan time is reduced by a factor equivalent to the number of k-space lines acquired (or echo train length) per rf excitation pulse. Double inversion-recovery magnetization preparation ensures that the signal from blood is suppressed, yielding black-blood image contrast that allows 2-D visualization of the coronary vasculature [67]. This technique has been expanded to include imaging of the vessel wall for possible assessment of coronary artery plaque [68,69].

The bulk of coronary artery angiography, however, has been with traditional bright-blood image contrast using gradient recalled echo pulse sequences. To account for cardiac motion, data acquisition is segmented over several cardiac cycles, with the acquisition time for each data segment kept as short as possible, typically about 100 milliseconds [70]. Fast (short TR) gradient recalled echo imaging allows the acquisition of multiple k-space lines in a short period of time. By segmenting the acquisition over several cardiac cycles, images with high spatial and temporal resolution can be obtained easily. Although rf phase spoiling provides T1-weighted image contrast, allowing the suppression of myocardial tissue as in conventional MR angiography, there is a continued need to increase the vessel contrast-to-noise ratio. Recently, the development of true steady-state free-precession techniques (known variously as balanced-FFE, FIESTA, and True-FISP) have provided significant increases in S/N and enabled the acquisition of images with the high spatial resolution essential for coronary imaging. Although these strategies greatly increase the image S/N, they are sensitive to magnetic field inhomogeneities. This sensitivity is especially important for cardiac imaging at 3.0 T, because magnetic susceptibility effects increase at higher magnetic field strengths.

As in conventional body MR angiography, the use of contrast media (gadolinum chelates) can benefit coronary MR angiography [71,72]. A disadvantage with the use of gadolinium chelate is that the myocardial tissue enhances over time, together with the vascular signal. This myocardial enhancement imposes an additional requirement for greater background suppression to adequately visualize the coronary vasculature with a high vessel-to-myocardial image contrast-to-noise ratio. Several intravascular (also known as "blood pool") contrast agents are being investigated currently. These contrast agents persist within the vasculature for longer periods (eg, >30 minutes) and may be well suited for coronary MR angiography. The extended vascular residence time may allow better visualization with both breath-hold and free-breathing acquisitions [73].

As previously stated, two major challenges to imaging coronary arteries arise from the physiologic constraints of cardiac and breathing motion. An essential component of any acquisition strategy consists of cardiac triggering to ameliorate the effect of cardiac motion. Two fundamental strategies are used to address respiratory motion. First, a breath-hold acquisition strategy may be implemented that is designed to acquire the MR data while the patient suspends breathing, typically for 20 seconds or less [74–76]. As shown in Fig. 12, breath-held scans can produce excellent images of the coronary vessels, provided the patient is able to maintain a breath-hold. Alternatively, a free-breathing strategy can be employed in which a respiratory gating method (eg, navigator echo gating) is applied so that the acquisitions are acquired only in the quiescent periods during free breathing, typically the end-expiratory phase of the respiratory cycle [77–80]. These two strategies can be assessed in terms of their spatial resolution and scan efficiency, but the choice of one strategy over another may depend on individual patient characteristics. Relatively healthy patients may be able to tolerate

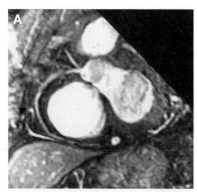

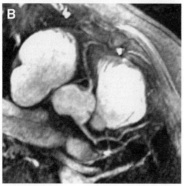

Fig. 12. Planar reformations of (*A*) the right coronary artery and (*B*) the left anterior descending coronary arteries in a patient using breath-held 3-D steady-state free-precession (FIESTA) pulse sequences. The breath-hold time was 22 seconds. Scan parameters were TE/TR/flip = 1.1 ms/4.1 ms/60° flip, 28 cm FOV; 256 × 192 matrix; 2-mm slice thickness (1.1 × 1.4 × 2.0 mm³ acquired spatial resolution). (Courtesy of Prof. J. Gao, Chinese PLA General Hospital, Beijing, China.)

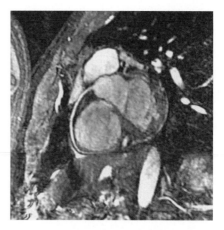

Fig. 13. Planar reformations from free-breathing navigator 3-D volume acquisition illustrating the right coronary artery and using a FIESTA pulse sequence. The scan time for the targeted volume acquisition was 1.5 minutes. Scan parameters were TE/TR/flip = 1.8 ms/4.4 ms/60°; 29 cm FOV; 256 × 256 matrix; 2-mm slice thickness. Spatial resolution was 1.1 × 1.1 × 2.0 mm³ (acquired).

breath-hold requirements and therefore be suitable for the more scan-efficient strategies. Very sick patients may not be able to tolerate even the shortest period of suspended respiration and therefore may be limited to free-breathing navigator strategies. Even so, inconsistent respiratory patterns may render suboptimal images with free-breathing navigator techniques [81]. Fig. 13 shows how a free-breathing navigator study can provide a vessel S/N and spatial resolution sufficient to assess proximal coronary arteries.

Free-breathing coronary MR angiography is the preferred imaging technique for assessing the major cardiac vessels, especially in patients with compromised respiratory function. Respiratory cycles can be monitored with either an external bellows or an MR-based navigator strategy [82]; the latter technique has been established as more

robust and reliable. Fig. 14 shows one such implementation at 3.0 T using a diastolic-triggered ECG delay with a 2-D selective pencil-beam navigator for prospective adaptive 3-D real-time motion correction [83]. Using the column excitation, the respiratory motion can be

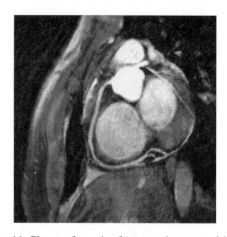

Fig. 14. Planar reformation from a navigator-gated 3-D gradient recalled echo MR angiography (TR/TE/flip = 7.8 ms/2.2 ms/20°, 27 cm FOV, 256 × 384 matrix; 3-mm slice thickness) with linear volumetric shimming at 3.0 T. Total scan time was 7 minutes per acquisition with an in-plane spatial resolution of 1.0 × 0.7 × 3.0 mm³. (Courtesy of A Gharib, MD, and M Stuber, MD, Johns Hopkins University, Baltimore, MD.)

monitored by noting the superior-inferior displacement of the right hemidiaphragm in real time to accept or reject data acquisition prospectively based on position in the respiratory cycle.

With free-breathing coronary artery imaging techniques, two basic strategies have emerged. The first is a targeted-volume approach in which a separate, thin-slab volume acquisition is made for each major coronary artery vessel [84,85]. Typically, a thin (2–3 cm) slab is acquired for each coronary artery. Each slab should be prescribed so that the acquired volume encompasses as much of the length of the vessel as possible. Although this strategy is relatively straightforward, it places a responsibility on the operator to locate and position the necessary imaging volumes from preliminary scout images. An alternative and simpler approach is to acquire axial data from the entire heart in a single acquisition and use postprocessing to extract the coronary artery vessel segments [86]. This whole-heart coverage is an easier alternative to the targeted-volumes strategy, because the operator needs only to prescribe sufficient slices in the axial plane to cover the entire heart. The disadvantage of whole-heart coverage is that the overall scan time is much longer than in targeted strategies, leaving this technique susceptible to irregular or inconsistent respiratory patterns or to bulk patient movement during or between acquisitions that may degrade image quality.

As in body MR angiography, parallel imaging can reduce the overall image-acquisition time for both the targeted and whole-heart approaches. The loss in image S/N with parallel imaging is somewhat offset by the use of contrast media or 2-D parallel acceleration [87,88]. The substantial reduction in scan time provides a choice of either short breath-holds (10- to 12-seconds for targeted-volume or 24 seconds for whole-heart coverage) or increased reliability of free-breathing scans achieved by minimizing overall scan time.

Summary

Advances in technology continue to enrich MR angiography. New techniques are being explored to address the primary goals of specificity and sensitivity in diagnosing vascular disease. To gain widespread acceptance, emerging techniques must demonstrate clinical efficacy and be robust and easy to use. Increasing the complexity of the examination does not necessarily increase the effectiveness of a technique. Development of improved MR angiographic techniques will ultimately converge to a "single-button" examination with high diagnostic accuracy and simplified operator-scanner interaction.

References

[1] Wedeen VJ, Meuli RA, Edelman RR, et al. Projective imaging of pulsatile flow with magnetic resonance. Science 1985;230(4728):946–8.

[2] Wehrli FW, Shimakawa A, Gullberg GT, et al. Time-of-flight MR flow imaging: selective saturation recovery with gradient refocusing. Radiology 1986; 160:781–5.

[3] Gullberg GT, Wehrli FW, Shimakawa A, et al. MR vascular imaging with a fast gradient refocusing pulse sequence and reformatted images from transaxial sections. Radiology 1987;165:241–6.

[4] Keller PJ, Drayer BP, Fram EK, et al. MR angiography with two-dimensional acquisition and three-dimensional display. Work in progress. Radiology 1989;173:527–32.

[5] Blatter DD, Parker DL, Robison RO. Cerebral MR angiography with multiple overlapping thin slab acquisition. Part I. Quantitative analysis of vessel visibility. Radiology 1991;179:805–11.

[6] Blatter DD, Bahr AL, Parker DL, et al. Cervical carotid MR angiography with multiple overlapping thin-slab acquisition: comparison with conventional angiography. AJR Am J Roentgenol 1993;161: 1269–77.

[7] Kanal E, Talagala SL, Applegate GR, et al. Fast 3D TOF MRA with timed contrast injection [abstract]. Radiology 1991;181(P):119.

[8] Prince MR, Yucel EK, Kaufman JA, et al. Dynamic gadolinium-enhanced three-dimensional abdominal MR arteriography. J Magn Reson Imaging 1993;3: 877–81.

[9] Talagala SL, Jungreis CA, Kanal E, et al. Fast three-dimensional time-of-flight MR angiography of the intra-cranial vasculature. J Magn Reson Imaging 1995;5:317–23.

[10] Maki JH, Prince MR, Londy FJ, et al. The effects of time varying intravascular signal intensity and k-space acquisition order on three-dimensional MR angiography image quality. J Magn Reson Imaging 1996;6:642–51.

[11] Hany TF, Carroll TJ, Omary RA, et al. Aorta and runoff vessels: single-injection MR angiography with automated table movement compared with multiinjection time-resolved MR angiography— initial results. Radiology 2001;221:266–72.

[12] Schoenberg SO, Bock M, Knopp MV, et al. Renal arteries: optimization of three-dimensional gadolinium-enhanced MR angiography with bolus-timing-independent fast multiphase acquisition in a single breath hold. Radiology 1999;211:667–79.

[13] Schoenberg SO, Essig M, Hallscheidt P, et al. Multiphase magnetic resonance angiography of the abdominal and pelvic arteries: results of a bicenter multireader analysis. Invest Radiol 2002;37:20–8.

[14] Foo TK, Saranathan M, Prince MR, et al. Automated detection of bolus arrival and initiation of data acquisition in fast, three-dimensional, gadolinium-enhanced MR angiography. Radiology 1997; 203:275–80.

[15] Prince MR, Chenevert TL, Foo TK, et al. Contrast-enhanced abdominal MR angiography: optimization of imaging delay time by automating the detection of contrast material arrival in the aorta. Radiology 1997;203:109–14.

[16] Huston J III, Fain SB, Riederer SJ, et al. Carotid arteries: maximizing arterial to venous contrast in fluoroscopically triggered contrast-enhanced MR angiography with elliptic centric view ordering. Radiology 1999;211:265–73.

[17] Riederer SJ, Fain SB, Kruger DG, et al. 3D contrast-enhanced MR angiography using fluoroscopic triggering and an elliptical centric view order. Int J Card Imaging 1999;15:117–29.

[18] Riederer SJ, Bernstein MA, Breen JF, et al. Three-dimensional contrast-enhanced MR angiography with real-time fluoroscopic triggering: design specifications and technical reliability in 330 patient studies. Radiology 2000;215:584–93.

[19] Hany TF, McKinnon GC, Leung DA, et al. Optimization of contrast timing for breath-hold three-dimensional MR angiography. J Magn Reson Imaging 1997;7:551–6.

[20] Levy RA, Prince MR. Arterial-phase three-dimensional contrast-enhanced MR angiography of the carotid arteries. AJR Am J Roentgenol 1996;167:211–5.

[21] Lee VS, Rofsky NM, Krinsky GA, et al. Single-dose breath-hold gadolinium-enhanced three-dimensional MR angiography of the renal arteries. Radiology 1999;211:69–78.

[22] Wang Y, Johnston DL, Breen JF, et al. Dynamic MR digital subtraction angiography using contrast enhancement, fast data acquisition, and complex subtraction. Magn Reson Med 1996;36:551–6.

[23] Hennig J, Scheffler K, Laubenberger J, et al. Time-resolved projection angiography after bolus injection of contrast agent. Magn Reson Med 1997;37: 341–5.

[24] van Vaals JJ, Brummer ME, Dixon WT, et al. "Keyhole" method for accelerating imaging of contrast agent uptake. J Magn Reson Imaging 1993;3: 671–5.

[25] Korosec FR, Frayne R, Grist TM, et al. Time-resolved contrast-enhanced 3D MR angiography. Magn Reson Med 1996;36:345–51.

[26] Doyle M, Walsh EG, Blackwell GG, et al. Block regional interpolation scheme for k-space (BRISK): a rapid cardiac imaging technique. Magn Reson Med 1995;33:163–70.

[27] Wilman AH, Riederer SJ. Performance of an elliptical centric view order for signal enhancement and motion artifact suppression in breath hold three-dimensional gradient echo imaging. Magn Reson Med 1997;38:793–802.

[28] Wilman AH, Riederer SJ, King BF, et al. Fluoroscopically triggered contrast-enhanced three-dimensional MR angiography with elliptical centric view order: application to the renal arteries. Radiology 1997;205:137–46.

[29] Zhou Y, Carroll TJ, Grist TM, et al. Time-resolved MRA with elliptical centric view ordering [abstract]. In: Proceedings of the International Society of Magnetic Resonance Medicine Ninth Scientific Meeting. Berkeley, CA; 2001. p. 1938.

[30] Goyen M, Laub G, Ladd ME, et al. Dynamic 3D MR angiography of the pulmonary arteries in under four seconds. J Magn Reson Imaging 2001;13: 372–7.

[31] Peters DC, Korosec FR, Grist TM, et al. Undersampled projection reconstruction applied to MR angiography. Magn Reson Med 2000;43:91–101.

[32] Vigen KK, Peters DC, Grist TM, et al. Undersampled projection reconstruction imaging for time-resolved contrast-enhanced imaging. Magn Reson Med 2000;43:170–6.

[33] Du J, Carroll TJ, Wagner HJ, et al. Time-resolved, undersampled projection reconstruction imaging for high-resolution CE-MRA of the distal runoff vessels. Magn Reson Med 2002;48:516–22.

[34] Mazaheri Y, Carroll TJ, Du J, et al. Combined time-resolved and high-spatial-resolution 3D MRA using an extended adaptive acquisition. J Magn Reson Imaging 2002;15:291–301.

[35] Barger AV, Block WF, Toropov Y, et al. Time-resolved contrast-enhanced imaging with isotropic resolution and broad coverage using an undersampled 3D projection trajectory. Magn Reson Med 2002;48:297–305.

[36] Sodickson DK, McKenzie CA, Li W, et al. Contrast-enhanced 3D MR angiography with simultaneous acquisition of spatial harmonics: a pilot study. Radiology 2000;217:284–9.

[37] Weiger M, Pruessmann KP, Kassner A, et al. Contrast-enhanced 3D MRA using SENSE. J Magn Reson Imaging 2000;12:671–7.

[38] Golay X, Brown SJ, Itoh R, et al. Time-resolved contrast-enhanced carotid MR angiography using sensitivity encoding (SENSE). Am J Neuroradiol 2001;22:1615–9.

[39] Ohno Y, Kawamitsu H, Higashino T, et al. Time-resolved contrast-enhanced pulmonary MR angiography using sensitivity encoding (SENSE). J Magn Reson Imaging 2003;17:330–6.

[40] Muthupillai R, Vick GW III, Flamm SD, et al. Time-resolved contrast-enhanced magnetic resonance angiography in pediatric patients using sensitivity encoding. J Magn Reson Imaging 2003;17: 559–64.

[41] Wang Y, Lee HM, Khilnani NM, et al. Bolus-chase MR digital subtraction angiography in the lower extremity. Radiology 1998;207:263–9.

[42] Ho KY, Leiner T, de Haan MW, et al. Peripheral vascular tree stenoses: evaluation with moving-bed infusion-tracking MR angiography. Radiology 1998;206:683–92.

[43] Foo TK, Ho VB, McCann RB, et al. Single bolus contrast enhanced peripheral 3D MRA using automated table motion integrated with automated bolus detection and acquisition triggering (MR SMART-PREP) [abstract]. In: Proceedings of the International Society of Magnetic Resonance Medicine Sixth Scientific Meeting. Berkeley, CA; 1998. p. 67.

[44] Czum JM, Ho VB, Hood MN, et al. Bolus-chase peripheral 3D MRA using a dual-rate contrast media injection. J Magn Reson Imaging 2000;12: 769–75.

[45] Herborn CU, Ajaj W, Goyen M, et al. Peripheral vasculature: whole-body MR angiography with midfemoral venous compression–initial experience. Radiology 2004;230:872–8.

[46] Lee HM, Wang Y. Dynamic k-space filling for bolus chase 3D MR digital subtraction angiography. Magn Reson Med 1998;40:99–104.

[47] Morasch MD, Collins J, Pereles FS, et al. Lower extremity stepping-table magnetic resonance angiography with multilevel contrast timing and segmented contrast infusion. J Vasc Surg 2003;37:62–71.

[48] Maki JH, Wilson GJ, Eubank WB, et al. Utilizing SENSE to achieve lower station sub-millimeter isotropic resolution and minimal venous enhancement in peripheral MR angiography. J Magn Reson Imaging 2002;15:484–91.

[49] Bezooijen R, van den Bosch HC, Tielbeek AV, et al. Peripheral arterial disease: sensitivity-encoded multiposition MR angiography compared with intraarterial angiography and conventional multiposition MR angiography. Radiology 2004;231:263–71.

[50] Foo TKF, Ho VB, Hood MN, et al. High resolution multi-station imaging of lower-extremity peripheral vasculature with segmented volume acquisition: feasibility study. Radiology 2001;219:835–41.

[51] Sodickson DK, Manning WJ. Simultaneous acquisition of spatial harmonics (SMASH): fast imaging with radiofrequency coil arrays. Magn Reson Med 1997;38:591–603.

[52] Pruessmann KP, Weiger M, Scheidegger MB, et al. SENSE: sensitivity encoding for fast MRI. Magn Reson Med 1999;42:952–62.

[53] Sodickson DK, Hardy CJ, Zhu Y, et al. Twelve- to sixteen-fold accelerations of contrast-enhanced MRA using highly parallel MRI with a 32-element array [abstract]. Proceedings of the International Society of Magnetic Resonance Medicine Twelfth Scientific Meeting. Berkeley, CA; 2004. p. 327.

[54] Aksit PA, Ho VB, Hood ML, et al. Single-injection, semi-automated multi-station bolus timing for optimization for 3D peripheral MR angiography [abstract]. Proceedings of the International Society of Magnetic Resonance Medicine Twelfth Scientific Meeting. Berkeley, CA; 2004. p. 228.

[55] Maki JH, Wilson GJ, Eubank WB, et al. Predicting venous enhancement in peripheral MRA using a two station timing bolus [abstract]. Proceedings of the International Society of Magnetic Resonance Medicine Eleventh Scientific Meeting. Berkeley, CA; 2003. p. 91.

[56] Maki JH, Wilson GJ, William EB, et al. Single injection peripheral MRA: SNR and two station timing bolus [abstract]. Proceedings of the International Society of Magnetic Resonance Medicine Twelfth Scientific Meeting. Berkeley, CA; 2004. p. 227.

[57] Polzin JA, Frayne R, Grist TM, et al. Frequency response of multi-phase segmented k-space phase-contrast. Magn Reson Med 1996;35:755–62.

[58] Beerbaum P, Korperich H, Gieseke J, et al. Rapid left-to-right shunt quantification in children by phase-contrast magnetic resonance imaging combined with sensitivity encoding (SENSE). Circulation 2003;108:1355–61.

[59] Muthupillai R, Vick GW III, Flamm SD, et al. Time-resolved contrast-enhanced magnetic resonance angiography in pediatric patients using sensitivity encoding. J Magn Reson Imaging 2003;17: 559–64.

[60] Thunberg P, Karlsson M, Wigstrom L. Accuracy and reproducibility in phase contrast imaging using SENSE. Magn Reson Med 2003;50:1061–8 [erratum in Magn Reson Med 2004;51:223].

[61] Foo TK, Polzin JA, Derbyshire JA. Method for phase contrast reconstruction for partial Fourier acquisitions [abstract]. Proceedings of the International Society of Magnetic Resonance Medicine Eighth Scientific Meeting. Berkeley, CA; 2000. p. 1718.

[62] Szarf G, Dori Y, Tekes A, et al. Evaluation of partial Fourier phase contrast acquisition in velocity measurements [abstract]. Proceedings of the International Society of Magnetic Resonance Medicine Eleventh Scientific Meeting. Berkeley, CA; 2003. p. 1675.

[63] Foo TK, Ho VB, Hood MN, et al. Preferential arterial imaging using gated thick-slice gadolinium-enhanced phase-contrast acquisition in peripheral MRA. J Magn Reson Imaging 2001;13:714–21.

[64] Manning WJ, Edelman RR. Coronary MR angiography. Radiology 1995;195:875–6.

[65] Danias PG, Stuber M, Botnar RM, et al. Coronary MR angiography clinical applications and potential for imaging coronary artery disease. Magn Reson Imaging Clin N Am 2003;11:81–99.

[66] Riederer SJ. Coronary artery MR angiography: are we there yet? Radiology 2004;231:302–4.

[67] Simonetti OP, Finn JP, White RD, et al. "Black blood" T2-weighted inversion-recovery MR imaging of the heart. Radiology 1996;199:49–57.

[68] Stuber M, Botnar RM, Kissinger KV, et al. Free-breathing black-blood coronary MR angiography: initial results. Radiology 2001;219:278–83.

[69] Botnar RM, Bucker A, Kim WY, et al. Initial experiences with in vivo intravascular coronary vessel wall imaging. J Magn Reson Imaging 2003;17:615–9.

[70] Atkinson DJ, Edelman RR. Cineangiography of the heart in a single breath hold with a segmented turbo-FLASH sequence. Radiology 1991;178:357–60.

[71] Goldfarb JW, Edelman RR. Coronary arteries: breath-hold, gadolinium-enhanced, three-dimensional MR angiography. Radiology 1998;206:830–4.

[72] Goldfarb JW, Holland AE, Edelman RR. Single breath-hold multi-slab and cine cardiac-synchronized gadolinium-enhanced three-dimensional angiography. Magn Reson Imaging 2001;19:1267–74.

[73] Herborn CU, Barkhausen J, Paetsch I, et al. Coronary arteries: contrast-enhanced MR imaging with SH L 643A—experience in 12 volunteers. Radiology 2003;229:217–23.

[74] Wielopolski PA, van Geuns RJ, de Feyter PJ, et al. Breath-hold coronary MR angiography with volume-targeted imaging. Radiology 1998;209:209–19.

[75] van Geuns RJ, Wielopolski PA, Wardeh AJ, et al. Volume coronary angiography using targeted scans (VCATS): a new strategy in MR coronary angiography. Int J Cardiovasc Imaging 2001;17:405–10.

[76] Li D, Carr JC, Shea SM, et al. Coronary arteries: magnetization-prepared contrast-enhanced three-dimensional volume-targeted breath-hold MR angiography. Radiology 2001;219:270–7.

[77] Wang Y, Rossman PJ, Grimm RC, et al. Navigator-echo-based real-time respiratory gating and triggering for reduction of respiration effects in three-dimensional coronary MR angiography. Radiology 1996;198:55–60.

[78] Li D, Kaushikkar S, Haacke EM, et al. Coronary arteries: three-dimensional MR imaging with retrospective respiratory gating. Radiology 1996;201:857–63.

[79] McConnell MV, Khasgiwala VC, Savord BJ, et al. Prospective adaptive navigator correction for breath-hold MR coronary angiography. Magn Reson Med 1997;37:148–52.

[80] Stuber M, Botnar RM, Danias PG, et al. Submillimeter three-dimensional coronary MR angiography with real-time navigator correction: comparison of navigator locations. Radiology 1999;212:579–87.

[81] Taylor AM, Jhooti P, Wiesmann F, et al. MR navigator-echo monitoring of temporal changes in diaphragm position: implications for MR coronary angiography. J Magn Reson Imaging 1997;7:629–36.

[82] Ehman RL, Felmlee JP. Adaptive technique for high-definition MR imaging of moving structures. Radiology 1989;173:255–63.

[83] Stuber M, Botnar RM, Fischer SE, et al. Preliminary report on in vivo coronary MRA at 3 Tesla in humans. Magn Reson Med 2002;48:425–9.

[84] Kim WY, Danias PG, Stuber M, et al. Coronary magnetic resonance angiography for the detection of coronary stenoses. N Engl J Med 2001;345:1863–9.

[85] Sommer T, Hofer U, Hackenbroch M, et al. Hochauflösende 3D-MR-Koronarangiographie in Echt-Zeit-Navigatortechnik: Ergebnisse aus 107 Patientenuntersuchungen [Submillimeter 3D coronary MR angiography with real-time navigator correction in 107 patients with suspected coronary artery disease]. Rofo 2002;174:459–66 [in German].

[86] Weber OM, Martin AJ, Higgins CB. Whole-heart steady-state free precession coronary artery magnetic resonance angiography. Magn Reson Med 2003;50:1223–8.

[87] Park J, McCarthy R, Li D. Feasibility and performance of breath-hold 3D true-FISP coronary MRA using self-calibrating parallel acquisition. Magn Reson Med 2004;52:7–13.

[88] Niendorf T, Sodickson DK, Hardy CJ, et al. Towards whole heart coverage in a single breath-hold: coronary artery imaging using a true 32-channel phased array MRI system [abstract]. Proceedings of the International Society of Magnetic Resonance Medicine Twelfth Scientific Meeting. Berkeley, CA: 2004. p. 703.

ELSEVIER
SAUNDERS

Magn Reson Imaging Clin N Am
13 (2005) 23–40

MAGNETIC
RESONANCE
IMAGING CLINICS
of North America

MR Angiography Interpretation: Techniques and Pitfalls

James F. Glockner, MD, PhD

Department of Radiology, Mayo Clinic, 200 First Street SW, Rochester, MN 55905, USA

In recent years three-dimensional contrast-enhanced (3-D CE) MR angiography has become a common examination. This increased use in part reflects a trend away from conventional diagnostic X-ray catheter angiography and its associated risks, costs, inconveniences, and radiation exposure. On current MR scanners, 3-D CE MR angiographic examinations can be performed easily and quickly, and their interpretation using standard commercial software is fast and straightforward. Moreover, MR angiographic images are easily understood by referring clinicians. A growing body of literature has demonstrated the efficacy of 3-D contrast enhancement in many vascular territories, including the aorto-iliac, renal, and lower extremity arteries [1–7]. Improvements in gradient hardware and novel techniques allow faster acquisitions with improved spatial resolution.

The enormous amount of data generated by these examinations, however, does present a problem to the busy radiologist: hundreds or even thousands of images must be examined and stored, and the results must be presented in a concise and understandable manner. Few clinicians enjoy sorting through MR angiography source images, and most would prefer to see the results presented in a few attractive images in addition to reading the report.

3-D reconstruction techniques offer an elegant solution to the information overload. They are an efficient means of evaluating MR angiography data sets, and available 3-D reconstruction methods actually can improve diagnostic accuracy or at least diagnostic confidence, especially when the

vascular anatomy is complex or overlapping. Several 3-D techniques are now commercially available and are used widely by radiologists. All have strengths and weaknesses, and it is probably best to become familiar with as many as possible rather than relying exclusively on a single method.

The successful interpretation of MR angiograms involves a number of distinct elements. The examination must be performed correctly, with sufficient spatial resolution and signal-to-noise ratio (S/N) to evaluate the vascular territory of interest. The data must be reconstructed in a manner that accurately conveys the anatomic findings. Furthermore, the radiologist must be able to recognize the findings and avoid common pitfalls in interpretation, and his or her report must accurately convey this information to the referring clinician. This article briefly surveys all these elements but concentrates primarily on what to do after the MR angiography has been performed, that is, on data reconstruction, presentation, and analysis.

MR angiography technique

Reconstruction and interpretation of MR angiograms is much easier when the examination has been tailored to the vascular territory and clinical question of interest. Spatial resolution is a vital and frequently overlooked consideration and is related directly to the size of the vascular bed to be studied. Although submillimeter resolution probably is not critical for evaluation of the aorta, it is necessary for adequate visualization of atherosclerotic lesions in the coronary arteries and other vessels of similar size. As a rule, accurate diagnosis of significant (>50%) stenosis requires at least four pixels spanning the vessel. These

E-mail address: glockner.james@mayo.edu

considerations are complicated by the fact that voxel size is often nonuniform—for instance, in-plane resolution is often superior to resolution along the slice direction—and therefore stenoses are identified more easily if they occur in a particular orientation.

A related consideration is the field-of-view (FOV). A relatively simple means of improving spatial resolution (ie, without increasing acquisition time) is to employ a smaller FOV with an identical phase and frequency matrix. This solution is ideal when the FOV can be made very small easily (eg, in renal MR angiography). On the other hand, a small FOV does not always allow sufficient coverage of the region of interest (eg, in the abdominal aorta and iliac arteries). In such cases, a large FOV is necessary for complete coverage, and spatial resolution must be improved by the use of thinner slices or a higher phase and frequency matrix. An alternative approach is the multistation examination, in which multiple sequentially acquired small FOVs track a single contrast bolus. This examination is technically more difficult, and it is important to scan the individual stations fast enough to keep up with the contrast bolus and avoid venous contamination. The smaller the FOV for an individual station, the more stations are needed to cover the volume completely, and the longer is the resulting acquisition time.

Spatial resolution is not the only determinant of image quality. Temporal resolution is a critical and often opposing consideration. Temporal resolution is important for several reasons: in the chest and abdomen, 3-D CE MR angiography must be performed with suspended respiration to avoid motion artifact. Breath-hold capacity is notoriously variable in any patient population, so a great deal of flexibility is necessary in determining acquisition times for 3-D CE MR angiography. Compromise often is required between achieving optimal spatial resolution and acquiring motion-free data [8]. Temporal resolution also is a critical factor in avoiding venous contamination, particularly in multistation lower extremity run-off examinations in which venous contamination in the calves is a frequent occurrence.

Many strategies to reduce motion artifact have been described. The most notable is the use of elliptic centric phase encoding or one of its variants, in which views of the central k-space are acquired at the beginning of the scan and the views of the periphery of k-space are acquired at the end [9]. This technique has the effect of acquiring the central, low-spatial-frequency portion of the k-space data (ie, center of k-space), which is also the portion most responsible for the resulting image contrast, at the beginning of the acquisition, presumably the most successful portion of the breath-hold. The remaining peripheral, high-spatial-frequency k-space data, which is responsible primarily for image detail, are acquired at the end of the breath hold. A number of strategies can be employed to reduce acquisition times without necessarily decreasing spatial resolution: parallel imaging, partial excitations, partial-phase FOVs, and keyhole imaging techniques [10–12].

The S/N is a final consideration. As voxel size decreases and spatial resolution improves, there is a corresponding decline in S/N, and often this decline is compounded when techniques to increase acquisition speed are employed. A number of imaging parameters can be adjusted to improve S/N, but most of these also lead to increased acquisition times.

In summary, successful interpretation of an MR angiography examination depends largely on obtaining good data. The interpretative skills are central to proper diagnosis, and the ability to perform 3-D data processing of MR angiography data often can be valuable. None of these skills, however, matters if the MR angiography is performed poorly.

Data processing and presentation

Data processing is an important aspect of 3-D CE MR angiography for accurate interpretation and also for widespread clinical acceptance. The ability to present a large volume of data concisely is greatly appreciated by referring physicians, who often are more familiar with images from conventional angiography and would much prefer a presentation similar of MR angiography data rather than examination of source images.

Filters and zero-filling

Image or data filters can be applied before or after the 3-D reconstruction has been performed. Sharpening or smoothing filters are common, and some vendors apply filters automatically to all MR images. The application of a filter may or may not enhance the usefulness of a particular examination, and therefore the choice of filters is probably best left to the judgment of the individual radiologist.

Zero-filling techniques to improve 3-D reconstruction involve data interpolation either in the slice-select or in-plane direction. Zero-filling techniques involve filling out the peripheral lines of k-space with zeroes before performing the Fourier transform. In the most common applications, a 256 in-plane matrix is interpolated to 512, and in the slice direction twice as many images are reconstructed with 50% overlap. Although not improving the "true" or inherent spatial resolution of the acquisition, zero-filling results in smoother representation of vascular structures on 3-D reconstructions, especially when viewing the data in oblique orientations.

Subtraction

Subtraction of a mask precontrast 3-D data set from the 3-D CE MR angiography is a common technique and often is useful in eliminating background signal for improved vascular image contrast. This technique is applied most often to examinations of the lower extremities, where motion between the mask and postcontrast acquisitions is usually not problematic, and where background signal (namely, that of bone marrow and adjacent fat) is especially troublesome in evaluating the small vessels of the calf (Fig. 1) [13–14]. Subtraction can be applied either before Fourier transform (complex subtraction) or on an image-by-image basis after Fourier transform

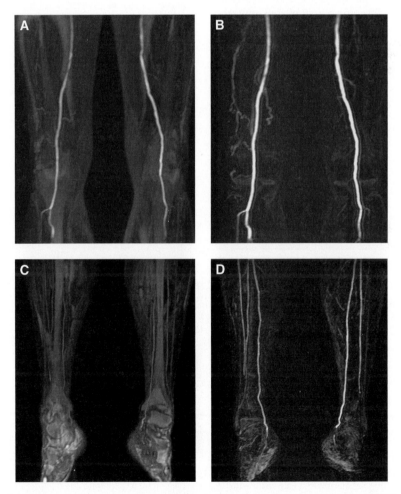

Fig. 1. Value of subtraction in lower extremity runoff examinations. (*A* and *C*). Non-subtracted MIP images from the thigh and calf stations of lower extremity runoff MRA are limited by overlying soft tissue. (*B* and *D*). MIP images from data set obtained by subtracting arterial phase from mask acquisition. Note markedly improved visualization of calf vessels.

(magnitude subtraction). Both methods are employed commonly. There probably is a slight consensus in favor of complex subtraction because of its superior elimination of background signal [15].

Subtraction in thoracic or abdominal CE MR angiography is more problematic, because exact registration of the pre- and postcontrast data sets is not guaranteed, and significant artifacts occasionally appear. Nevertheless, subtraction in well-coached patients is usually successful and may be particularly useful in MR venography, where the contrast-to-noise ratio (C/N) is inherently lower, and where superimposed arterial structures may interfere with adequate visualization of veins. Alternative strategies are also available. Fat suppression or partial fat suppression adds slightly to the total acquisition time but eliminates subtraction artifact and generally results in improved S/N relative to subtracted data sets (Fig. 2).

Three-dimensional reconstruction techniques

A variety of 3-D reconstruction techniques are now commercially available, and it is important to be well versed in as many of these as possible. Each technique has its own strengths and weaknesses that can lead to artifacts and interpretation errors in inexperienced hands.

Multiplanar reformation

Multiplanar reformation (MPR) is perhaps the simplest and most widely available method for visualization of 3-D data. In this technique, the 3-D volume is cut along a user-defined plane with variable thickness. Reformatted images are commonly displayed in axial, coronal, and sagittal planes, but oblique planes are often useful, and curved reformatted images can be generated along user-specified paths. Thin-section reformatted images are valuable for evaluating vascular lesions from multiple perspectives and are particularly important for eccentric stenoses, which may be seen well in only one plane.

Maximum intensity projection

Maximum intensity projection (MIP) images are probably the most common method for displaying 3-D MR angiography data. In this technique, a ray is projected along the data set in the desired direction, and the highest voxel value along the ray becomes the pixel value of the two-dimensional (2-D) MIP image (Fig. 3) [16]. This method is well suited to 3-D CE MR angiography, because background signal is typically low, and arterial contrast is high. Nevertheless, MIP images obtained from the entire 3-D data set usually are contaminated to some extent by wraparound or edge artifacts that can limit visualization of vessels. Image quality can be improved by obtaining subvolume MIP images or by manually editing the entire data set. The generation and postprocessing of MIP images is rapid and straightforward on most commercially available workstations. A standard 3-D CE MR angiography examination

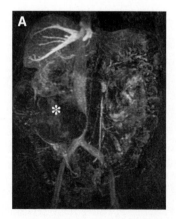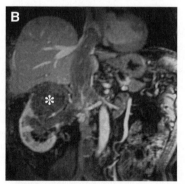

Fig. 2. Subtraction and fat-saturation techniques for MR venography. (*A*). MIP image from subtracted data set (arterial phase subtracted from venous phase) in a patient with large paraganglioma (*) compressing the inferior vena cava. Note the excellent visualization of the inferior vena cava without arterial overlap, but reduced S/N. (*B*) Subvolume MIP image from fat-saturated CE MR venogram in patient with renal cell carcinoma (*) and extensive renal vein and inferior vena cava thrombus. Although arterial structures minimally limit visualization of the inferior vena cava, there is improved S/N relative to the subtracted technique.

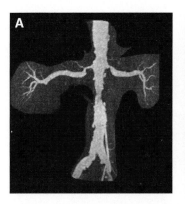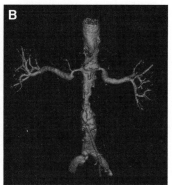

Fig. 3. 3-D CE MR angiography in a patient with severe aortic atherosclerosis and bilateral renal artery stenosis. (*A*) MIP image. (*B*) Volume rendered image.

can be edited to remove artifact and extraneous signal within a few minutes (Fig. 4).

Advantages of the MIP technique include wide availability, versatility, and speed. The ability to generate subvolume MIP images in a variety of projections and thicknesses often aids in interpretation of difficult cases. Some standard pitfalls of reliance only on MIP images are well known, however. When viewing MIP images in only one or two projections, it is possible to underestimate the severity of stenosis caused by an eccentric plaque. On the other hand, evaluation of a thick subvolume MIP image may result in overestimation of the degree of stenosis in a small vessel. Dissections without thick intimal flaps are easily missed when viewing only MIP images, and the true diameters of aneurysms are underestimated when only the patent lumen, and not the thrombosed portion of the vessel, can be seen (Fig. 5).

Surface rendering

Surface rendering employs a user-prescribed threshold level that is applied to the selected volume of data. Voxels with signal intensity levels above or below the threshold are eliminated from the final display. Voxels with attenuation levels within the threshold are joined, creating a surface display of the vessels of interest. An imaginary light source is applied to illuminate the display. Surface rendering techniques give a 3-D appearance to data not appreciated with MIP images.

Volume rendering

Volume rendering employs an algorithm in which each voxel makes two contributions to the final image: it emits light and blocks light from the voxels behind it. The color, or amount of emitted light, and opacity (the degree to which a voxel blocks light) are determined by a transfer function that maps signal intensity to brightness, color, and opacity. The user can manipulate the transfer function to a greater or lesser degree, depending on which commercially available software version is employed. The resulting images have a more 3-D appearance than MIP images and contain more information than MIP or surface-rendered images (see Fig. 3) [16]. Some investigators have found that volume-rendered images resulted in the most accurate measurement of stenoses in comparison to MIP images and source images [17–18]. It also is possible, however, to generate volume-rendered data in which stenoses are over- or underestimated by an injudicious choice of transfer function, color maps, threshold parameters, or opacity. An additional limitation of volume rendering is that it is computationally intensive. Powerful computers are necessary to permit real-time manipulation of 3-D MR angiography data sets with volume-rendering algorithms, and such computers are not universally available.

Virtual vascular endoscopy

Virtual vascular endoscopy (VVE) is the computer-generated simulation of endoscopic images derived from 3-D MR angiography. VVE allows the viewer to explore the inner surfaces of anatomic structures from a unique perspective (Fig. 6) [19]. This technique is essentially a specialized application of surface or volume rendering. In VVE, thresholding is performed to assure that only the vessel wall is included in the reconstruction (in the case of surface rendering) or that voxels with high intensities within the vessel are rendered transparent (in volume rendering). Most

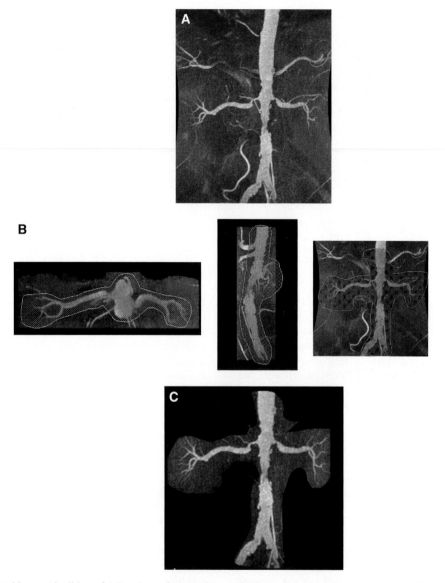

Fig. 4. Rapid manual editing of 3-D volume from patient with bilateral renal artery stenosis. (*A*) MIP image from original data is limited slightly by artifact and overlying vessels. (*B*) Manual editing performed in axial, sagittal, and coronal planes. (*C*) Resultant coronal MIP image.

commercially available software allows the user to navigate through the vessel in a fly-through mode (moving the camera within the vessel lumen with the computer mouse) or by movement of the cursor on axial, sagittal, and coronal reformatted images. Navigation also can be performed on a semiautomatic basis by asking the computer to select the next step, which generally is chosen based on the longest available open path. At present VVE is primarily an interesting novelty. It also is a computationally and user-intensive application, and there is little evidence that the time and effort currently needed to generate these images lead to improvements in diagnostic accuracy. Nevertheless, VVE often is attractive to both clinicians and patients, and it may prove useful in future specialized applications of 3-D CE MR angiography.

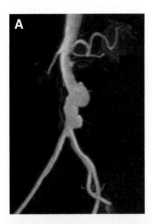

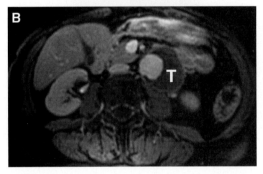

Fig. 5. Underestimation of aneurysm diameter on MIP image. (*A*) Coronal MIP image from 3-D CE MR angiography reveals eccentric infrarenal aortic aneurysm. (*B*) Axial postcontrast spoiled gradient echo image reveals true diameter of aneurysm, which contains abundant peripheral thrombus (T).

Vascular segmentation

Vascular segmentation may be helpful for distinguishing vessels from background tissue or arteries from veins. These techniques rely on a variety of algorithms, typically based on signal intensity, designed to follow the course of a vessel from one or more seed points placed by the user. The vessels are tracked, usually with mechanisms for crossing stenoses or occlusions, and then the vascular volume can be removed from the 3-D data set and analyzed separately [20–23]. Images also must have sufficient spatial resolution for proper segmentation of structures, however.

Segmentation can be useful in special regions such as carotid MR angiography or possibly coronary MR angiography. In the case of coronary MR angiography, the coronary arteries and veins are often in close proximity and may be equally opacified. Intravascular contrast agents for MR angiography are nearing approval by the

US Food and Drug Administration, and many of the most interesting applications will involve long, high-resolution MR angiography during the equilibrium phase of the bolus when both arteries and veins are enhanced. For these applications, effective segmentation techniques will be essential to separate arteries from veins.

Multiple-station image stitching

One final innovation in 3-D reconstruction, particularly helpful for presenting results of multi-station runoff examinations, is stitching software, which allows seamless merging of the data from each station. These techniques are becoming commercially available and have varying levels of sophistication. Some applications simply merge the MIP or volume-rendered images. Others merge the entire 3-D data sets and correct for differences in FOV and orientation.

Interpretation of MR angiograms

Successful interpretation of MR angiograms depends on a number of elements. Most important is obtaining the best possible examination from a technical standpoint: it is much easier to interpret an MR angiography that is not degraded by artifact. As noted previously, avoiding artifact often requires great flexibility on the part of the technologist and radiologist to adapt protocols to the abilities of a particular patient or to the goals of a particular examination.

Recognizing pathology is usually straightforward if the examination is of high quality. MR angiograms are best evaluated at an independent computer workstation where the radiologist has access to the source images and a host of image-processing tools (particularly MPR, MIP, and volume rendering). These tools enable real-time reformation of image sets to variable thicknesses and orientations that can aid interpretation. Reliance on only a standard set of MIP images, for example, is not advisable for interpretation of body MR angiography, because important findings can be missed occasionally. Pre- and postcontrast axial images are also useful for assessing atherosclerotic plaque, intraluminal thrombus, and the presence of vessel wall thickening or enhancement in patients with suspected vasculitis (Fig. 7).

An important question often encountered in 3-D CE MR angiography is the functional significance of an atherosclerotic lesion. A severe (>90%) or critical stenosis is almost always significant, but the importance of a moderate lesion is much less certain. In these situations,

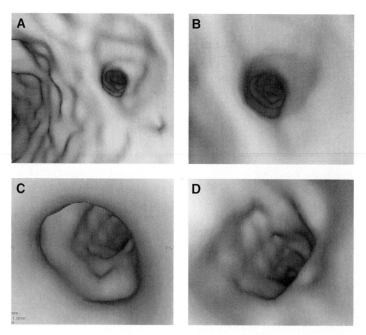

Fig. 6. VVE. (*A*) Image from the perspective of an observer inside the aorta just above the renal artery orifice. (*B–D*) The renal artery is approached and entered.

additional findings beyond the percentage of stenosis may be helpful in guiding management. For example, in the evaluation of renal artery stenosis, the findings of renal parenchymal atrophy or poststenotic dilatation support the presence of a hemodynamically significant narrowing of the renal artery (Fig. 8).

MR imaging also offers potential for functional evaluation of blood vessels. Phase-contrast techniques, for example, can measure blood flow and velocity profiles across stenotic lesions, and this information might be valuable for assessing severity, monitoring therapy, or predicting whether an intervention will be successful [24–26].

Common pitfalls and artifacts

Although the interpretation of 3-D CE MR angiographic examinations is generally straightforward, there are several pitfalls and artifacts to bear in mind. Some of the most common problems involve coordinating data acquisition with arrival of the contrast bolus. If the scan is initiated before the contrast bolus arrives or after it has passed, the arterial S/N is low, and the examination is difficult to interpret (Fig. 9).

The contrast bolus must arrive at the proper time, and it must also remain relatively stable during acquisition of the central lines of k-space. Rapid variation of arterial contrast can lead to ringing artifact (Fig. 10), which is occasionally encountered when elliptic centric acquisitions are initiated just before the arterial concentration has peaked [27]. Ringing artifact occurs secondary to the early acquisition of central k-space data during the period of rapid rise in gadolinium within the vessel and can be identified as alternating black and white lines paralleling vessels on CE MR angiography. Ringing artifact can be minimized by ensuring that the delay between the bolus arrival and data acquisition is long enough to ensure that the central k-space data acquisition occurs several seconds after the immediate arrival of contrast, during a more stable or plateau phase of the bolus. When using a test bolus for timing CE MR angiography, the addition of 2 or 3 seconds to the arrival time of the contrast test bolus (which represents the peak of the test bolus) assures that this problem is minimized. Alternatively, recessed elliptic centric k-space acquisition schemes have been described in which acquisition of the center of k-space is delayed for a few seconds from the beginning of data acquisition [28].

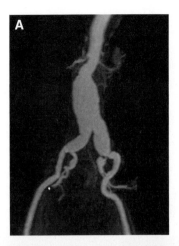

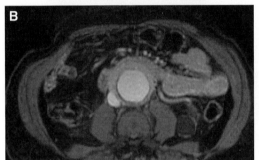

Fig. 7. Inflammatory aneurysm. (*A*) MIP image demonstrates aneurismal dilatation of the aorta and common iliac arteries. (*B*) Postcontrast fat-saturated spoiled gradient echo image reveals thickening and intense enhancement of the wall of the distal aorta. An inflammatory aneurysm was found at surgery.

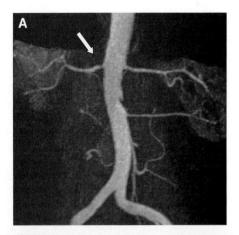

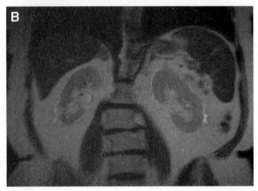

Fig. 8. Functional significance of moderate renal artery stenosis. (*A*) Renal MR angiography reveals a moderate stenosis in the proximal right renal artery (*arrow*). (*B*) Coronal single-shot fast spin echo image demonstrates mild atrophy of the right kidney, suggesting that the stenosis is functionally significant. Note incidental right adrenal mass.

The arrival of contrast usually is determined either by a test bolus or by fluoroscopic triggering. Fluoroscopic triggering is more efficient, because a separate series is not required to determine the circulation time, but orchestrating patient breath-holding with bolus arrival and scan initiation can be difficult, particularly for patients who are hard-of-hearing or who have limited breath-holding capacity. The test bolus allows greater flexibility in preparing the patient to suspend respiration, but occasionally discrepancies between the circulation time of the test bolus and the larger bolus for CE MR angiography lead to poor results. The test bolus also can be used as a visual gauge of the potential S/N of the MR angiography. If a 1- or 2-mL dose of contrast yields a long peak with high S/N, then probably the MR angiography will be of excellent quality with a relatively small dose of contrast. If the contrast peak is barely visible and fades rapidly, it might be worth considering a higher contrast dose. Errors in bolus timing are difficult to eliminate, but fortunately a second attempt at the MR angiography is usually possible.

Timing and coordination are perhaps most challenging in multistation run-off examinations. In these examinations the bolus timing must be correct for all stations, and acquisition of the initial volumes must be fast enough to prevent venous contamination in the more distal stations while preserving an acceptable spatial resolution. A number of strategies have been described to overcome some of these challenges, including the use of parallel imaging in the upper stations, mid-thigh venous compression, and continuously moving table acquisitions [3,11,29–31]. Time-resolved

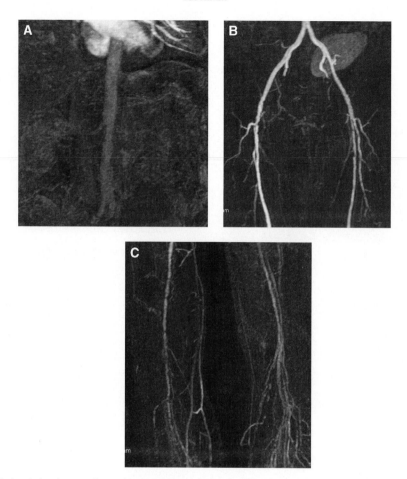

Fig. 9. Poor bolus timing in run-off examination. (*A*) The contrast bolus is too early for the abdominal station (most of the contrast remains in the heart). (*B*) Optimal contrast for the pelvic station. (*C*) The bolus is too late for the thigh station (poor arterial contrast and significant venous contamination).

techniques such as time-resolved imaging of contrast kinetics (TRICKS) also are useful and can be employed before the run-off, with a relatively small contrast dose, or as a corrective measure after the runoff, with a higher contrast dose to offset the effect of background gadolinium (Fig. 11) [32–33].

Poor breath-holding is another frequent source of artifact. For this reason, it usually is worthwhile to acquire a precontrast 3-D acquisition to assess the patient's breath-holding ability and to give the patient an opportunity to rehearse. In addition, the correct positioning of the 3-D volume can be verified, and the precontrast data can serve as a mask should subtraction be desired.

If the duration of MR angiography data acquisition is too long to ensure patient comfort and compliance, the operator has several options.

The easiest alternative is to change nothing and hope that the patient's performance improves. Although this strategy has the virtue of simplicity, it is, unfortunately, often ineffective. Acquisition times can be shortened in a number of ways. Spatial resolution can be decreased, or volumetric coverage can be reduced. Partial-phase FOV or partial echo acquisitions can also be performed. Increasing the receiver bandwidth will often reduce the minimum TR and thereby allow faster acquisitions. Parallel imaging is also an attractive option that allows gains in acquisition speed by factors of two to three (Fig. 12) [10,34–35]. Care must be taken, however, to avoid reconstruction artifacts associated with this technique.

Motion artifact also can occur even in the absence of poor breath-holding. It has been shown, for example, that significant motion of

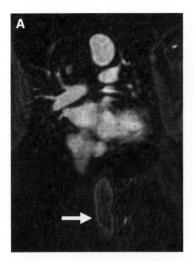
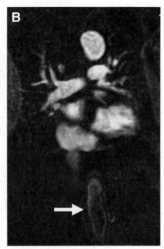

Fig. 10. (*A* and *B*) Two source images from a thoracic 3-D CE MR angiography demonstrate ringing artifact (*arrow*) in abdominal aorta caused by the acquisition of central k-space data during the initial arrival of the contrast bolus when the concentration of gadolinium is rising rapidly. The ringing artifact is identified by alternating bright and dark lines that parallel the vessel wall, in this case the abdominal aorta.

the kidneys occurs despite successfully suspended respiration [36]. In general, diaphragmatic motion is minimized when respiration is suspended at end-expiration rather than end-inspiration, but many patients find this maneuver difficult and unpleasant. Motion artifact also may be caused by peristalsis, vascular pulsation, cardiac motion, or other involuntary motion. Cardiac pulsation artifact can be particularly troublesome in the ascending aorta. If visualization of this region is important, it is often prudent to include cardiac-gated steady-state free-precession sequences, black-blood sequences, or non-gated fast sequential bright-blood acquisitions in addition to 3-D CE MR angiography to facilitate evaluation of the aortic root and ascending aorta (Fig. 13).

Artifacts can be particularly troubling when they mimic disease. Arterial pseudostenosis has been described as a result of high concentrations of gadolinium within an overlying vein. A high concentration of gadolinium can result in prominent T2* susceptibility artifacts, which in turn obscure proper visualization of the adjacent artery and may result in the erroneous appearance of an arterial stenosis [37–38]. This phenomenon probably occurs most frequently in the subclavian artery, particularly the left subclavian artery after a left antecubital venous injection of contrast medium. A second 3-D acquisition immediately following the arterial phase, after the concentrated venous gadolinium has dispersed, can help

to distinguish between artifact and a true lesion. On the second set of images, the arteries should have a normal caliber, and the pseudostenosis should have disappeared.

Metallic susceptibility artifact can easily obscure visualization of the vascular territory of interest. Relatively little can be done about large metal objects, although increasing the receiver bandwidth and flip angle and minimizing TE may help limit the amount of signal void [39]. Vascular stents are the most problematic source of metallic artifact. Although a few MR-transparent stents are manufactured now [40–42], most stents are not MR transparent and will cause artifact substantial enough to prevent determination of in-stent patency or stenosis. An additional problem is the presence of an unsuspected stent, which can mimic a vascular stenosis or a short segment occlusion. Inspection of source images is helpful, because most metallic stents have characteristic signal dropout from metallic susceptibility artifact. These findings are typically more obvious on 2-D pre- or postcontrast images (Figs. 14). Surgical clips present a similar dilemma: the artifact they generate can mimic stenosis, a particular problem in imaging the vascular supply to renal or hepatic transplants.

Overestimation of stenoses resulting from intravoxel dephasing is a well-known artifact of noncontrast time-of-flight techniques. Although this phenomenon is much less prominent in 3-D

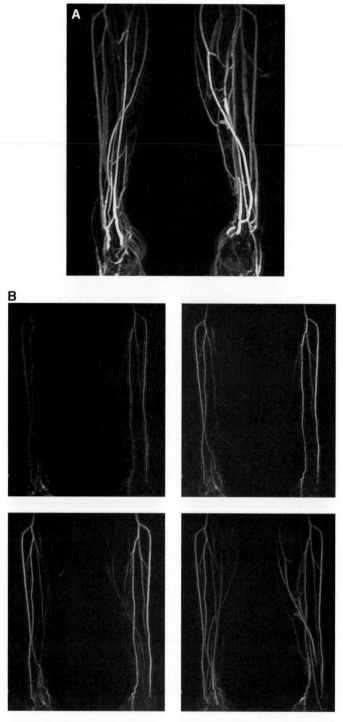

Fig. 11. Venous contamination in the calf station of a lower extremity runoff examination. (*A*) Thick-section MIP of the subtracted data from the final station of a multistation bolus-chase 3-D CE MR angiography examination. (*B*) Four MIP images from a separate time-resolved acquisition (TRICKS) performed with a temporal resolution of approximately 6 seconds. Note that the optimal arterial frame can be selected and this data set reconstructed to minimize venous contamination.

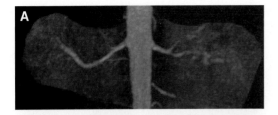

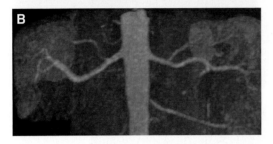

Fig. 12. Motion artifact reduction with parallel imaging. (*A*) Renal MR angiography is limited in a patient with poor breath-hold capacity. (*B*) Parallel imaging was applied to reduce acquisition time from 20 seconds to 10 seconds. Note improved visualization of distal renal arteries and accessory left renal artery.

CE MR angiography, it can occur, particularly in small vessels with severe stenoses.

Evaluation of renal arteries for fibromuscular dysplasia is a challenging application of 3-D CE MR angiography. Although severe lesions are usually detected, subtle cases are often overlooked. The sensitivity and specificity of 3-D CE MR angiography for fibromuscular dysplasia is not ideal. Both false-positive and false-negative examinations probably are related to insufficient spatial resolution as well as to subtle motion of the kidneys and renal arteries during acquisition of the MR angiography (Fig. 15) [43].

Subtraction artifacts are uncommon in vascular territories that are not affected by respiratory motion (ie, the head, neck, and extremities). When there is significant misregistration between the mask data and the CE MR angiography, subtraction artifacts are usually obvious. Subtle artifacts are more problematic, because stenoses in small vessels may be under- or overestimated. It is usually worth verifying that the lesions seen in

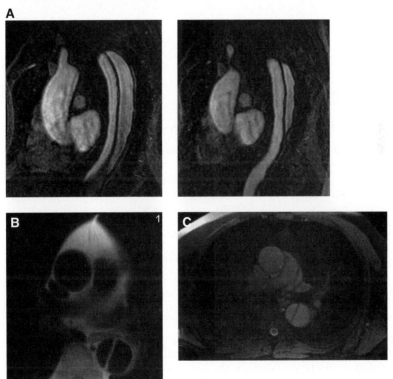

Fig. 13. (*A*) Source images from thoracic MR angiography reveal a dissection in the descending thoracic aorta. Evaluation of the proximal ascending aorta is limited by motion artifact. Cardiac-gated black-blood single-shot fast spin echo image (*B*) and non-gated steady-state free-precession image (*C*) eliminate artifact and provide improved visualization of the proximal aorta.

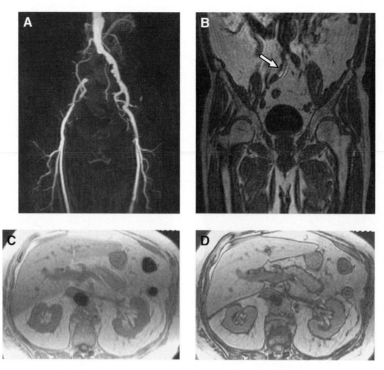

Fig. 14. Metallic susceptibility artifacts secondary to vascular stent grafts. (*A* and *B*) Pseudo-occlusion secondary to iliac artery stent. MR angiography reveals apparent short-segment occlusion of the right common iliac artery. (*B*) Subtle metallic susceptibility artifact (*arrow*) is demonstrated in a source image from the mask precontrast acquisition. (*C* and *D*) Renal artery stent. More extensive susceptibility artifact is seen on in-phase (*C*) and out-of-phase (*D*) spoiled gradient echo images in a patient with a right renal artery stent. Note that the in-phase image demonstrates more extensive artifact because of a longer TE.

a subtracted data set in the chest or abdomen also can be visualized on the unsubtracted images.

Interpretation errors can occur when only MIP or volume-rendered images are examined: eccentric stenoses can be missed, lesions in small vessels may be overestimated, and visualization of dissections is limited. Data from 3-D CE MR angiography should always be evaluated at the workstation where a range of 3-D reconstruction techniques is available simultaneously, and where the radiologist can examine a vessel from multiple perspectives.

Finally, it is important to realize the fundamental limitations of 3-D CE MR angiography. This technique visualizes the patent lumen of vessels, and therefore it is easy to overlook the true diameter of an aneurysm if it contains abundant thrombus (see Fig. 5). Likewise, 3-D CE MR angiography provides little information regarding the vessel wall. Thickening or enhancement in the setting of vasculitis often is missed, as are small

intramural hematomas (see Fig. 7). For this reason it is important to supplement the data acquired with 3-D CE MR angiography with pre- and postcontrast acquisitions to visualize the vessel wall.

Incidental findings

The radiologist must decide whether any additional imaging beyond the requested MR angiography should be performed to evaluate incidental findings, particularly in the chest and abdomen, where incidental pathology is much more likely to occur. For example, a standard protocol for renal MR angiography might include single-shot fast spin echo, in-phase/out-of-phase spoiled gradient echo, and postcontrast fat-saturated 2-D spoiled gradient echo acquisitions. All of these are useful to exclude renal masses, but they might also demonstrate renal atrophy,

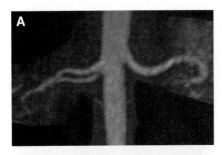

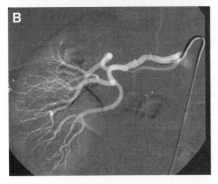

Fig. 15. Fibromuscular dysplasia missed on MR angiography. (*A*) Slight irregularity of the superior right renal artery was thought to be artifactual. (*B*) Conventional angiogram reveals mild fibromuscular dysplasia in the mid-distal artery. The left renal artery was normal at angiography.

asymmetric enhancement, or other findings relevant to the interpretation of the MR angiography. Postcontrast axial images, as noted previously, are important for characterizing aortic atherosclerotic disease as well as for obtaining accurate measurements of the true diameter of aneurysms. In-phase/out-of-phase images help characterize the incidental adrenal mass, which occurs with great frequency and might be an important finding in the patient with unexplained hypertension. These extra sequences fall short of a complete abdominal examination but usually can be accomplished quickly without adding unduly to the total examination time.

Indications for thoracic or abdominal MR angiography are often ambiguous, and it is worth noting that many of the symptoms prompting the requested MR angiography could be explained by other findings. Mesenteric ischemia, for example, can produce vague symptoms that mimic a great many other abdominal pathologies (Fig. 16). Axial imaging is useful in any case in this indication to evaluate the bowel wall for abnormal thickening or enhancement.

Reporting results

Results from MR angiography examinations should be reported clearly and concisely. The description of atherosclerotic lesions should at least be semiquantitative: a stenosis can be graded either as a percentage narrowing (ie, normal diameter – stenotic diameter/normal diameter) or with some descriptor of severity such as mild (<50%), moderate (50%–75%), or severe (>75%).

If the referring physician might not be familiar with the range of therapeutic options, it is helpful to state which lesions might be amenable to percutaneous angioplasty. MR angiographic examinations performed for vascular surgical planning should note whether there is adequate inflow into the vessel above the stenosis and, if a bypass procedure is being considered, whether a distal target vessel is present that is large enough to maintain patency of the graft and provide adequate flow to the limb.

Dissections should be characterized by their involvement of the ascending aorta and great vessels as well as by their inferior extent. Extension of flaps into great vessels, mesenteric arteries, renal arteries, or iliac vessels is information that it is important to convey. Differential perfusion of one kidney supplied by the false lumen, particularly in the setting of hypertension or renal insufficiency, may prompt surgery or fenestration.

Aneurysms should be described by their location, length, and diameter. Careful comparison with previous examinations is important to document interval growth. If stent graft placement is a therapeutic option, the distance of the aneurysm neck from the renal arteries should be measured, and any sharp angulations should be noted.

Summary

3-D CE MR angiography has become a versatile and effective technique that can be applied successfully to nearly any vascular territory. Although innovations in both hardware and pulse-sequence development continue unabated, there are a few persistent pitfalls and artifacts that must be recognized and avoided, if possible. Most can be minimized with careful attention to technique. Familiarity with the latest developments in parallel imaging and time-resolved MR angiography is not essential, but the commercially available applications of these techniques can be valuable in many situations.

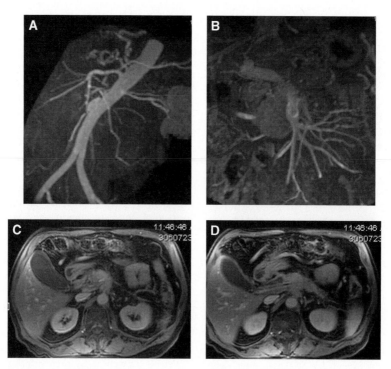

Fig. 16. Pancreatic cancer incidentally detected in a patient evaluated for mesenteric ischemia. (*A*) MIP image from arterial-phase MR angiography reveals irregular narrowing of the splenic and hepatic arteries, which have separate origins from the aorta. (*B*) Venous-phase MIP reveals occlusion of the splenic vein. (*C* and *D*) Postcontrast fat-saturated spoiled gradient echo images reveal ill-defined mass encasing the celiac and hepatic arteries. Pancreatic adenocarcinoma was diagnosed by needle biopsy.

3-D reconstruction techniques are increasing in complexity but, somewhat paradoxically, are also becoming easier and faster to employ. The wide availability of powerful computers has opened many interesting possibilities in 3-D visualization, and in all likelihood these techniques will continue to evolve rapidly. It is important to recognize, however, that even the most sophisticated techniques can do very little with poor data.

References

[1] Prince MR. Contrast-enhanced MR angiography: theory and optimization. Magn Reson Imaging Clin N Am 1998;6(2):257–68.

[2] Montgomery ML, Case RS. Magnetic resonance imaging of the vascular system: a practical approach for the radiologist. Top Magn Reson Imaging 2003; 14(5):376–85.

[3] Meaney JFM. Magnetic resonance angiography of the peripheral arteries: current status. Eur Radiol 2003;13:836–52.

[4] Tatli S, Lipton MJ, Davison BD, et al. MR imaging of aortic and peripheral vascular disease. Radiographics 2003;23:S59–78.

[5] Shetty AN, Bis KG, Kirsch M, et al. Contrast-enhanced breath-hold three-dimensional magnetic resonance angiography in the evaluation of renal arteries: optimization of technique and pitfalls. J Magn Reson Imaging 2000;12:912–23.

[6] Glockner JF. Three-dimensional gadolinium-enhanced MR angiography: applications for abdominal imaging. Radiographics 2001;21: 357–70.

[7] Fain SB, King BF, Breen JF, et al. High spatial resolution contrast-enhanced MR angiography of the renal arteries: a prospective comparison with digital subtraction angiography. Radiology 2001;218: 481–90.

[8] Maki JH, Chenevert TL, Prince MR. The effects of incomplete breath-holding on 3D MR image quality. J Magn Reson Imaging 1997;7(6): 1132–9.

[9] Willman AH, Riederer SJ. Performance of an elliptical centric view order for signal enhancement and motion artifact suppression in breath-hold three-dimensional gradient echo imaging. Magn Reson Med 1997;38(5):793–802.

[10] Weiger M, Pruessmann KP, Kassner A, et al. Contrast-enhanced MRA using SENSE. J Magn Reson Imaging 2000;12:671–7.

[11] Maki JH, Wilson GJ, Eubank WB, et al. Utilizing SENSE to achieve lower station sub-millimeter isotropic resolution and minimal venous enhancement in peripheral MR angiography. J Magn Reson Imaging 2002;15:484–91.

[12] Volk M, Strotzer M, Lenhart M, et al. Time-resolved contrast-enhanced MR angiography of renal artery stenosis: diagnostic accuracy and inter-observer variability. AJR Am J Roentgenol 2000; 174:1583–8.

[13] Ruehm SG, Nanz D, Baumann A, et al. 3D contrast-enhanced MR angiography of the run-off vessels: value of image subtraction. J Magn Reson Imaging 2001;13(3):402–11.

[14] Leiner T, de Weert TT, Nijenhuis RJ, et al. Need for background suppression in contrast-enhanced peripheral magnetic resonance angiography. J Magn Reson Imaging 2001;14(6):724–33.

[15] Naganawa S, Ito T, Iwayama E, et al. Magnitude subtraction vs complex subtraction in dynamic contrast-enhanced MR angiography: basic experiments and clinical evaluation. J Magn Reson Imaging 1999;10(5):813–20.

[16] Calhoun PS, Kuszyk BS, Heath DG, et al. Three-dimensional volume rendering of spiral CT data: theory and method. Radiographics 1999;19: 745–64.

[17] Malouhi A, Schocke M, Judmaier W, et al. 3D MR angiography of renal arteries: comparison of volume rendering and maximum intensity projection algorithms. Radiology 2002;223(2):509–16.

[18] Baskaran V, Perles FS, Nemcek AA, et al. Gadolinium-enhanced 3D MR angiography of renal artery stenosis: a bilateral comparison of maximum intensity projection, multiplanar reformatting, and 3D volume rendering post processing algorithms. Acad Radiol 2002;9(1):50–9.

[19] Glockner JF. Navigating the aorta: MR virtual vascular endoscopy. Radiographics 2003;23(2):E11.

[20] de Koning PJ, Schaap JA, Janssen JP, et al. Automated segmentation and analysis of vascular structures in magnetic resonance angiographic images. Magn Reson Med 2003;50(6):1189–98.

[21] Martel AL, Fraser D, Delay GS, et al. Separating arterial and venous components from 3D dynamic contrast-enhanced MRI studies using factor analysis. Magn Reson Med 2003;49(5):928–33.

[22] Flasque N, Desvignes M, Constans JM, et al. Acquisition, segmentation and tracking of the cerebral vascular tree on 3D magnetic resonance angiography images. Med Image Anal 2001;5(3):173–83.

[23] Bock M, Schoenberg SO, Floemer F, et al. Separation of arteries and veins in 3D MR angiography using correlation analysis. Magn Reson Med 2000; 43(3):481–7.

[24] Schoenberg SO, Rieger J, Nittka M, et al. Renal MR angiography: current debates and developments in imaging of renal artery stenosis. Semin Ultrasound CT MRI 2003;24(4):255–67.

[25] Schoenberg SO, Knopp MV, Londy F, et al. Morphologic and functional magnetic resonance imaging of renal artery stenosis: a multireader tricenter study. J Am Soc Nephrol 2002;13:158–69.

[26] Hood MN, Ho VB, Corse WR. Three-dimensional phase-contrast magnetic resonance angiography: a useful clinical adjunct to gadolinium-enhanced three-dimensional renal magnetic resonance angiography? Mil Med 2002;167(4):343–9.

[27] Svensson J, Petersson JS, Stahlberg F, et al. Image artifacts due to a time-varying contrast medium concentration in 3D contrast-enhanced MRA. J Magn Reson Imaging 1999;10(6):919–28.

[28] Watts R, Wang Y, Redd B, et al. Recessed elliptical-centric view-ordering for contrast-enhanced 3D MR angiography of the carotid arteries. Magn Reson Med 2002;48(3):419–24.

[29] Herborn CU, Ajaj W, Goyen M, et al. Peripheral vasculature: whole-body MR angiography with midfemoral venous compression—initial experience. Radiology 2004;230(3):872–8.

[30] Wentz KU, Frohlich JM, von Weymarn C, et al. High-resolution magnetic resonance angiography of hands with timed arterial compression. Lancet 2003;361:49–50.

[31] Madhuranthakam AJ, Kruger DG, Riederer SJ, et al. Time-resolved 3D contrast-enhanced MRA of an extended FOV using continuous table motion. Magn Reson Med 2004;51:568–76.

[32] Swan JS, Carroll TJ, Kennell TW, et al. Time-resolved three-dimensional contrast-enhanced MR angiography of the peripheral vessels. Radiology 2002;225(1):43–52.

[33] Hany TF, Carroll TJ, Omary RA, et al. Aorta and runoff vessels single injection MR angiography with automated table movement compared with multi-injection time-resolved MR angiography—initial results. Radiology 2001;221(1):266–72.

[34] Pruessmann KP, Weiger M, Scheidegger MB, et al. SENSE: sensitivity encoding for fast MRI. Magn Reson Med 1999;42:952–62.

[35] Ohno Y, Kawamitsu H, Higashino T, et al. Time-resolved contrast-enhanced pulmonary MR angiography using sensitivity encoding. J Magn Reson Imaging 2003;17:330–6.

[36] Vasbinder GB, Maki JH, Nijenhuis RJ, et al. Motion of the distal renal artery during three-dimensional contrast-enhanced breath-hold MRA. J Magn Reson Imaging 2002;16(6):685–96.

[37] Neimatallah MA, Chenevert TL, Carlos RC, et al. Subclavian MR arteriography: reduction of susceptibility artifact with short echo time and dilute gadopenetate dimeglumine. Radiology 2000;217: 581–6.

[38] Tirkes AT, Rosen MA, Siegelman ES. Gadolinium susceptibility artifact causing false positive stenosis isolated to the proximal common carotid artery in 3D dynamic contrast medium enhanced MR angiography of the thorax—a brief review of causes and

prevention. Int J Cardiovasc Imaging 2003;19(2): 151–5.

[39] Gonner F, Lovblad KO, Heid O, et al. Magnetic resonance angiography with ultrashort echo times reduces the artifact of aneurysm clips. Neuroradiology 2002;44(9):755–8.

[40] Buecker A, Spuentrup E, Ruebben A, et al. Artifact-free in-stent lumen visualization by standard magnetic resonance angiography using a new metallic magnetic resonance imaging stent. Circulation 2002;105(15):1772–5.

[41] van Holten J, Wielopolski P, Bruck E, et al. High flip angle imaging of metallic stents: implications for MR angiography and intraluminal signal interpretation. Magn Reson Med 2003;50(4):879–83.

[42] Spuentrup E, Ruebben A, Stuber M, et al. Metallic renal artery MR imaging stent: artifact-free lumen visualization with projection and standard renal MR angiography. Radiology 2003;227(3):897–902.

[43] Lee VS, Martin DJ, Krinsky GA, et al. Gadolinium-enhanced MR angiography: artifacts and pitfalls. AJR Am J Roentgenol 2000;175:197–205.

ELSEVIER
SAUNDERS

Magn Reson Imaging Clin N Am
13 (2005) 41–64

MAGNETIC
RESONANCE
IMAGING CLINICS
of North America

MR Angiography of the Thoracic Aorta

Julianna M. Czum, MD[a,*], William R. Corse, DO[b,c],
Vincent B. Ho, MD[c]

[a]Department of Radiology, Box 141, New York Presbyterian Hospital, Weill Medical College of Cornell University,
525 East 68th Street, New York, NY 10021, USA
[b]Department of Radiology, Doylestown Hospital, 595 West State Street, Doylestown, PA 18901, USA
[c]Department of Radiology and Radiological Sciences, Uniformed Services University of the Health Sciences,
4301 Jones Bridge Road, Bethesda, MD 20814, USA

Catheter-based diagnostic contrast angiography of the aorta has largely been replaced in clinical practice by its noninvasive counterparts, namely, CT angiography and MR angiography [1–12]. Compared with MR angiography, CT angiography has the benefits of greater general availability (and access) and ease of performance—features that frequently make it the modality of choice, especially in acute situations. Nevertheless, MR imaging has several distinct advantages over CT, which admittedly may not always be pertinent for every clinical evaluation. MR imaging does not require the use of ionizing radiation, which is a distinct advantage in vulnerable populations such as children or pregnant women. The lack of radiation also enables the performance of several different imaging techniques and repetitive dynamic imaging for improved characterization and definition of vascular lesions without radiation exposure concerns. MR imaging has the advantage of improved blood flow and tissue characterization that is distinctly better than that achieved by simple x-ray density and vascular "luminography" afforded by CT

angiography. MR imaging can provide a host of options beyond simple three-dimensional (3D) angiographic illustration [8–21]. Cine MR imaging can be performed to evaluate blood flow through structures; cine phase contrast (PC) can be used to quantify blood flow. Cine MR imaging can be used specifically to evaluate valvular and cardiac function.

Unlike CT angiography, MR angiography does not require the use of iodinated contrast media, which has well-known clinical concerns of nephrotoxicity and a higher rate of adverse reaction—concerns not associated with gadolinium (Gd)-chelate contrast media used for MR angiography. Nephrotoxicity is a particularly relevant issue, because renal insufficiency is often present in patients with aortic disease secondary to atherosclerosis or diabetes mellitus. In particular, MR angiography has benefits for patients undergoing percutaneous intervention. The use of MR angiography for pre-procedural planning removes the concerns related to iodine load and impaired renal function that are common when pre-planning with CT angiography, which may preclude same day or close scheduling of interventional procedures.

Recent advances in fast imaging, such as steady state free precession (SSFP) and subsecond contrast-enhanced (CE) MR angiography, enable quick thoracic examinations with initial screening evaluations of the aorta within 4 minutes [22]. These improvements in speed in addition to the global improvements in clinical availability of MR imaging and the aforementioned advantages of MR imaging over CT evaluation suggest an

The opinions or assertions contained herein are the private views of the authors and are not to be construed as official or reflecting the views of the Uniformed Services University of the Health Sciences or the Department of Defense.

* Corresponding author.

E-mail address: jmcz012@med.cornell.edu (J.M. Czum).

1064-9689/05/$ - see front matter. Published by Elsevier Inc.
doi:10.1016/j.mric.2004.12.009

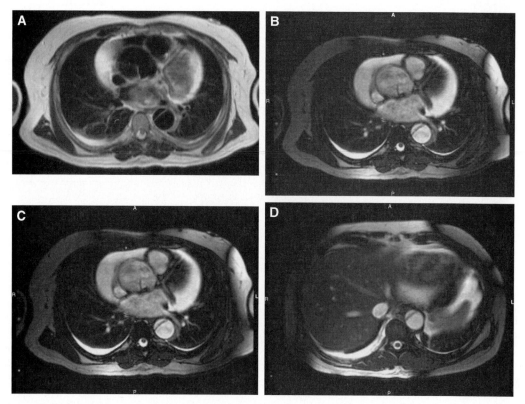

Fig. 1. Type A aortic dissection in a man with chest pain. (*A*) Axial breath hold ECG-gated black blood DIR FSE image demonstrates intimal tears within the ascending and descending aorta consistent with aortic dissection. (*B–E*) Free-breathing SSFP images (*B–D*, axial cranial to caudal; *E*, sagittal oblique) demonstrating the dissection and its involvement of the entire thoracic aorta with patency of the true and false lumens. (*F–J*) 3D contrast-enhanced (CE) MR angiography (*F*, sagittal thick MIP; *G*, oblique sagittal subvolume MIP; *H*, coronal subvolume MIP) shows the full extent of the aortic dissection. The intimal tear (ie, the ascending aorta and arch regions) is obscured on the MIP (*F*) by overlying signal within adjacent lumens. The common origin of the right innominate and left common carotid artery (*, bovine arch) is noted. On thinner subvolume MIP images (*G*, oblique coronal; *H*, coronal) of the same 3D data set, the intimal tear that separates the true (T) and false (F) channels is better visualized. The dissection is also noted to extend into the proximal right innominate artery (*G*), but the remaining great vessels arise from the true lumen (T). Because the renal arteries and the celiac axis were included within the 3D CE MR angiography volume, selective subvolume MIPs can be performed through the lower abdomen. On axial subvolume MIP through the celiac axis (*I*), the celiac artery (*arrow*) is noted to arise from the anterior true lumen. Slightly lower on another axial subvolume MIP (*J*), the right renal artery is seen arising from the anterior true lumen, and the left renal artery is seen arising from the false lumen (F). (*K–M*) VR views (*K*, left anterior oblique view; *L*, right posterior oblique view; *M*, left anterior oblique translucent view) well illustrate the extent of the aortic dissection. Note on the right posterior oblique view (*L*), the origin of the great vessels from the true lumen is more apparent, which is also well demonstrated on the translucent view (*M*). On the translucent VR image (*M*), the extension of the intimal flap into the right innominate artery is seen. Translucent VR views often enable an added appreciation of the spatial relationships when compared with MIP (compare the visualization of the ascending aorta, arch, and arch vessels in *M* with that in *F*).

increasing role for MR aortography, even in the evaluation of some acute conditions (Fig. 1).

This article reviews MR and MR angiographic techniques for evaluation of the thoracic aorta and the practical issues for their implementation. Common diseases of the thoracic aorta will be discussed focussing of their anticipated locations, and unique morphologic and functional features. An understanding of both the MR techniques and pathologic considerations will enable the formulation of tailored imaging strategies for a thorough, accurate and time-efficient aortic MR evaluation.

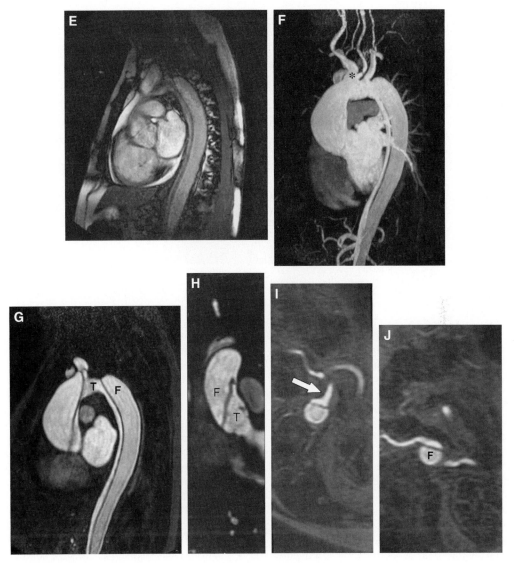

Fig. 1 (*continued*)

Basic considerations for thoracic MR angiography

Clinical issues

The thorax presents a unique challenge for successful vascular MR imaging because of the beating heart and breathing. Ever-present cardiac and respiratory motion must be overcome to minimize image-degrading blurring artifacts that can result from spatial misregistration of data. Such artifacts can decrease the homogeneity of high intraluminal signal on bright blood sequences or the desired dark intraluminal flow void on black blood imaging, producing false-positive intraluminal pathology. Moreover, the mismapping of signal may obscure bona fide abnormalities, resulting in false-negative interpretation. Fortunately, several MR techniques are available to minimize cardiac and respiratory motion artifacts. MR imaging can be performed using electrocardiogram (ECG) gating that exploits the rhythmicity of the cardiac cycle. This technique also enables a variety of additional imaging strategies (eg, cine MR) that can be employed to evaluate blood flow.

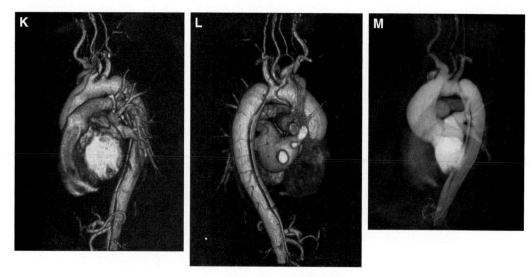

Fig. 1 (*continued*)

Using ECG gating, images can be acquired throughout the cardiac cycle (eg, cine MR) or targeted for acquisition during diastole, the more quiescent phase of the cardiac cycle. In the setting of significant dysrhythmias or ectopy or poor ECG signal amplitude, triggering is inconsistent (missed R waves and fewer valid R waves triggered); consequently, examination times can be prohibitively long and image quality poor. Peripheral gating is a viable option for cardiac synchronization in these patients.

Respiratory motion must also be overcome. In many cases, respiratory compensation or triggering using respiratory bellows can successfully synchronize image acquisition if the patient has regular tidal respiration. With newer faster pulse sequences, imaging can be performed during a single breath hold. Supplemental oxygen administration and hyperventilation can extend the length of breath holding, even in patients with chronic pulmonary disease [23]. Most individuals should be able to breath hold for 20 to 30 seconds, the length needed for standard Gd-enhanced 3D MR angiography. When the patient is unable to hold his or her breath for long periods, the use of multiple averages (eg, the number of signal averages [NSA] or the number of excitations [NEX] equals two to four) will provide adequate image quality during free-breathing acquisitions. This method is particularly valuable when imaging patients such as sedated children in whom the tidal respiratory pattern and rate are stable.

Alternatively, a faster imaging sequence such as SSFP can provide adequate image quality, even if acquired during free breathing (see Fig. 1).

In addition to assessing the patient's cardiac and respiratory limitations for MR angiography, one must consider the venous access. In many cases, 3D CE MR angiography is helpful if not essential for proper aortic diagnosis [2–12]. When performing CE MR angiography, the intravenous catheter should be placed in a right antecubital vein. Administration of a Gd-chelate contrast agent via the left upper extremity can result in pseudostenosis or pseudo-occlusion of the proximal aortic arch vessels (Fig. 2) [4,12,24]. This appearance results from the T2* effect (also called T2* susceptibility artifact) of the high concentration of Gd within the left bracheocephalic vein during the initial first pass of the bolus. It can be avoided by preferentially administering the contrast via the right upper extremity antecubital vein, as the venous return through the right brachiocephalic vein does not cross anterior to the aortic arch branch arteries as it courses to the superior vena cava. When left upper extremity contrast administration is unavoidable, multiphase imaging (ie, imaging the arterial and delayed phases) will confirm the presence of artifactual narrowing seen on the initial arterial phase images. In general, it is best to perform 3D CE MR angiography using multiple postcontrast acquisitions or phases (eg, arterial and one or more delayed phase MR angiography) [4,12]. A multiphase 3D CE MR

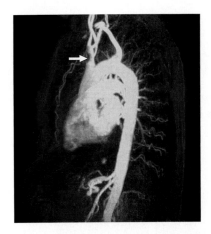

Fig. 2. T2* artifact from left antecubital venous Gd-chelate contrast media injection. Sagittal arterial phase MIP image of 3D contrast-enhanced MR angiography depicts an apparent defect along the anterior aspect of the proximal innominate artery (*arrow*), suggesting an eccentric anterior stenosis. This defect occurred secondary to the high concentration of Gd in the left brachiocephalic vein coursing anterior to the proximal arch vessel that results in T2* susceptibility artifact. Subsequent delayed image (not shown) demonstrated normal caliber of the innominate artery.

angiographic examination enables not only the proper recognition of artifacts but also allows for proper identification of late- or slow-filling vascular structures, such as false channels or very stenotic arterial segments. Typically, multiphase imaging is performed with each high-spatial resolution 3D acquisition (20 to 30 seconds) during an individual breath hold with brief interscan pauses (20 to 30 seconds) to yield an acquisition every minute and a total time requirement of 3 to 4 minutes. Using newer pulse sequences such as time resolved imaging of contrast kinetics [25] and subsecond 3D MR angiography [26], it is possible to perform time-resolved imaging using faster lower-spatial resolution scans for multiphase imaging during a single breath hold (eg, five low-spatial resolution 3D MR angiographic studies during a single 25-second breath hold). For proper illustration of smaller branch vessels, higher spatial resolution imaging is often necessary.

MR techniques: pulse sequences and image interpretation

Three-dimensional contrast-enhanced MR angiography

3D CE MR angiography is arguably the singular most profound advancement in vascular

MR imaging in the last decade, virtually replacing diagnostic conventional invasive angiography [2–12]. Technically, it has the advantage of being fast, reliable, and easy to perform. Diagnostically, it has the benefit of providing high-spatial resolution 3D data sets for improved advanced postprocessing multiplanar reformation (MPR), maximum intensity projection (MIP), and volume rendering (VR) (see Fig. 1). In contemporary MR imaging algorithms, 3D CE MR angiography forms the foundation upon which most comprehensive aortic evaluation is constructed.

Gadolinium-chelate contrast media increases vascular signal by the T1-shortening effects that it exerts on adjacent blood-pool hydrogen protons [27–29]. To optimize this benefit, CE MR angiography is generally performed using a T1-weighted pulse sequence, typically, a 3D spoiled-gradient echo using the shortest possible echo time (TE), repetition time (TR), and a 20- to 45-degree flip angle. The imaging volume is typically placed as a sagittal or oblique sagittal acquisition that includes the long axis of the aorta. This placement minimizes the overall imaged volume size and corresponds to a left anterior oblique radiographic projection, that is, a "candy cane" view of the aorta (Figs. 1 and 3). A coronal acquisition is sometimes preferred for evaluation of the arch vessels (ie, carotid, vertebral, or subclavian arteries) (Fig. 4), or for evaluation of patients with aortic dissection with suspected distal renal artery involvement. On most 1.5 Tesla MR scanners, a spatial resolution of roughly 1.5 to 2 mm voxel dimension can be achieved in 20 to 30 seconds. To decrease the imaging time (and patient breath hold requirements), a variety of scanning adjustments can be made, including the use of a rectangular field of view, partial Fourier (eg, 0.5 NEX or NSA), increased receiver bandwidth (eg, ±128 kHz), and parallel imaging.

Parallel imaging techniques deserve additional comment [30–32]. These techniques (eg, sensitivity encoding, Philips Medical Systems, Best, The Netherlands; array spatial sensitivity encoding technique, General Electric Health Care, Waukesha, Wisconsin; integrated parallel acquisition techniques, Siemens Medical Solutions, Erlangen, Germany) require the use of phased-array surface coils and allow the operator to decrease image acquisition times significantly while maintaining spatial resolution, but at the expense of signal-to-noise ratio. Properly performed arterial phase Gd-enhanced MR angiography typically provides sufficient arterial signal to noise for diagnostic

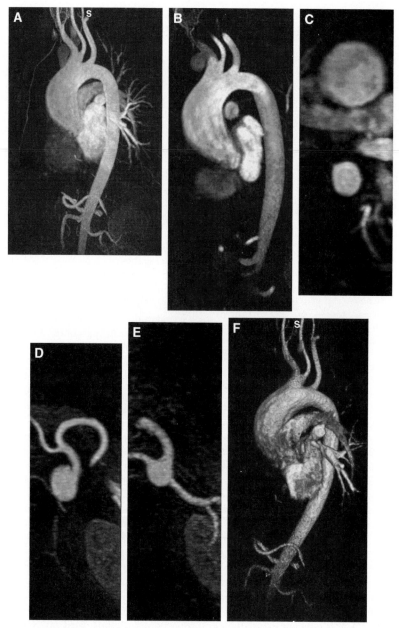

Fig. 3. Oblique sagittal 3D contrast-enhanced (CE) MR angiography acquisition in a patient with a large 5- to 6-cm ascending aortic aneurysm. (A–E) The dilated ascending aorta is well visualized on arterial phase 3D CE MR angiography (A, oblique sagittal MIP; B, oblique sagittal subvolume MIP; C, axial MPR through ascending aorta). There is no intimal tear to suggest a dissection. In addition, the field of view included the upper abdomen so that the celiac axis (D, axial subvolume MIP), superior mesenteric artery (E, axial subvolume MIP), and renal arteries (E, axial subvolume MIP) could also be evaluated. (F) VR image also demonstrates the dilated ascending aorta. As previously mentioned, VR viewing allows improved visualization of depth as can be seen by the ability to differentiate the overlapping left pulmonary arteries and veins on the VR image. Note also the common origin of the innominate and left common cartoid artery from the aortic arch (so-called, "bovine arch").

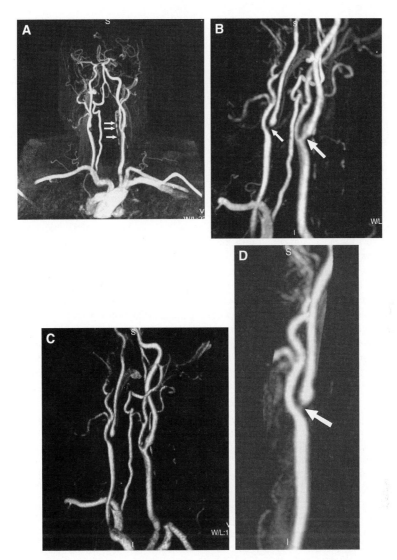

Fig. 4. Coronal 3D contrast-enhanced MR angiography of the aortic arch and great vessels in a patient with atherosclerotic disease. (*A*, coronal MIP; *B*, oblique MIP; *C*, oblique VR) Severe stenoses of the right internal carotid artery (*B*, *small arrow*) and moderate stenosis of the left internal carotid artery (*B*, *large arrow*) are shown. On VR (*C*) and to a lesser extent on oblique MIP (*B*), the right internal carotid artery appears to be occluded owing to an artifact of the thickness of the volume. Thinner subvolume MIP (*D*) shows the right internal carotid to be significantly narrow but with continuity of its luminal signal intensity (*arrow*) across the lesion. This appearance highlights the need for image interpretation not to rely solely on large volume MIP but also to include a review of thinner source data or preferably thin section MPR and subvolume MIP images as well. On MIP, multiple stenoses of the left vertebral artery (*A*, *arrows*) were also seen.

quality images using parallel imaging. As a result of faster scan times, the contrast bolus injection time and dose can be adjusted downward along with a shorter breath hold period, with even greater guarantees for imaging free of respiratory motion artifacts. Alternatively, a faster imaging speed can be used to increase the spatial resolution of MR angiography while keeping the acquisition time constant.

CE MR angiography can be performed using a contrast media dose that is weight based (ie, 0.1–0.2 mmol/kg) or volume based (eg, 20 or 30 mL).

Although diagnostic CE MR angiography can be achieved using 0.1 mmol/kg, a slightly higher dose is often helpful (ie, 0.15 mmol/kg), because it reduces the margin of error for timing. In practice, many sites have converted to a volume-based dosing (eg, 20 or 30 mL) for simplicity. Nevertheless, in small individuals, especially children, weight-based dosing (eg, 0.1–0.2 mmol/kg) is more commonly applied. Contrast injections are typically performed at a rate of 2 mL/s [33]. Use of a large saline flush (eg, 20–30 mL) is also beneficial for 3D CE MR angiography [34]. The reliability of contrast delivery is improved if an MR-compatible injector is used.

For successful first-pass imaging, the study must be synchronized with the peak and preferably the plateau portion of arterial enhancement [27–29]. Because most of the resultant image contrast is determined by the data in the center of k-space, this portion of the data acquisition should be timed for peak arterial enhancement by the contrast bolus. Four methods are generally available to achieve this: (1) a fixed scan delay (eg, 10-second imaging delay from initiation of contrast injection), (2) a timing bolus scan [35], (3) the use of automatic bolus detection software [36,37], and (4) fluoroscopic triggering [38–40]. Although using a fixed delay time can result in successful thoracic MR angiography, it is not advised, because larger contrast doses (eg, 40 mL) are generally required to achieve routine reliability of the image quality. In most instances, properly timed CE MR angiography using a test bolus or real-time automated algorithm or MR fluoroscopic trigger will result in superior reliability of vascular signal and optimization of the contrast dose.

On most MR scanners, a test bolus scan can be performed [29,35]. This timing technique requires a 1- to 2-mL dose of Gd-chelate contrast media injected at 2 mL/s and a T1-weighted fast two-dimensional (2D) spoiled-gradient echo pulse sequence (SPGR) capable of imaging at a frame every 1 to 2 seconds. Imaging should be centered in the midthorax and should include the ascending and descending aorta, for example, an axial image centered at the level of the right pulmonary artery below the aortic arch but above the aortic valve. If an axial acquisition is used, saturation bands should be placed on either side of the imaging plane to ensure that only contrast arrival will result in an increase in aortic signal. Without the saturation bands, the normal pulsatility of the aortic flow may result in an increase in aortic signal from flow-related enhancement (also known as "in-flow" or

the "time-of-flight" [TOF] effect). To perform the timing bolus scan, the injection and imaging should be initiated simultaneously. From the resulting series of images, the frame with the highest signal can be determined and represents the arrival time for the contrast bolus. This information can be used to calculate the scan delay for the resulting CE MR angiography acquisition. If the study is performed using a centric or elliptical centric k-space acquisition scheme, the scan delay used should be roughly equivalent to the contrast arrival time. To avoid potential ringing artifacts [41] that may occur when central k-space views are acquired during the initial rise time of Gd arrival, 2 to 3 seconds should be added to the scan delay (ie, for elliptical centric acquisition, the bolus scan arrival equals 11 seconds and the scan delay, 13 seconds).

On most current high-field MR scanners, special real-time software is available for timing CE MR angiography. The two forms are an automated bolus detection algorithm (eg, Smart-Prep, General Electric Health Care) and an MR fluoroscopic trigger (eg, CareBolus, Siemens Medical Solutions; BolusTrak, Philips Medical Systems; FluoroTrigger, General Electric Health Care). Both systems have the benefit of requiring a single contrast injection. The automated trigger algorithm [36,37] consists of a single pulse sequence that can detect the arrival of the contrast column and that automatically begins the 3D MR angiography data acquisition upon exceeding two operator-determined thresholds (typically set at signal increases of 20% and 2 standard deviations over baseline signal). For this scheme, the operator is required to prescribe a monitoring volume to detect the contrast arrival and an imaging volume for the actual diagnostic 3D CE MR angiography. For CE MR angiography of the thoracic aorta, the monitoring volume is best placed in the aortic arch or descending aorta. In addition, breath holding is preferable. When using this automated detection scheme, a change in pitch between the monitoring phase and imaging phase can be used as an audible cue for the patient to initiate breath holding. An interscan delay between monitoring and the 3D imaging phase of 5 seconds is usually sufficient to enable proper patient breath holding.

The MR fluoroscopic triggering scheme is somewhat similar in that it also has a monitoring and 3D imaging phase [38–40]; however, using this real-time scheme, the operator is presented with 2D fluoroscopic images from which he or she must visually detect the contrast arrival into the aorta and initiate the data acquisition manually from the operator's console. Both methods have been shown to produce high-quality 3D CE MR angiography.

3D CE MR angiography is primarily interpreted on an independent computer work station equipped with specialized postprocessing software to perform MPR or one of various image postprocessing techniques, such as MIP or VR. These tools (see Figs. 1, 3, and 4) are critical for proper interpretation of MR angiography, and such soft copy interpretation should be included in all cases. MIP or VR display with variable degrees of rotation is the standard display format and is typically well suited for review with clinicians, because it presents a projectional viewing of data similar to a conventional angiogram. Subvolume MIP (a thinner slab MIP reconstruction) or MPR (a single voxel reconstruction through the 3D data) should be used to evaluate cross-sections of the lumen orthogonal to the long axis along the various levels. MPR and subvolume MIP are particularly helpful for evaluating the aorta and its branch vessels (see Figs. 1, 3, and 4). In addition, these thinner reconstructions allow improved visualization of subtle luminal defects such as intimal flaps that may not be evident on larger projectional viewing using MIP alone (see Fig. 1). VR reconstruction has emerged as an additional method for excellent image display. Unlike MIP views, which illustrate the brightest pixel in a ray projection, VR viewing retains pixel depth information. Translucent VR provides the operator the added ability to "see through" the data set, revealing intraluminal and overlapping extraluminal detail (see Fig. 1).

Adjunctive MR techniques

Bright blood

In addition to 3D CE MR angiography, several other bright blood techniques can be performed without the need for contrast agents [13–22]. These techniques are flow-based methods that rely on the differential behavior of moving protons (in flowing blood) and stationary protons (in adjacent background tissue). One of the oldest techniques is the TOF effect (also known as "flow-related enhancement" or in-flow effect). This method has limited usefulness for high-resolution aortic MR angiography, mainly because of the numerous image-degrading effects of constant cardiac pulsation and the complex flow pattern of aortic blood (and, to a lesser degree, in-plane saturation at the level of the aortic arch). With cardiac gating, arterial signal can be improved, but imaging times are long, and arterial signal often remains inhomogeneous and unreliable on TOF MR angiography for proper illustration of the thoracic aorta and its branch vessels. For targeted applications such as coronary artery imaging [21,42], several TOF-based techniques, such as 2D spiral, 2D fast gradient echo, and 3D fast gradient echo, have had some early success.

The TOF effect can be useful when acquired in a 2D cine mode, for example, cine gradient echo (cine GRE) or cine fast gradient echo (cine fGRE), because dynamic evaluation of blood flow in an individual slice location can be helpful in evaluating the aorta. More recently, a particularly robust form of bright blood cine MR, SSFP (also known as trueFISP, Siemens Medical Solutions; FIESTA, General Electric Health Care; and balanced FFE, Philips Medical), has become more widely available [21,22]. On SSFP, intraluminal signal is generally not only very high but also homogeneous, resulting in excellent vascular image quality. Although also a gradient echo pulse sequence, the signal of SSFP images is largely a function of the T2/T1 ratio, resulting in its improved ability to illustrate blood vessels, even those with slower flow. In urgent situations, SSFP can be used to demonstrate aortic caliber quickly, as well as findings consistent with dissection [22], such as the intimal flap and its two vascular channels (see Fig.1).

One critical advantage of flow-based bright blood techniques is that they offer the ability to perform a functional assessment of blood flow [13–16]. On cine GRE (and cine fGRE), signal loss occurs from intravoxel dephasing of spins, which is most commonly seen as flow jets extending distal to or downstream from the lesion. The presence of flow jets can be exploited to produce meaningful clinical information concerning an arterial stenosis or valvular function. For example, a flow jet on cine GRE in a patient with coarctation of the aorta suggests the presence of a significant pressure gradient across the narrowing (Fig. 5). A similar systolic flow jet may be seen on cine GRE extending from the aortic valve into the ascending aorta in a patient with aortic stenosis. Similarly, a regurgitant diastolic flow jet can be seen extending from the aortic valve into the left ventricle in a patient with aortic insufficiency (Fig. 6). The size of the flow jet has been shown to approximate the severity in aortic valvular stenosis and regurgitation. With the use

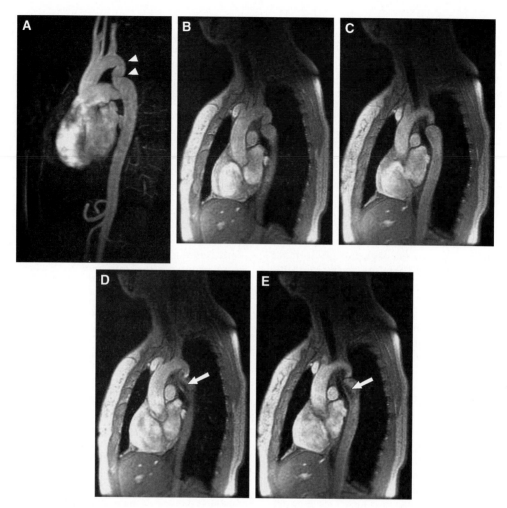

Fig. 5. Adult with a prior history of coarctation of the aorta. (*A*) On oblique sagittal MIP of 3D contrast-enhanced (CE) MR angiography, a very tortuous coarctation of the aorta (*arrowheads*) is clearly seen in the juxtaductal region, which bridges the posterior aortic arch and proximal descending aorta. No dilated collateral vessels are seen. (*B–E*) On cine fGRE images (*B* and *C*, diastole; and *D* and *E*, systole), a flow jet is noted distal to the narrowing during systolic phases (*D* and *E*, *arrows*). The presence of a flow jet suggests some turbulence and a pressure gradient across the coarctation; however, the absence of dilated collateral vessels on 3D CE MR angiography argues against the narrowing currently having hemodynamic significance in this adult patient.

of newer fGRE pulse sequences with an ultrashort TR and TE, a flow jet may not be present despite the presence of a significant flow disturbance. The very short TE times may be insufficient for a sizeable flow jet to form on this faster sequence. In cases of high suspicion, standard gradient echo pulse sequences (eg, TE greater than 10 ms) can be performed during free breathing. The longer TE will allow intravoxel dephasing to develop, and a flow jet should be seen if flow is turbulent.

Cine PC is another bright blood tool for dynamic evaluation of blood flow [16–20]. Unlike cine GRE, which relies on flow-related enhancement, cine PC depends on the phase shifts that flowing protons experience as they travel along the gradient field. These phase shifts can be used to determine flow velocity and direction. Phase map images from a cine PC acquisition display the direction of flow as bright or dark pixels, with their relative signal intensity (ie, intensity of their brightness or blackness) representing their velocity. Phase map images can be used to assess flow direction, which may be important information for proper identification of a vascular structure or for

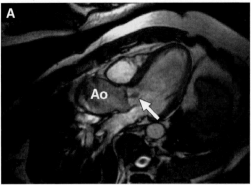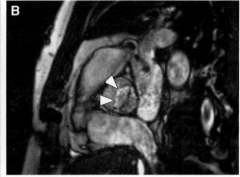

Fig. 6. Cine MR in a patient with a 5.2-cm ascending aortic aneurysm, bicuspid aortic valve, and mild aortic insufficiency. On a diastolic image from a cine SSFP acquisition (*A*) performed in a "three-chamber" view, a small flow jet (*arrow*) consistent with mild aortic insufficiency is seen arising from the aortic valve and projecting back into left ventricle. On a separate oblique cine SSFP acquisition performed through the aortic valve (*B*), the characteristic lens or "fish-mouth" appearance (*arrowheads*) of a bicuspid aortic valve is seen in systole. Ao, aorta.

quantifying blood flow. PC acquisitions can be performed for the evaluation of flow in one or more directions. Unidirectional flow evaluation using cine PC requires the least amount of time, but care must be taken to ensure that the blood flow being evaluated is primarily unidirectional; otherwise, it may be underestimated using a single flow direction encoding. Using specialized flow analysis software that is commercially available from the scanner manufacturer or a third-party vendor, flow can be measured by an operator. Using phase map images, the operator can determine peak and average flow. Because the information is ECG gated, actual flow across a vessel or location can be determined. Flow volumes can be calculated using the flow equation, $Q = $ velocity $\times$ area, where Q is flow (mL/min), *velocity* is measured on phase map images (cm/s), and *area* (cm^2) is that of an operator-defined region of interest around the vessel used to measure flow. By tracing the cross-sectional area of the ascending aorta on a cine PC acquisition perpendicular to the aortic flow, the blood flow volume (cm^3 or mL) across through the aorta can be determined over the cardiac cycle (mL/cardiac cycle) or, because the patient's heart rate is also known, over a time period (eg, mL/min).

The main pitfall for cine PC flow measurements is proper selection of the velocity encoding (VENC) for the acquisition. The VENC must be sufficiently high to avoid aliasing of the signal, which will invalidate flow measurement. Setting the VENC slightly above the peak velocity of the flow within the vessel being evaluated can minimize this. Understandably, it is often difficult to known the peak velocity a priori. For a patient with a normal aorta, a VENC of 250 cm/s is usually sufficient, but higher VENC settings may often be necessary.

Cine PC can be used in a variety of non-quantitative applications to identify flow direction properly for differentiation of an artery versus a vein, or for determination of reversed flow direction, as may be seen in the vertebral artery in subclavian steal syndrome. Alternatively, cine PC can be used to confirm luminal patency, such as in aortic dissection, when patency versus thrombosis of the false channel may be in question. Cine PC can be used to establish flow direction within the false channel (ie, antegrade, retrograde, or bidirectional). Intraluminal thrombus will appear as fixed or stationary defects.

Black blood

The aorta can also be well illustrated using black blood methods, namely, ECG-gated spin echo (and fast spin echo [FSE]) that exploits the inherent contrast between rapidly flowing blood and the aortic wall [43–48]. Unlike in bright blood imaging, luminal signal void or a black lumen occurs owing to high velocity signal loss (or "wash out" of spins) and spin dephasing seen with turbulent flow. Spin echo imaging has been employed to gain basic anatomic information, particularly on morphology and relationships between vascular and extravascular structures in the setting of a congenital vascular anomaly and for aneurysm detection and surveillance. Spin echo imaging not only depicts the vessel wall and perivascular structures but also is useful for the assessment of aortic caliber and mural features, such as wall thickening or edema. Wall thickness can be readily demonstrated on T1-weighted imaging, and edema is seen as hyperintense intramural signal on T2-weighted imaging. Mural enhancement of the vessel wall on T1-weighted images after contrast administration is considered evidence of active inflammation (eg, aortitis). ECG-gated double inversion recovery (DIR) FSE, (see Fig. 1) is a more recent black blood method that permits breath hold acquisition [48]. By applying a nonspecific inversion pulse and a slice-specific inversion pulse, DIR FSE improves the reliability of the intraluminal signal void. The major advantages of DIR FSE are not only the homogeneity of the luminal signal void but also its speed, which enables breath hold acquisitions for "freeze-frame" images. For targeted applications, such as aortic valve imaging, the temporal resolution permits direct visualization of aortic valve morphology and pathology, such as the bicuspid aortic valve, as well as thickening of valve leaflets and vegetations. A main consideration in black blood imaging is that the images are not dynamic but specific for a cardiac phase, typically with gating targeted for diastole, which is the more quiescent period of the cardiac cycle. This difference is important to keep in mind mainly when one is correlating the measurements obtained on spin echo images with those of a dynamic examination such as echocardiography.

Coronary artery imaging

The techniques discussed previously are primarily used for imaging the thoracic aorta. MR imaging of the coronary arteries continues to be challenging, with no single technique being widely successful or universally accepted as best. The MR techniques used for coronary artery imaging continue to evolve, with preferred techniques varying by vendor. A more detailed discussion of the various coronary imaging methods can be found elsewhere in this issue in the article by Foo et al. Current techniques are primarily reliable for imaging congenital anomalies of the proximal coronary artery origins. Although recent research by Kim et al [49] has been promising for the detection of coronary artery stenoses, this continues to be a work in progress [50]. Identification of the coronary artery origins can be performed using any of the available bright blood MR angiography methods (eg, 3D SSFP, 2D spiral,

or ECG-gated T2-prepped 3D) or black blood methods (eg, DIR FSE). The key to illustration of the coronary artery origins is proper scan plane prescription, good cardiac and respiratory motion compensation, and sufficient signal to noise to achieve adequate spatial resolution.

MR imaging evaluation of selected conditions of the thoracic aorta

Designing an MR imaging strategy for evaluating the thoracic aorta typically requires a combination of black and bright blood techniques. In addition, the protocol must be targeted for the primary regions of disease involvement, include proper imaging of the disease's extent and pattern, and provide proper visualization of associated extravascular findings.

Like real estate sales, the approach to MR imaging of thoracic aortic pathology is perhaps best represented by the three-word mantra "location, location, location." Beginning at the aortic valve, the thoracic aorta can be divided into three distinct regions in the proximal-to-distal direction, namely, the aortic root, ascending aorta, aortic arch, and descending aorta. In addition, anatomic landmarks that flank these segments serve as discrete boundaries that impact clinical decision making and imaging strategy. Classic clinical conditions in each of these segments and boundaries serve as examples of tailored imaging strategy.

Aortic root

Sinuses of Valsalva

Discrete aneurysms (Fig. 7) involving one or more sinuses of Valsalva occur below the sinotubular ridge [51,52]. The clinical presentation is typically secondary to consequences of rupture, such as heart failure or a new murmur from an aortocardiac fistula. When such presentation is not acute and dramatic, MR may be used in the imaging evaluation to demonstrate not only the aneurysm but also the donor sinus and recipient chamber of a small fistula. Bright blood techniques are particularly well suited for these evaluations [52]. Although an aneurysm can be readily displayed on morphologic imaging, a small fistula tract may be better demonstrated with bright blood techniques, especially cine MR.

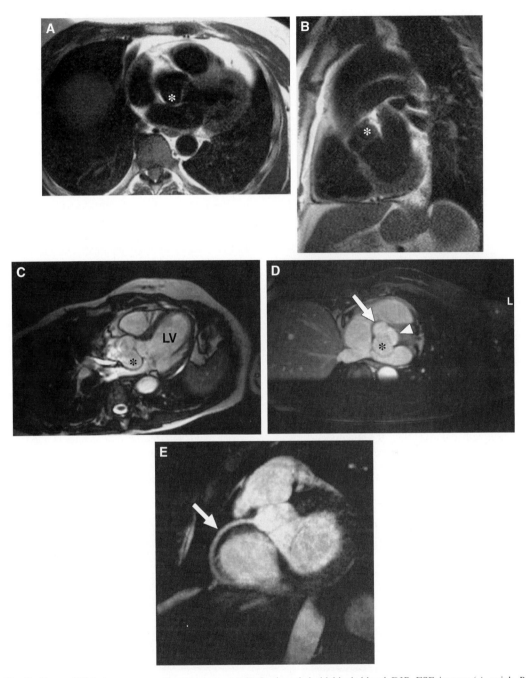

Fig. 7. Sinus of Valsalva aneurysm in a woman. (*A,B*) On breath hold black blood DIR FSE images (*A*, axial; *B*, sagittal), there is the suggestion of an enlarged noncoronary sinus of Valsalva (*). (*C*) On cine SSFP images performed in the three-chamber view, the dilated noncoronary sinus of Valsalva (*) is noted. (*D*) The aneurysm of the noncoronary sinus of Valsalva (*) is confirmed on navigator echo-gated T2-prepped coronary 3D MR angiography (oblique subvolume MIP through the sinuses of Valsalva). On this same image, note the normal appearance of the right coronary sinus of Valsalva (*arrow*) and left coronary sinus of Valsalva (*arrowhead*). (*E*) The patient's normal right coronary artery (*arrow*) was also imaged using navigator echo-gated T2-prepped coronary 3D MR angiography (subvolume MIP). LV, left ventricle.

Coronary arteries

One of the more common cardiac MR referrals is the patient with a suspected anomalous coronary artery [53,54]. Typically, this anomaly is considered in young patients who present with chest pain. Although there are several anomalous routes, the interarterial course of an anomalous left or right coronary artery is the most concerning. In this situation, the coronary artery arises from the contralateral sinus of Valsalva and passes between the ascending aorta and pulmonary artery (the so-called "interarterial" course). During exercise or periods of increased cardiac output, the anomalous coronary may be "pinched" by the two great arteries, resulting in myocardial ischemia or possibly infarction. The role of MR imaging in this case is primarily to identify the proximal coronary arteries, which typically are well evaluated using a combination of black blood DIR FSE and bright blood methods. The route of an anomalous coronary artery may also be circumaortic, coursing from an anterior (Fig. 8) or posterior sinus of Valsalva.

Sinotubular junction

Diseases involving the tubular portion of the ascending aorta typically spare the sinotubular junction with the exception of annuloaortic ectasia [55,56]. Cystic medial necrosis is characterized histologically as myxomatous change of cardiac valves, with enlargement of the sinuses of Valsalva

and annular dilatation of the ascending aorta with a return to normal caliber by the innominate artery origin. Effacement of the sinotubular ridge and dilatation of all three sinuses of Valsalva are the imaging hallmarks that create the aptly named "spring onion" or "tulip bulb" appearance (Fig. 9). A careful search for another potential consequence of cystic medial necrosis, dissection (Fig. 10), should be conducted.

Ascending aorta

The ascending thoracic aorta extends from the sinotubular ridge to immediately proximal to the innominate artery origin. One of the most serious and potentially life-threatening conditions involving the aortic root and ascending aorta is aortic dissection [43,55,57–59]. The DeBakey and Stanford criteria divide aortic dissections into those that involve the ascending aorta or aortic arch (Stanford type A or DeBakey I and II, see Fig. 1) and those that are delimited to only the descending thoracic aorta beyond the left subclavian artery origin (Stanford type B or DeBakey III, Fig. 10). This distinction is critical for the determination of whether surgery or medical treatment is warranted. The first goal of imaging, especially in the acute setting, is to determine the most proximal site of involvement. Dissection may be fatal if it extends proximally into the aortic root, the aortic valve, and the coronary arteries, potentially resulting in intrapericardial hemorrhage and cardiac tamponade,

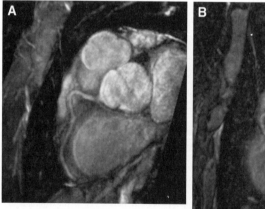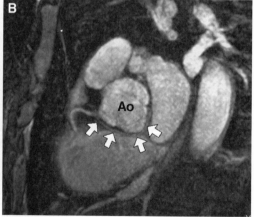

Fig. 8. Anomalous left circumflex coronary artery. Double oblique navigator echo-gated T2-prepped coronary 3D MR angiography (*A*, thicker subvolume MIP; *B*, thinner subvolume MIP) performed through the aortic sinuses of Valsalva demonstrates an anomalous left circumflex coronary artery, which arises anteriorly from the right sinus of Valsalva and passes posteriorly behind the aorta (*arrows*). Ao, aorta.

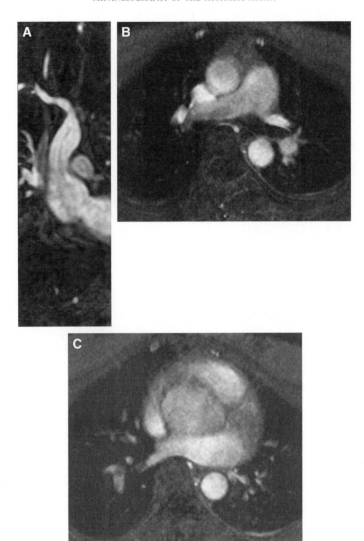

Fig. 9. A 12-year-old girl with Marfan's syndrome. (*A*) Coronal oblique 3D contrast-enhanced MR angiography (MIP) demonstrates the "spring onion" bulb appearance of annuloaortic ectasia, with effacement of the sinotubular junction. (*B,C*) Axial 2D postcontrast GRE images (cranial to caudal) demonstrate the relative cross-sectional dimensions of the aortic root (*C*) compared with the ascending and descending thoracic aorta (*B*), which measured 4.6, 2.9, and 2.3 cm in maximum diameter, respectively.

acute aortic insufficiency, and myocardial ischemia, respectively. Additionally, extension of the intimal flap into one or more of the aortic arch vessels may produce cerebral ischemia or infarction. For this reason, Stanford type A dissections typically warrant acute surgical repair. Type B aortic dissections tend to be more stable and can be managed medically.

Intramural hematoma represents bleeding within the aortic wall from vasa vasorum of the media, in effect, a forme fruste of dissection [60,61]. The time-varying appearance of hematoma reflects the known evolution of signal intensity of blood breakdown products from acute to subacute to chronic. Subacute hemorrhage (methemoglobin) appears as crescentic or lentiform high intramural signal with adjacent normal signal void on non-CE T1-weighted sequences.

On MR imaging, a variety of artifacts may erroneously lead to the appearance of an intimal

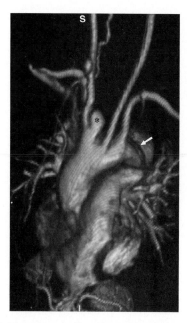

Fig. 10. Type B aortic dissection in a woman with cystic medial necrosis. On VR projection of 3D contrast-enhanced MR angiography, the type B aortic dissection (*arrow*) is well seen. In addition, the patient is noted to have a saccular aneurysm (*) of the innominate artery.

tear or conversely obscure it. Artifacts within the aortic root and ascending aorta can occur secondary to a number of concerns, such as the normal pulsatility of aortic blood flow, the movement of the aortic valve leaflets, and cardiac motion. The use of current bright blood techniques, namely, SSFP and 3D CE MR angiography, will result in an accurate diagnosis (see Fig. 1). One additional aid in the recognition of an intimal flap is its configuration. Type A dissections typically spiral along the outer greater curvature of the aorta, with the false channel usually rightward in the ascending aorta and posterolateral in the descending aorta.

When performing 3D CE MR angiography, the upper abdominal aorta should be included in the field of view. In patients who are small or when the image acquisition can be accelerated using parallel imaging, it may be advantageous to use a coronal volume to include the renal arteries, especially the left, which are commonly involved in dissections that extend into the abdomen. Coronal acquisitions generally require the prescription of thicker volumes for adequate coverage of the thoracic aorta than typically recommended oblique sagittal images ("candy cane" or left anterior oblique acquisition); therefore, this option

is generally reserved for smaller patients or accelerated acquisition schemes. Note that an oblique sagittal acquisition using a large field of view will usually enable reasonable coverage of the upper abdominal aorta, including the renal arteries (see Fig. 1).

Another common indication for thoracic MR imaging is the evaluation of a suspected or known aortic aneurysm [2,6,9,45,46,55]. The normal aortic diameter on ECG-gated black blood images has been reported [56] to be as follows: aortic root, 3.3 cm; midascending aorta, 3.0 cm; aortic arch, 2.7 cm; and descending aorta, 2.4 cm. Aneurysms that measure greater than 5 to 6 cm, that are expanding rapidly, or that are symptomatic will generally be repaired. Care must be taken to obtain aortic diameter measurements in a plane perpendicular to the aorta. On an axial image, measurement at the level of the horizontal portion of the right pulmonary artery will ensure that the aorta is generally vertical, and that diameter measurements accurately reflect the aorta's cross-sectional size. Use of an axial MR image will also enable comparisons with dimensions measured on CT. There may be discrepancies with measurements obtained on echocardiography secondary to technical differences in measurement, such as the plane of measurement or cardiac phase. In children, the ascending aorta is aneurysmal if the ratio of the ascending aorta to the descending aorta diameter is greater than 1.5 [62]. Dilatation of the ascending thoracic aorta can occur from intrinsic pathology that is acquired, such as atherosclerotic disease (see Fig. 3), or congenital, such as connective tissue disorders such as Marfan's syndrome (see Fig. 9). Dilatation of the ascending aorta can also occur owing to aortic valve disease. Aortic stenosis and aortic regurgitation (see Fig. 6) can be demonstrated on MR imaging. By exploiting the spin-dephasing effects of flow turbulence across stenotic and regurgitant valves, qualitative and quantitative data can be generated to assess the severity of valve dysfunction. A parameter frequently assessed by echocardiography, the regurgitant fraction, is also readily obtainable with axial 2D cine PC at the level of the aortic root and is calculated by dividing the regurgitant volume by the stroke volume.

Aortic arch

The aortic arch begins at the brachiocephalic, or innominate artery, and extends to the ligamentum arteriosus [55]. The arterial supply to both upper extremities as well as the head and neck regions arises from this relatively short, albeit, critical segment. The classic configuration of three aortic arch vessels, namely, the innominate artery, the left common carotid artery, and the left subclavian artery, in the proximal-to-distal direction is found in about two-thirds to three-quarters of individuals. Variant anatomy is common, particularly a common origin of the innominate and left common carotid arteries (so-called "bovine arch," see Figs. 1 and 3), which has been reported in up to 22% of the population [55]. Other variants to consider are a separate origin of the left vertebral artery from the arch.

Failure of the primitive aortic arches to fuse or regress can result in anomalous arch configurations called vascular rings that can encircle the trachea or esophagus and result in stridor, wheezing, or dysphagia [9,16,47,63]. The most common vascular rings are a left aortic arch with an aberrant right subclavian artery, a right aortic arch with an aberrant left subclavian artery, and a double aortic arch. Aberrant subclavian arteries may also be associated with a diverticulum of Kommerell and are typically retroesophageal. An aberrant subclavian artery is more likely to be symptomatic in the setting of an atretic vascular segment that produces a complete ring, such as a persistent ductus ligament with a right aortic arch and aberrant left subclavian artery. Vascular rings are usually well demonstrated on black blood imaging with supplemental cine MR. 3D CE MR angiography is often not necessary for diagnosing vascular rings but may be helpful for surgical planning. The presence of an aortic anomaly (eg, vascular ring or coarctation of the aorta) is particularly common with many congenital heart diseases, and the inclusion of an aortic assessment during the MR evaluation of cardiac morphology is often prudent.

Entities that involve the ascending aorta may also affect the arch and its branches, either as an extension with a type A dissection (see Fig. 1) or a large ascending aortic aneurysm (see Fig. 2), or as its primary location (see Fig. 10). Atherosclerosis is a systemic process that can commonly result in aneurysms (see Fig. 3) or branch vessel stenoses (see Fig. 4). When performing 3D CE MR angiography for evaluation of the arch vessels, it is generally preferable to use a coronal acquisition to ensure adequate coverage of the carotid, vertebral, and subclavian arteries within the imaging volume (see Fig. 4).

Ligamentum arteriosum

The juxtaductal region is defined by the ligamentum arteriosum, the remnant of the fetal

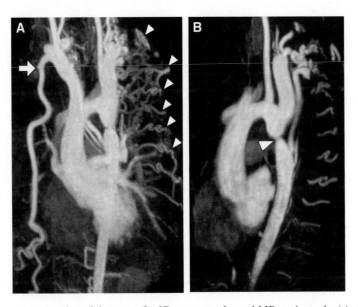

Fig. 11. Man with severe coarctation of the aorta. On 3D contrast-enhanced MR angiography (*A*, oblique sagittal VR; *B*, oblique sagittal subvolume MIP), a high-grade stenosis of the juxtaductal aorta is well seen (*B, arrowhead*). Marked dilatation of the collateral vessels (*A, arrow*, dilated internal mammary artery; *arrowheads*, dilated posterior intercostal arteries) is noted, consistent with a severe (and hemodynamically significant) coarctation of the aorta.

ductus arteriosus, and approximates a boundary between the aortic arch and descending thoracic aorta. One of the most common entities to involve this region is coarctation of the aorta (Figs. 5 and 11) [9,13,16,47,64]. Typically, a discrete area of narrowing just distal to the left subclavian artery origin region, aortic coarctation represents an infolding of juxtaductal aortic tissue. Cine bright blood imaging in a sagittal oblique plane parallel to the long axis of the aorta can demonstrate a downstream flow jet (see Fig. 5) in the presence of a pressure gradient. The presence of prominent collateral circulation, such as retrograde flow through the intercostal arteries, is readily depicted on 3D CE MR angiography and is present in older children and adults with hemodynamically significant stenosis. Single-slice 2D cine PC performed at two locations, specifically, the proximal and distal descending thoracic aorta, can be performed to calculate the incremental contribution of collateral circulation to the descending aorta and to quantify the hemodynamic severity of the lesion [65]. Cine MR can also be performed to detect the presence of an associated bicuspid aortic valve, as well as its consequences, including aortic valvular stenosis or insufficiency. In contrast, pseudocoarctation represents buckling at the isthmus owing to abnormal elongation with kinking at the fixed point of attachment, namely, the ligamentum arteriosum, with no associated collateral circulation and no pressure gradient (ie, no flow jet on cine MR).

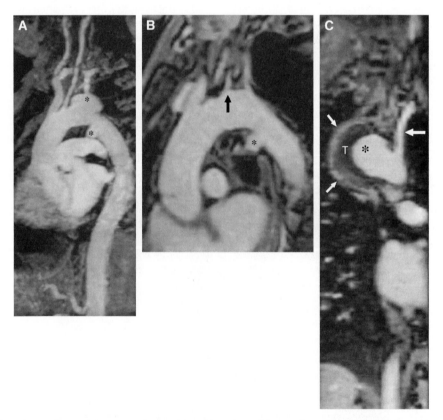

Fig. 12. Saccular aortic pseudoaneurysms in a patient with a remote history of a severe motor vehicle accident. (*A*) Two saccular pseudoaneurysms (*) are noted on arterial phase 3D contrast-enhanced MR angiography. Oblique sagittal MPR image (*B*) from the delayed phase shows the neck of the smaller saccular aneurysm (*) and aberrant origin of the left vertebral artery (*arrow*) from the aortic arch. On coronal MPR (*C*) of the delayed phase, the neck of the larger superior saccular aneurysm (*) and its relationship to the origin of the left subclavian artery (*large arrow*) can be evaluated en face. On the delayed-phase images, perianeurysmal enhancement (*C*, *small arrows*) aids in the identification of thrombus (T) within the larger superior saccular aneurysm. (*From* Ho VB, Prince MR. Thoracic MR angiography: imaging techniques and strategies. Radiographics 1998;18:287–309; with permission.)

Pseudoaneurysms are typically posttraumatic and affect the lesser curvature of the aorta at the fixed point of attachment to the left pulmonary artery by the ligamentum arteriosum, the vestigial remnant of the ductus arteriosus [9,55]. The risk of delayed rupture remains high even in stable patients with remote trauma. Pseudoaneuryms are typically saccular and can be well evaluated using 3D CE MR angiography (Fig. 12). Thinner image reconstruction of the data sets using MPR and subvolume MIP is particularly useful for visualization of individual branch vessel origins, which is critical for preoperative planning.

Descending aorta

The descending thoracic aorta extends from the ligamentum to the aortic hiatus of the diaphragm. True aortic aneurysms involve all three layers (intima, media, and adventitia) of the aortic wall and are typically atherosclerotic in nature or related to connective tissue disorders.

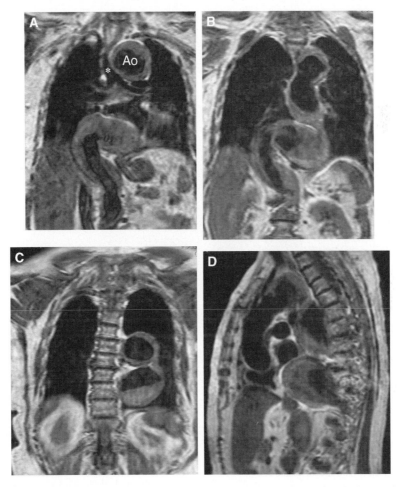

Fig. 13. Thoracic aortic aneurysm in an 81-year-old woman. (*A–E*) On black blood spin echo images (*A* to *C*, coronal anterior to posterior; *D* to *E*, sagittal right to left), a fusiform aneurysm of the aorta is noted beginning in the midarch region and extending down the descending thoracic aorta. On image *A*, note the displacement of the trachea (*) by the enlarged aortic arch (Ao). (*F*) Sagittal 3D contrast-enhanced (CE) MR angiography was also performed and documented normal arch vessels (not shown), but the overall caliber of the aorta (ie, wall to wall diameter) and mural features were generally better appreciated on the black blood images (compare *F* with *E*). (*G*) It is often beneficial to perform supplemental postcontrast acquisitions in an additional plane following 3D CE MR angiography. In this case, axial postcontrast GRE imaging (*G*) was obtained and confirmed the presence of atherosclerotic plaque (*arrowhead*) within the aortic aneurysm.

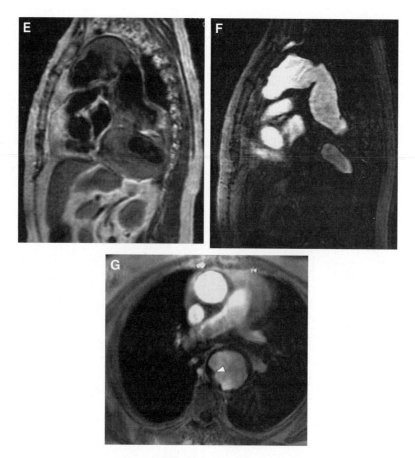

Fig. 13 (*continued*)

Atherosclerotic aneurysms occur most typically in the descending thoracic aorta and may be fusiform (Fig. 13) or saccular in morphology [2,6,9,45,46,55].

A penetrating aortic ulcer [9,55,66] is another entity that tends to present in the descending aorta where the bulk of atherosclerosis occurs. The natural history of penetrating atherosclerotic ulcers remains controversial, and its treatment generally parallels that of dissection. Penetrating atherosclerotic ulcers need to be differentiated from focal saccular aneurysm and intramural hematoma. In patients with a suspicion of a penetrating ulcer and aortic dissection, it is generally advisable that precontrast T1-weighted images be performed. Intramural hematomas (also called aortic dissection without an intimal flap) are often subtle and may only be evident on precontrast images as hemorrhage within thickened regions of the aortic wall.

Aortic hiatus of the diaphragm

Descending thoracic aortic pathology that may traverse the threshold of the aortic hiatus to extend below the diaphragm and involve the abdominal aorta includes atherosclerotic aneurysm and dissection. Imaging of thoracoabdominal aortic pathology requires a larger cranial-caudal field of view to include at least the aortic bifurcation but often the proximal iliac vessels owing to potential involvement. Unlike in CT, in which the cranial-caudal extent can be scanned in one breath hold as the table moves continuously through the scanner bore, MR imaging requires an extended field of view (see Fig. 1) or, possibly, two contiguous (slightly overlapping) fields of view (ie, two stations) [67]. The body coil of the magnet can be used if a longer multiple phased-array peripheral vascular coil is not available. Automated (or manual) table translation can be

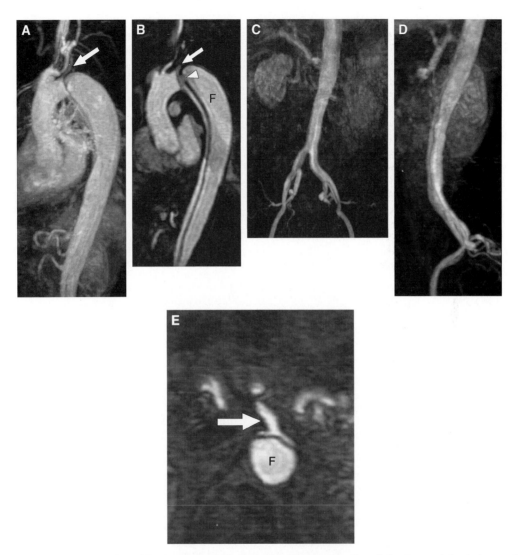

Fig. 14. Two-station moving table 3D contrast-enhanced (CE) MR angiography of the thoracoabdominal aorta in a patient with type B aortic dissection. (*A,B*) Study of the thorax (*A*, sagittal MIP; *B*, sagittal MPR) demonstrates a type B aortic dissection with the intimal tear arising beyond the left subclavian artery (*arrow*). On the thinner MPR (*B*), the entry tear (*arrowhead*) and intimal flap separating the two lumens (F, false lumen) is well seen. (*C–E*) The second-station 3D CE MR angiography performed immediately after table translation of the abdominal station into the isocenter shows continuation of the dissection into the abdominal aorta (*C*, coronal MIP; *D*, sagittal MIP). As previously shown, thinner subvolume MIP and MPR can be used to evaluate individual vessel origins. On axial MPR (*E*) of the abdominal data, the superior mesenteric artery (*arrow*) is noted to arise from the smaller anterior true lumen.

employed to scan sequentially two contiguous imaging stations for evaluation of the entire length of the thoracoabdominal aorta (Fig. 14).

Summary

The thoracic aorta can be evaluated comprehensively using MR imaging. 3D CE MR angiography, in particular, can provide angiographic and high spatial resolution images of the aorta. Diagnostic accuracy and speed can be improved by using a variety of postprocessing tools, such as MPR, MIP, and VR. MR angiography also has the ability to image blood flow quickly, especially using SSFP pulse sequences. The prudent combination of traditional black blood and bright blood techniques will adequately and accurately evaluate most diseases of the thoracic aorta. Knowledge of the salient clinical and technical concerns will optimize scanning efficiency and enable timely completion of most MR evaluations.

References

[1] Hartnell GG, Finn JP, Zenni M, et al. MR imaging of the thoracic aorta: comparison of spin echo, angiographic, and breath-hold techniques. Radiology 1994;191:697–704.

[2] Prince MR, Narasimham DL, Jacoby WT, et al. Three-dimensional gadolinium-enhanced MR angiography of the thoracic aorta. AJR Am J Roentgenol 1996;166:1387–97.

[3] Krinsky G, Rofsky N, Flyer M, et al. Gadolinium-enhanced three-dimensional MR angiography of acquired arch vessel disease. AJR Am J Roentgenol 1996;167:981–7.

[4] Neimatallah MA, Ho VB, Dong Q, et al. Gadolinium-enhanced 3D magnetic resonance angiography of the thoracic vessels. J Magn Reson Imaging 1999;10:758–70.

[5] Flamm SD, VanDyke CW, White RD. MR imaging of the thoracic aorta. Magn Reson Imaging Clin N Am 1996;4:217–35.

[6] Krinsky GA, Rofsky NM, DeCorato DR, et al. Thoracic aorta: comparison of gadolinium-enhanced three-dimensional MR angiography with conventional MR imaging. Radiology 1997;202:183–93.

[7] Leung DA, Debatin JF. Three-dimensional contrast-enhanced MRA of the thoracic vasculature. Eur Radiol 1997;7:981–9.

[8] Krinsky G, Reuss PM. MR angiography of the thoracic aorta. Magn Reson Imaging Clin N Am 1998; 6:293–320.

[9] Ho VB, Prince MR. Thoracic MR angiography: imaging techniques and strategies. Radiographics 1998;18:287–309.

[10] Czum JM, Ho VB. MR of the thoracic aorta: a pulse sequence approach to discrete feature analysis. Crit Rev Diagn Imaging 1999;40:23–61.

[11] Reddy GP, Higgins CB. MR imaging of the thoracic aorta. Magn Reson Imaging Clin N Am 2000;8: 1–15.

[12] Ho VB, Corse WR, Hood MN, et al. MRA of the thoracic vessels. Semin Ultrasound CT MR 2003; 24:192–216.

[13] Simpson IA, Chung KJ, Glass RF, et al. Cine magnetic resonance imaging for evaluation of anatomy and flow relations in infants and children with coarctation of the aorta. Circulation 1988;78:142–8.

[14] Plugfelder PW, Landzberg JS, Cassidy MM, et al. Comparison of cine MR imaging with Doppler echocardiography for the evaluation of aortic regurgitation. AJR Am J Roentgenol 1989;152:729–35.

[15] Didier D, Ratib O, Friedli B, et al. Cine gradient-echo MR imaging in the evaluation of cardiovascular diseases. Radiographics 1993;13:561–73.

[16] Ho VB, Kinney JB, Sahn DJ. Contributions of newer MR imaging strategies for congenital heart disease. Radiographics 1996;16:43–60.

[17] Bogren HG, Klipstein RH, Firmin DN, et al. Quantification of antegrade and retrograde blood flow in the human aorta by magnetic resonance velocity mapping. Am Heart J 1989;117:1214–22.

[18] Mostbeck GH, Caputo GR, Higgins CB. MR measurement of blood flow in the cardiovascular system. AJR Am J Roentgenol 1992;159:453–61.

[19] Pelc LR, Pelc NJ, Rayhill SC, et al. Arterial and venous blood flow: noninvasive quantification with MR imaging. Radiology 1992;185:809–12.

[20] Rebergen SA, van der Wall EE, Doornbos J, et al. Magnetic resonance measurement of velocity and flow: technique, validation, and cardiovascular applications. Am Heart J 1993;126:1439–56.

[21] Earls JP, Ho VB, Foo TK, et al. Cardiac MRI: recent progress and continued challenges. J Magn Reson Imaging 2002;16:111–27.

[22] Pereles FS, McCarthy RM, Baskaran V, et al. Thoracic aortic dissection and aneurysm: evaluation with nonenhanced true FISP MR angiography in less than 4 minutes. Radiology 2002;223:270–4.

[23] Marks B, Mitchell DG, Simelaro JP. Breath-holding in healthy and pulmonary-compromised populations: effects of hyperventilation and oxygen inspiration. J Magn Reson Imaging 1997;7:595–7.

[24] Neimatallah MA, Chenevert TL, Carlos RC, et al. Subclavian MR arteriography: reduction of susceptibility artifact with short echo time and dilute gadopentetate dimeglumine. Radiology 2000;217:581–6.

[25] Korosec FR, Frayne R, Grist TM, et al. Time-resolved contrast-enhanced 3D MR angiography. Magn Reson Med 1996;36:345–51.

[26] Finn JP, Baskaran V, Carr JC, et al. Thorax: low-dose contrast-enhanced three-dimensional MR angiography with subsecond temporal resolution—initial results. Radiology 2002;224(3):896–904.

[27] Prince MR. Gadolinium-enhanced MR aortography. Radiology 1994;191:155–64.

[28] Prince MR. Contrast-enhanced MR angiography: theory and optimization. Magn Reson Imaging Clin N Am 1998;6:257–67.

[29] Ho VB, Foo TK, Czum JM, et al. Contrast-enhanced magnetic resonance angiography: technical considerations for optimized clinical implementation. Top Magn Reson Imaging 2001;12:283–99.

[30] Weiger M, Pruessmann KP, Kassner A, et al. Contrast-enhanced 3D MRA using SENSE. J Magn Reson Imaging 2000;12:671–7.

[31] van den Brink JS, Watanabe Y, Kuhl CK, et al. Implications of SENSE MR in routine clinical practice. Eur J Radiol 2003;46(1):3–27.

[32] Maki JH, Wilson GJ, Eubank WB, et al. Utilizing SENSE to achieve lower station sub-millimeter iso-

tropic resolution and minimal venous enhancement in peripheral MR angiography. J Magn Reson Imaging 2002;15(4):484–91.

[33] Kopka L, Vosshenrich R, Rodenwaldt J, et al. Differences in injection rates on contrast-enhanced breath-hold three-dimensional MR angiography. AJR Am J Roentgenol 1998;170(2):345–8.

[34] Boos M, Scheffler K, Haselhorst R, et al. Arterial first pass gadolinium-CM dynamics as a function of several intravenous saline flush and Gd volumes. J Magn Reson Imaging 2001;13:568–76.

[35] Earls JP, Rofsky NM, DeCorato DR, et al. Breath-hold single dose Gd-enhanced three-dimensional MR aortography: usefulness of a timing examination and MR power injector. Radiology 1996; 201(3):705–10.

[36] Foo TKF, Saranathan M, Prince MR, et al. Automated detection of bolus arrival and initiation of data acquisition in fast, three-dimensional, gadolinium-enhanced MR angiography. Radiology 1997; 203:275–80.

[37] Ho VB, Foo TKF. Optimization of gadolinium-enhanced magnetic resonance angiography using an automated bolus-detection algorithm (MR Smart-Prep). Invest Radiol 1998;33:515–23.

[38] Wilman AH, Riederer SJ, King BF, et al. Fluoroscopically triggered contrast-enhanced three-dimensional MR angiography with elliptical centric view order: application to the renal arteries. Radiology 1997;205:137–46.

[39] Riederer SJ, Fain SB, Kruger DG, et al. Real-time and triggering of 3D contrast-enhanced MR angiograms using MR fluoroscopy. MAGMA 1999;8: 196–206.

[40] Riederer SJ, Bernstein MA, Breen JF, et al. Three-dimensional contrast-enhanced MR angiography with real-time fluoroscopic triggering: design specifications and technical reliability in 330 patient studies. Radiology 2000;215:584–93.

[41] Maki JH, Prince MR, Londy FJ, et al. The effects of time varying intravascular signal intensity and k-space acquisition order on three-dimensional MR angiography image quality. J Magn Reson Imaging 1996;6:642–51.

[42] Foo TK, Saranathan M, Hardy CJ, et al. Coronary artery magnetic resonance imaging: a patient-tailored approach. Top Magn Reson Imaging 2000;11:406–16.

[43] Amparo EG, Higgins CB, Hricak H, et al. Aortic dissection: magnetic resonance imaging. Radiology 1985;155:399–406.

[44] Geisinger MA, Risius B, O'Donnell JA, et al. Thoracic aortic dissections: magnetic resonance imaging. Radiology 1985;155:407–12.

[45] Glazier HS, Gutierrez FR, Levitt G, et al. The thoracic aorta studied by MR imaging. Radiology 1985;157:149–55.

[46] Link KM, Lesko NM. The role of MR imaging in the evaluation of acquired diseases of the thoracic aorta. AJR Am J Roentgenol 1992;158:1115–25.

[47] Gomes AS. MR imaging of congenital anomalies of the thoracic aorta and pulmonary arteries. Radiol Clin North Am 1989;27:1171–81.

[48] Simonetti OP, Finn JP, White RD, et al. "Black blood" T2-weighted inversion recovery MR imaging of the heart. Radiology 1996;199:49–57.

[49] Kim WY, Danias PG, Stuber M, et al. Coronary magnetic resonance angiography for the detection of coronary stenoses. N Engl J Med 2001;345(26): 1863–9.

[50] Flamm SD, Muthupillai R. Coronary artery magnetic resonance angiography. J Magn Reson Imaging 2004;19:686–709.

[51] Tomita T, Hanaoka T, Owa M. Images in cardiology. Unruptured aneurysm of the sinus of Valsalva obstructing the right ventricular outflow tract: magnetic resonance imaging findings. Heart 2002; 88:42.

[52] Ho VB, Kinney JB, Sahn DJ. Ruptured sinus of Valsalva aneurysm: cine phase-contrast MR characterization. J Comput Assist Tomogr 1995;19: 652–6.

[53] McConnell MV, Ganz P, Selwyn AP, et al. Identification of anomalous coronary arteries and their anatomic course by magnetic resonance coronary angiography. Circulation 1995;92:3158–62.

[54] Taylor AM, Thorne SA, Rubens MB, et al. Coronary artery imaging in grown up congenital heart disease: complementary role of magnetic resonance and x-ray coronary angiography. Circulation 2000; 101(14):1670–8.

[55] Valji K. Vascular and interventional radiology. Philadelphia: WB Saunders; 1999. p. 61–79.

[56] Kerting-Sommerhoff BA, Schtem UP, Schiller NB, et al. MRI of the thoracic aorta in Marfan patients. J Comput Assist Tomogr 1987;11:633–9.

[57] DeBakey ME, Henley WS, Cooley DA, et al. Surgical management of dissecting aneurysms of the aorta. J Thorac Cardiovasc Surg 1965;49: 130–49.

[58] Crawford ES. The diagnosis and management of aortic dissection. JAMA 1990;264:2537–41.

[59] Nienaber CA, von Kodolitsch Y, Nicholas V, et al. The diagnosis of thoracic aortic dissection by non-invasive imaging procedures. N Engl J Med 1993; 328:1–9.

[60] Yamada T, Tada S, Harada J. Aortic dissection without intimal rupture: diagnosis with MR imaging and CT. Radiology 1988;168:347–52.

[61] Murray JG, Manisali M, Flamm SD, et al. Intramural hematoma of the thoracic aorta: MR image findings and their prognostic implications. Radiology 1997;204:349–55.

[62] Bank ER. Magnetic resonance of congenital disease: an update. Radiol Clin North Am 1993;31: 553–72.

[63] Bisset GS III, Strife JL, Kirks DR, et al. Vascular rings: MR imaging. AJR Am J Roentgenol 1987; 149:251–6.

[64] von Schulthess GK, Higashino SM, Higgins SS, et al. Coarctation of the aorta: MR imaging. Radiology 1986;158:469–74.

[65] Steffens JC, Bourne MW, Sakuma H, et al. Quantification of collateral blood flow in coarctation of the aorta by velocity encoded cine magnetic resonance imaging. Circulation 1994;90:937–43.

[66] Welch TJ, Stanson AW, Sheedy PF 2nd, et al. Radiologic evaluation of penetrating aortic atherosclerotic ulcer. Radiographics 1990;10:675–85.

[67] Earls JP, DeSena S, Bluemke DA. Gadolinium-enhanced three-dimensional MR angiography of the entire aorta and iliac arteries with dynamic manual table translation. Radiology 1998;209:844–9.

ELSEVIER
SAUNDERS

Magn Reson Imaging Clin N Am
13 (2005) 65–89

**MAGNETIC
RESONANCE
IMAGING CLINICS**
of North America

MR Angiography of the Abdominal Aorta

Elizabeth A. McGuigan, MD[a,b,*], Stephen T. Sears, MD[b],
William R. Corse, DO[a,c], Vincent B. Ho, MD[a]

[a]Department of Radiology and Radiological Sciences, Uniformed Services University of the Health Sciences,
4301 Jones Bridge Road, Bethesda, MD 20814, USA
[b]Department of Radiology, National Naval Medical Center, 8901 Wisconsin Avenue, Bethesda, MD 20889-5600, USA
[c]Department of Radiology, Doylestown Hospital, 595 West State Street, Doylestown, PA 18901, USA

In a remarkably short time, MR angiography has become a robust and reliable diagnostic tool for the noninvasive evaluation of the abdominal aorta and its branches [1–3]. This advancement has been greatly due to the innovation of three-dimensional (3D) contrast-enhanced (CE) MR angiography in the early 1990s [4,5] and the numerous technical improvements in MR angiography since its initial description. Current commercially available software and equipment enable the rapid and reliable performance of accurate MR angiography, using 3D CE MR angiography in almost all clinical abdominal applications. These techniques are easily adaptable to patients of all ages, providing an accurate, detailed, and often dramatic display of pathology. Its speed, reliability, and diagnostic accuracy have contributed to the integration of MR angiography into clinical care pathways at many centers. Improvements in image processing speed and tools have facilitated image interpretation and timely diagnosis that have allowed the referring clinician to make relevant and informed decisions about a patient's course of treatment. This article reviews the technical and common clinical applications for MR angiography in the abdomen and discusses various methods for MR angiography optimization and possible pitfalls to be avoided.

Basic considerations for abdominal MR angiography: clinical issues

Evaluation of the abdominal aorta and its branch vessels is one of the most common MR angiography indications in the body. 3D CE MR angiography is well suited for evaluation of most abdominal aortic pathologies and overcomes the numerous flow-related limitations of traditional time-of-flight and phase-contrast (PC) MR angiography [1–10]. 3D CE MR angiography is particularly helpful for imaging the abdominal vasculature, where blood flow within the various vessels is inherently multidirectional and the geometry is complex (Fig. 1). The range of flow velocities and their variable directions in the different abdominal vessels make flow-based (ie, non–contrast-enhanced) MR angiography techniques usually suboptimal for comprehensive abdominal angiographic illustration. Because 3D CE MR angiography often is essential for optimal illustration of the abdominal vessels, it is important first to determine that 3D CE MR angiography can be performed successfully. Proper preliminary screening of patients enables the tailoring of the study to avoid potential pitfalls and allows for a more efficient experience for the patient and the operator. In addition, a foreknowledge of potential problems provides a more realistic diagnostic expectation for the MR angiography request in advance, which cannot be

The opinions or assertions contained herein are the private views of the authors and are not to be construed as official or reflecting the views of the Uniformed Services University of the Health Sciences or the Department of Defense.

* Corresponding author. Department of Radiology and Radiological Sciences, Uniformed Services University of the Health Sciences, 4301 Jones Bridge Road, Bethesda, MD 20814.
   E-mail address: EAMcGuigan@bethesda.med.navy.mil (E.A. McGuigan).

1064-9689/05/$ - see front matter. Published by Elsevier Inc.
doi:10.1016/j.mric.2004.12.010

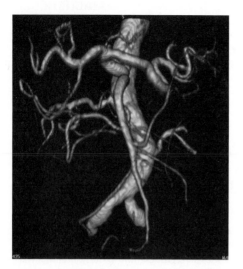

Fig. 1. An 82-year-old woman suspected to have mesenteric ischemia. Coronal VR projection of 3D CE MR angiography shows normal caliber and orientation of the celiac artery and superior mesenteric artery. The normal tortuosity and complex relationships of the abdominal aorta and the celiac and superior mesenteric arteries are evident. (*Adapted from* Ho VB, Corse WR. MR angiography of the abdominal aorta and peripheral vessels. Radiol Clin North Am 2003;41:115–44; with permission.)

underemphasized for any clinical practice. In most cases, abdominal MR angiography yields pertinent clinical information that in many cases may not be possible otherwise (Fig. 2).

To enable 3D CE MR angiography, the patient first must have good venous access; generally an antecubital 20G or 22G intravenous catheter is sufficient. Even in patients without good venous access, however, the aorta still can be evaluated using a host of noncontrast MR techniques, notably steady-state free precession (SSFP) (also known as TrueFISP, Siemens Medical Solutions, Erlangen, Germany); FIESTA, General Electric Healthcare (Waukesha, Wisconsin); balanced FFE, Philips Medical Systems (Best, The Netherlands)). Pereles et al [11] described the ability to perform a rapid aortic screening examination for dissection and aneurysm in 4 minutes using SSFP pulse sequences. Second, the patient must be able to hold his or her breath comfortably for at least 20 seconds. Breath holding can be accomplished in most patients with the assistance of supplemental oxygen and hyperventilation [12]. In patients incapable of breath holding, 3D CE MR angiography during free breathing can be performed, but generally respiratory motion artifacts degrade image quality, precluding the confident diagnosis of more subtle

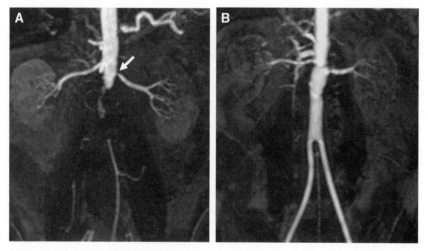

Fig. 2. A 56-year-old man with Leriche syndrome presented with hypertension and buttock claudication. (*A*) Preoperative 3D CE MR angiography (coronal MIP) show the characteristic occlusion of the distal abdominal aorta below the renal arteries. A high-grade stenosis also was noted in the proximal left renal artery (*arrow*). (*B*) Postoperative 3D CE MR angiography (coronal MIP) shows the aortobifemoral graft, which included revascularization of the left renal artery at the proximal anastomosis. (Courtesy of Qian Dong, MD, and Martin R. Prince, MD, PhD, Ann Arbor, MI. *Adapted from* Ho VB, Corse WR. MR angiography of the abdominal aorta and peripheral vessels. Radiol Clin North Am 2003;41:115–44; with permission.)

vascular diseases, such as renal fibromuscular dysplasia (FMD). Respiratory motion effect can be minimized by using multiple signal averages (eg, number of excitations [NEX] or number of signal averages [NSA] = ≥2) or possibly employing faster imaging techniques, such as SSFP. Vascular signal on SSFP relies primarily on T2-to-T1 ratio and is generally less flow dependent, resulting in its ability to depict vessels well even during free breathing (Fig. 3) [8,11]. Infants and children present additional clinical issues (see the article by Chung and Krishnamurthy elsewhere in this issue) [13].

It also is important to obtain a good clinical history concerning a patient's prior interventional history and the referring clinician's specific clinical query. The presence of surgical clips is well known to cause T2* metallic susceptibility artifacts,

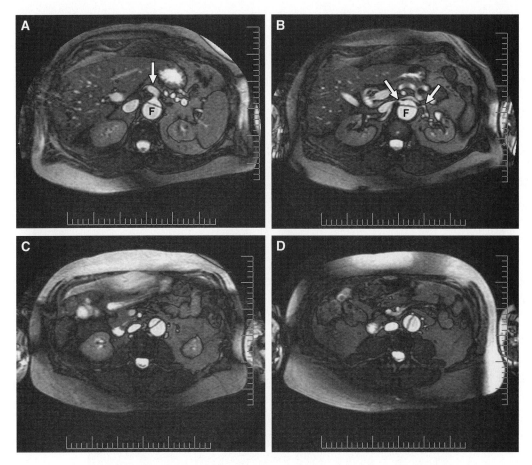

Fig. 3. (*A–J*) Type B aortic dissection with extension through the abdominal aorta into the iliac arteries. (*A–G*) Free-breathing axial 2D SSFP imaging can be used as a fast screening examination. In this case, it was used to determine the distal extent of a type B dissection of the thoracic aortic. On select axial images (*A–G,* cranial to caudal), two channels—true and false (F)—separated by the dissection flap are seen throughout the entire length of the abdominal aorta and are noted to extend into the common iliac arteries. On the upper abdominal images (*A* and *B*), the celiac artery (*arrow* in *A*) and the renal arteries (*arrows* in *B*) are noted to arise from the anterior true lumen. On the mid and lower abdominal images (*C–G*), the intimal flap is noted to spiral counterclockwise down the aorta through the aortic bifurcation into both iliac arteries. (*H–J*) VR reconstruction of 3D CE MR angiography shows the abdominal extent of the dissection well (*H,* large field of view oblique frontal VR image). (*I*) On subvolume VR reconstruction of the upper abdominal aorta, the anterior true (T) and posterior false (F) lumens are well seen separated by the intimal tear (*arrowheads*). On a VR view from the left side (*I*), the celiac artery (*upper large arrow*) and superior mesenteric artery (*lower smaller arrow*) are seen to originate from the true (T) lumen. (*J*) On a VR view from above, the renal arteries (*arrows*) are noted also to arise from the anterior true lumen, as does the celiac artery (C).

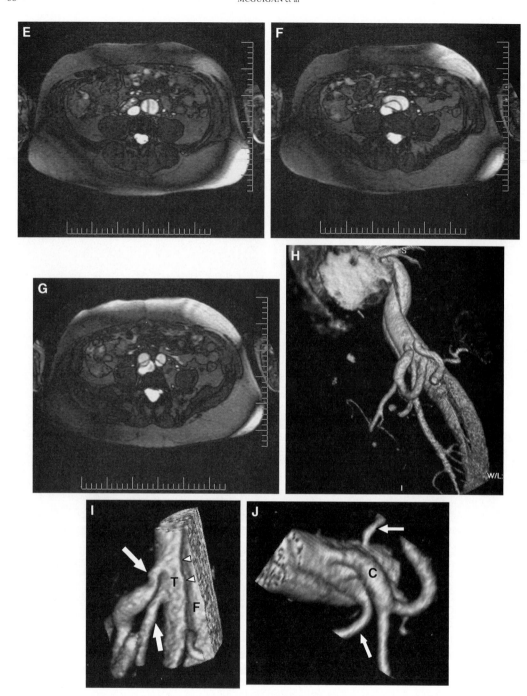

Fig. 3 (*continued*)

which if unrecognized may result in erroneous interpretation as a focal stenosis or occlusion. Patients who have undergone prior bypass graft or shunt procedures (eg, aortoiliac, aortofemoral, splenorenal) present additional concerns, and it is important to note the type and location of the donor and recipient vessels. This is particularly true for extra-anatomic bypass grafts (eg, axillary-femoral bypass), which may be peripheral or superficial in location. It is important to know about a patient's history of an endovascular procedure, which now is becoming more widely performed. Most current stents and endografts contain substances that cause some degree of T2* metallic susceptibility artifacts, which may preclude arterial illustration even using 3D CE MR angiography. Attempts to optimize 3D CE MR angiography for imaging within newer stents are promising, however [14]. In general, a thorough knowledge of a patient's past interventional history ensures better optimization and tailoring of the MR angiography examination for answering the relevant clinical questions properly.

MR techniques: pulse sequences and image interpretation

Three-dimensional contrast-enhanced MR angiography

The abdominal aorta is best evaluated using 3D CE MR angiography [1–6]. This technique, first used in the early 1990s for MR angiography of the abdominal aorta [4,5], has been modified for imaging most vascular territories within the body, which speaks to the versatility of the technique. The underlying principles for the technique remain the same, however. CE MR angiography relies on the T1 shortening effects of a circulating gadolinium (Gd)-chelate contrast agent [4–8]. The key is to synchronize the imaging with the transit of the contrast bolus through the target vascular territory. The important technical issues for 3D CE MR angiography are detailed in the sections that follow.

Patient positioning and preparation

As with most abdominal MR imaging, patient position is typically supine with feet first. With 3D CE MR angiography, however, it is preferable to elevate the patient's arms outside of the potential imaging volume. 3D CE MR angiography of the abdominal aorta typically is performed using a coronal or oblique coronal prescription, and modest elevation of the arms using pads or towels under the patient's arms is sufficient. By removing the arms from the field of view (FOV), aliasing artifacts (also known as "wraparound" artifacts) of peripheral signal into the target regions are minimized. The use of the smallest possible FOV inherently yields the highest possible spatial resolution for individual 3D CE MR angiography.

Although not necessary for 3D CE MR angiography, the placement of respiratory bellows is often helpful because it not only enables respiratory-triggered acquisitions for adjunctive visceral imaging, but also provides the operator with a real-time visualization of the patient's respiratory status and pattern, an additional tool to confirm patient compliance with breath-holding instructions before initiation of breath-held acquisitions. Cardiac gating is an additional consideration but is not necessary for 3D CE MR angiography. In more complicated cases, in which flow direction may be important or flow quantification is desired, cardiac-gated cine MR acquisitions usually are required. In these cases, it is often helpful to perform the suitable setup for cardiac gating in advance of the scanning. In more tenuous patients, it is always preferable to have cardiac gating for proper patient monitoring. Setup for physiologic monitoring during the initial patient preparation minimizes scan delays and potential for bulk patient motion when scanning is initiated. When imaging the upper central abdominal aorta and its visceral branches, it is preferable to use a torso phased array coil [6,8]; as with other body applications, this increases overall signal-to-noise ratio (SNR) but will limit the superior-to-inferior dimension of the FOV. In tall patients or patients in whom a longer FOV is desired, the standard body coil is typically sufficient for 3D CE MR angiography. Newer, longer phased array coils (with eight or more coils) and newer multichannel MR scanner platforms provide interesting new opportunities, for improved CE MR angiography over larger territories. If parallel imaging is implemented, a phased array coil must be used.

MR angiography pulse sequence selection and scan prescription

Because CE MR angiography technique relies on the T1 shortening effects of Gd, a T1-weighted fast 3D spoiled gradient echo pulse sequence typically is used [6–9]. Use of a 3D acquisition yields the highest possible spatial resolution, improves background suppression, and facilitates better data sets for image postprocessing. The use of radiofrequency spoiling and a higher flip angle (eg, 45°) accentuates the T1 weighting and optimizes the signal gains from contrast enhancement. Ideally, 3D CE MR angiography is performed during a breath hold, so the shortest possible repetition time (TR) and echo time (TE) should be used for CE MR angiography. The actual TR and TE depend on scanner field strength and gradient subsystem. In addition to TR and TE, a variety of other parameters may be modified to improve imaging speed, which may be particularly important when imaging patients with limited breath-hold capacity. Imaging time can be decreased by using partial Fourier (eg, 0.5 NEX), increased receiver bandwidth (eg, ±128 kHz), and parallel imaging. All these result in slight reductions in overall SNR; however, arterial SNR is typically sufficient if 3D CE MR angiography is performed correctly.

Parallel imaging techniques (eg, sensitivity encoding, or SENSE, Philips Medical Systems; array spatial sensitivity encoding technique, or ASSET, General Electric Healthcare; GRAPPA, Siemens Medical Solutions) [15–18] take advantage of spatial information intrinsic to the receiver coil to allow a decrease in the number of phase-encoding steps and provide faster image acquisition, acquiring an entire volume in 5 to 20 seconds depending on the selected acceleration factor [8,15–18]. Individualized selection of the acceleration factor allows the acquisition to be tailored to the patient's breath-holding ability. The reconstruction algorithm for the imaging system takes into account the encoding effect of coil sensitivities to obviate the aliasing artifact that otherwise would result. These techniques allow the operator to optimize scan parameters within patient limits for breath hold, but, as mentioned previously, require the use of a phased array coil. The main downside of parallel imaging is a reduction in SNR by a factor of approximately the square root of the acceleration factor. This reduction generally is not significant because this signal loss is seen in the vessel and background tissues, and the loss is small compared with the high SNR intrinsic to 3D CE MR angiography.

On most current high-field MR scanners, judicious adjustment of imaging parameters should yield a 20- to 30-second 3D MR angiography acquisition with spatial resolution adequate for diagnostic visualization of the abdominal aorta and its branch vessel origins (Fig. 4) [6,9]. Faster scanning can be performed, but typically at a reduced spatial resolution, which may not be adequate for imaging smaller vessels. Most patients, especially with assistance of supplemental oxygen and hyperventilation, should be able to hold their breath for 20 to 30 seconds [12]. The use of supplemental oxygen in patients with severe chronic obstructive pulmonary disease is problematic, but the use of oxygen at no more than 2 L/min with close monitoring is safe. Marks et al [12] reported successful use of supplemental oxygen in pulmonary compromised patients, which

resulted in a 97.8% increase in breath-hold time without oxygen-induced apnea in patients with chronic obstructive pulmonary disease.

3D CE MR angiography also is best performed as a dynamic series of 3D acquisitions. Initial precontrast 3D MR angiography should be performed to ensure proper placement of the imaging volume; this also serves as a good practice for patient (and operator) for the actual contrast-enhanced scans. Two or more 3D MR angiography scans should be performed after contrast administration; the first typically is timed for arteries with delayed phases more adequately showing venous structures. Delayed phase 3D MR angiography scans (ie, second and third dynamic acquisitions) are particularly useful to illustrate slow-filling structures, such as a large capacious abdominal aortic aneurysm (AAA), collateral vessels, the false channel of an aortic dissection, or vessels with diffuse of high-grade stenoses. Parenchymal enhancement of end organs also can be evaluated [19]. The use of multiple acquisitions (ie, multiphase imaging) further ensures a diagnostic result and overall reliability of the study because occasionally unexpected technical problems or timing artifacts may occur during the arterial phase acquisition that may not be present on subsequent scanning. Delayed phase imaging also can provide excellent venous illustration (Fig. 5).

It is important to evaluate the balance of spatial and temporal resolution in breath-hold imaging techniques [8]. In general, faster image acquisition would be better because it minimizes motion-related blurring artifacts, but this must be balanced with the need for sufficient spatial resolution; in smaller caliber vessel areas, such as the renal and mesenteric arteries, this is particularly important. For renal 3D CE MR angiography, spatial resolution of at least 1.5 mm (or at least approaching this) should be sought [20]. With the use of parallel imaging, high spatial resolution renal 3D CE MR angiography is possible (Fig. 6).

Although a reduction in the FOV would improve spatial resolution, and minimizing spatial coverage potentially would improve imaging speed, care must be taken to ensure proper inclusion of the target vessels. In general, the imaging volume and the acquisition plane should be adapted to the vascular territory of interest. In most cases, a coronal or oblique coronal imaging plane is best for performing 3D CE MR angiography of the abdominal aorta and its major branches [6]. Occasionally, alternative imaging

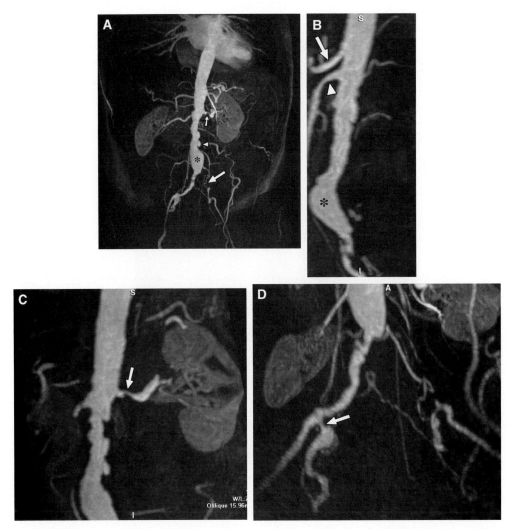

Fig. 4. (*A–G*) 3D CE MR angiography in a patient with diffuse atherosclerosis. (*A*) On coronal MIP, a large infrarenal AAA (*) is seen just above the aortic bifurcation with the remainder of the infrarenal abdominal aorta having an irregular contour consistent with atherosclerotic plaque with ulceration (*arrowhead*). Occlusion of the left common iliac artery (*large arrow*) and a severe stenosis of the left renal artery (*small arrow*) also are seen. (*B*) On sagittal subvolume MIP, the large AAA (*) and irregular contour of the infrarenal abdominal aorta is again noted. The celiac artery (*arrow*) and the superior mesenteric artery (*arrowhead*) are normal. (*C* and *D*) Thinner subvolume MIP viewing of 3D data would improve visualization of arterial stenoses. In this case, subvolume MIP reconstruction shows the severe stenosis of the left renal artery (*arrow* in *C*) and proximal right internal iliac artery (*arrow* in *D*). (*D*) The left common iliac artery occlusion is again seen. (*E–G*) VR viewing of 3D CE MR angiography (*E*, coronal; *F*, oblique coronal; *G*, oblique) also illustrates the aforementioned lesions. One major advantage of VR viewing is the preservation of depth information, which is not present on standard MIP viewing. Depth information allows improved viewing of overlapping arterial segments, as is shown in these VR images.

planes, such as an axial acquisition, may be beneficial because the anterior-to-posterior dimension is typically the smallest, enabling a smaller rectangular FOV prescription for a further reduction in scan time. Axial prescriptions necessarily limit the length of aortic visualization, however.

Contrast agent considerations

3D CE MR angiography of the abdominal aorta and its primary branches typically is performed using one of the commercially available extracellular Gd-chelate contrast agents [1–6]. Although the use of contrast agents for MR

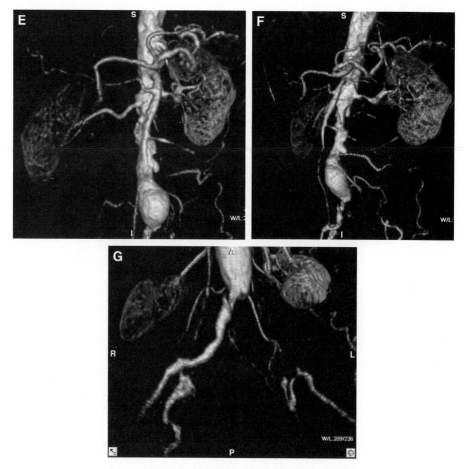

Fig. 4 (*continued*)

angiography continues to be an "off-label" application [21,22], it has become standard clinical practice in most centers and has been widely recognized as a diagnostic standard for imaging the abdominal aorta [1–6]. Typically a 20- or 30-mL contrast agent dose (approximately 0.1–0.2 mmol/kg dose) injected at 2 mL/sec [23] provides sufficient arterial signal on 3D CE MR angiography. In smaller patients, a weight-based dose (eg, 0.15 or 0.2 mmol/kg dose) would be prudent. Experience and ability to synchronize imaging properly with timing can enable the use of a lower dose [24], but the use of low doses risks inadequate signal for illustration of a large aortic aneurysm or of subtle vascular detail as may be expected in a patient with renal artery FMD. In cases in which illustration of the venous anatomy is important, such as the evaluation of a potential renal donor, use of a higher contrast dose (ie,

30–40 mL) often is helpful to ensure adequate venous signal for venous evaluation. Similarly, extending the duration of the contrast bolus using a biphasic injection (eg, half of the dose administered at 2 mL/sec followed by the remaining dose at 1 or 1.5 mL/sec) improves venous visualization on delayed-phase 3D CE MR angiography. In all cases, a large saline flush is beneficial (eg, 20–30 mL) because it ensures that the entire dose is delivered centrally, and it prolongs the duration of arterial enhancement for improved arterial-phase 3D CE MR angiography [25].

Timing options for three-dimensional contrast-enhanced MR angiography

Proper synchronization of imaging with contrast transit through the vascular bed is essential for optimized vascular illustration on 3D CE MR

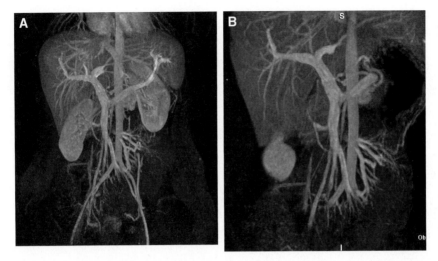

Fig. 5. Portography on delayed phase 3D CE MR angiography. (*A*) On a delayed phase of 3D CE MR angiography (coronal MIP), the abdominal venous system is well shown. (*B*) In this case, a normal portal venous system is well seen on the subvolume MIP of the delayed phase 3D data set.

angiography [7–9]. In the initial implementation of CE MR angiography, 3D data acquisition required 3 to 4 minutes, and the contrast material was administered via slow infusion to match the prolonged data acquisition period [4,5]. With the introduction of fast 3D spoiled gradient echo pulse sequences, imaging was shortened significantly, enabling breath-hold acquisition but requiring more attention to timing and bolus delivery. One of the simplest, but also the least reliable methods is to use a fixed time delay (eg, 15 seconds) between initiation of the contrast bolus and beginning of imaging. This fixed time delay results in wide variation in arterial illustration, however, because circulatory times can vary significantly. Earls et al [26] reported transit times from the antecubital fossa injection site to the abdominal aorta that ranged from 10 to 50 seconds. Variations in circulatory time depend on multiple factors, including the patient's gender, age, cardiovascular status, hydration status, and intervening arterial anatomy [27]. These variations result in inconsistency in contrast bolus arrival time between patients and accounts for the inconsistency in arterial visualization that is seen when using a fixed timing delay for 3D CE MR angiography.

Fixed timing schemes generally have been abandoned for timed 3D CE MR angiography using a bolus timing scan or a real-time timing algorithm. Timed acquisitions result in optimized arterial signal, more efficient use of contrast media

dose, and overall improvement in the reliability of arterial signal [7–9,26,28–33]. Test bolus scans can be achieved using a small dose (1–2 mL) of a Gd-chelate contrast agent injected at 2 mL/sec and followed by a large saline flush (eg, 20–30 mL) at the same rate [8,26,28]. Arrival of the contrast material in the abdominal aorta can be determined by rapid sequential imaging of the aorta using a fast T1-weighted two-dimensional (2D) spoiled gradient echo pulse sequence. Temporal resolution of one image every 1 to 2 seconds for a period of 40 to 50 seconds is adequate. A potential pitfall of this technique is confusion of normal bright signal from vascular inflow related to normal aortic pulsatility (time-of-flight effect into the imaging slice) with the arrival of contrast agent. Placement of superior and inferior saturation bands on an axial timing scan through the aorta can be used. Alternatively, this problem can be overcome by using a sagittal acquisition for the timing scan because this minimizes inflow effects as aortic flow is primarily in-plane. When performing a test bolus scan, it is helpful to have an MR-compatible injector because this ensures consistency between bolus deliveries and minimizes additional timing variations related to bolus administration. Timing differences still may be present if there are changes in the patient's heart rate or cardiac output, but these are unusual because scan delays are often negligible if patient preparation and setup are correct. The use of a test bolus also contributes to background signal,

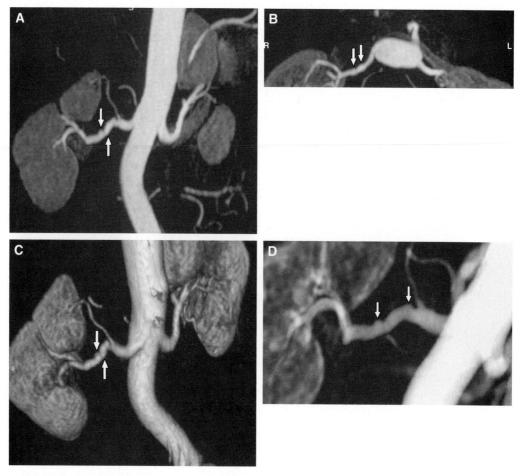

Fig. 6. (*A–G*) A 50-year-old woman with hypertension. On 3D CE MR angiography (*A*, oblique coronal subvolume MIP; *B*, axial subvolume MIP; *C*, coronal VR projection; *D*, coronal transparent VR projection), the "string of beads" appearance (*arrows*) characteristic of FMD is noted in the right renal artery, which looks comparable to that of conventional x-ray angiography (*E*). The beaded appearance was well seen in the right renal artery on 3D CE MR angiography, especially on the VR projections (*C* and *D*). (*F*) Mild FMD also was noted on conventional x-ray angiography in the proximal left renal artery (*arrow*). (*G*) FMD was suggested on 3D CE MR angiography but less clearly seen, probably secondary to the inherent spatial resolution limitations of MR angiography. (*Adapted from* Ho VB, Corse WR. MR angiography of the abdominal aorta and peripheral vessels. Radiol Clin North Am 2003;41:115–44; with permission.)

notably in the urinary collecting system. This may make evaluation of some renal or pelvic branch vessels more challenging, but typically not impossible.

There are two methods for real-time timing or triggering of 3D CE MR angiography. One method, known as automatic bolus detection algorithm (SmartPrep, General Electric Healthcare), is composed of two phases [29–40]. The initial phase monitors the signal in an operator-defined volume of interest (typically placed in the abdominal aorta at the level of the renal arteries).

When signal within the monitoring volume exceeds two operator-defined thresholds (typically a signal increase of >20% and 2 SDs over baseline signal), the pulse sequence initiates the 3D MR angiography acquisition. A scan delay between phases of 5 seconds typically is sufficient for proper coaching of the patient to hold his or her breath for 3D CE MR angiography. For this technique, the operator must prescribe the monitoring volume and the 3D imaging volume. The monitoring volume ideally is placed in the middle of the FOV, typically in the abdominal aorta at

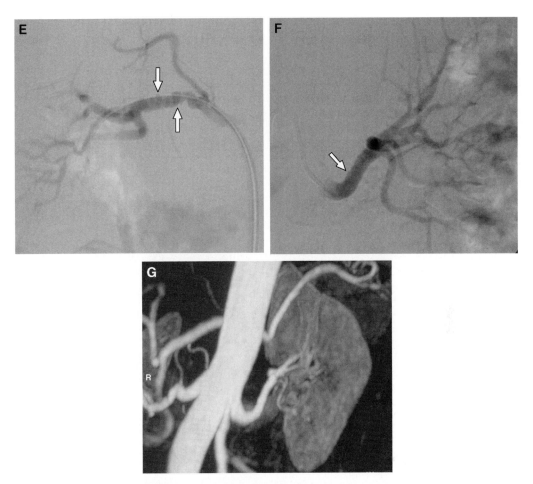

Fig. 6 (*continued*)

the level of the renal arteries. Placement of the monitoring volume is best on an axial scan because this minimizes the possibility of erroneous placement in the inferior vena cava, which on sagittal images may be confused with the aorta because of their proximity and similar vertical orientations. The prescription of the monitoring volume does not preclude prescription of 3D MR angiography on a sagittal localizer, which is generally best for abdominal aortic scan prescription.

The second technique for real-time triggering of 3D CE MR angiography uses MR fluoroscopy (eg, CareBolus, Siemens Medical Solutions; Bolus-Trak, Philips Medical Systems; FlouroTrigger, General Electric Healthcare) [31–33]. Similar to the aforementioned scheme, this technique has a monitoring phase and 3D MR angiography phase. Monitoring of contrast material arrival is performed, however, by the operator, who

monitors a series of fast 2D gradient echo images during the actual contrast bolus injection and manually triggers the 3D acquisition on visualization of the contrast arrival on the fluoroscopic images. Real-time triggering by either MR fluoroscopic trigger or the previously mentioned automated bolus detection algorithm is easy to learn and when mastered results in diagnostic quality 3D CE MR angiography of the abdominal aorta in most cases.

One final method for achieving arterial phase 3D CE MR angiography is by using a time-resolved technique, such as time-resolved acquisition imaging of contrast kinetics (TRICKS) [34] or subsecond 3D MR angiography [35]. These techniques rely on the continuous imaging of the FOV, which theoretically includes the arterial phase of the contrast bolus. Aortic visualization by either technique still is improved by the acquisition during a breath hold, and the practical issue of when to initiate the breath hold still must be determined, or else a longer than usual breath hold is used to ensure proper timing. TRICKS is more practical for imaging regions such as the lower extremities, where breath holding is not necessary. Subsecond 3D MR angiography, which provides relatively lower spatial resolution images, can be useful as the initial bolus timing scan or as an adjunct to higher spatial resolution 3D CE MR angiography. Subsecond 3D MR angiography can provide insight for illustration of more complex anatomic relationships (eg, arteries and veins in an arteriovenous malformation) or to identify entry or reentry tears in patients with dissection.

k-Space acquisition schemes

One special consideration for 3D CE MR angiography is a k-space sampling scheme [8,29,31]. Most image contrast is determined by the data from the central k-space region (also known as the low spatial frequency data). Because the duration of preferential arterial enhancement is transient, signal on 3D CE MR angiography also is variable with optimal signal achieved if central k-space data are timed to coincide with peak enhancement of the target vessel. Using conventional linear 3D k-space acquisition schemes, the central k-space data are acquired during the middle of the imaging period (eg, about 10 seconds into a 20-second acquisition). With the introduction of real-time timing schemes, it became advantageous to acquire these crucial central k-space data earlier in the scan because this would afford improved coordination with contrast bolus arrival. That is to say, use of a traditional linear acquisition scheme for a 20-second acquisition would require real-time detection of the bolus 10 seconds "upstream" to the target vascular bed for proper initiation of the scan to begin. For this reason, alternate centric [29] and elliptical centric [31] phase ordered acquisition schemes have been implemented for 3D CE MR angiography. These k-space schemes acquire the central k-space data early in the acquisition period, enabling real-time monitoring of the contrast bolus arrival in the actual target vascular territory. One pitfall of using centric and elliptical centric phase ordered k-space schemes is the potential for acquiring the central k-space data too early during the actual arrival of contrast material, during which the Gd concentration is rapidly rising. "Ringing" artifact [36], which appears as alternating black and white linear lines that parallel the vessel walls (Fig. 7), results. This can be avoided by starting the imaging slightly after the actual contrast arrival (eg, 5 seconds)

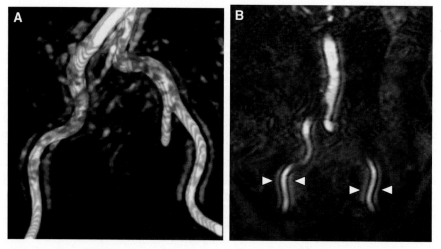

Fig. 7. "Ringing" artifact. (*A* and *B*) The premature performance of 3D CE MR angiography during the actual arrival of the contrast bolus into the aortoiliac arteries results in a distinctive "ringing" artifact (*A*, VR view; *B*, coronal source image). This artifact consists of alternating dark and bright bands that parallel the arterial contours and are identified more easily on source (*B*) or thin reconstruction of the data set. This artifact occurs because of the acquisition of central k-space data during the rapid rise in Gd concentration in the target vessel. To avoid this artifact, central k-space data should be sampled during the more stable plateau phase of peak arterial enhancement.

when the Gd concentration is high but stable (ie, plateau phase of the bolus) [8].

Three-dimensional contrast-enhanced MR angiography image processing and interpretation

As with other radiographic procedures, it is most important to develop a personal technique to ensure that all of the sequences and anatomy included in the study are evaluated. Interpretation of 3D CE MR angiography is described in more detail in the article by Glockner [37], but some additional suggestions for interpretation of abdominal 3D CE MR angiography data sets are presented here. The most commonly used image processing tools are multiplanar reformation (MPR), maximum intensity projection (MIP), and volume rendering (VR). Global visualization of the aorta and its branches is best performed using a thicker MIP (see Figs. 2, 4, and 6) or VR reconstruction (see Figs. 1, 3, 4, and 6), but subtle intraluminal detail is best seen on thinner sub-volume MIP (see Figs. 3, 4, and 6) or MPR, which is a single-voxel planar reconstruction through the 3D volume. The origins of the branch vessels, such as the renal arteries, celiac arteries, and mesenteric arteries, are best visualized in subvolume MIPs (see Fig. 4). A difference between VR and MIP display merits comment. In VR, the computer algorithm uses a weighted sum of data from all voxels along a ray projected through the 3D data set, resulting in better depth perception that is absent in MIP projections (see Fig. 4). When processing image data, one must be mindful of reconstruction thickness because use of too thick of a thickness results in volume averaging and potentially an overestimate of the severity of a vascular stenosis. The use of subvolume MIP or MPR can improve the visualization of smaller vessels, but requires a skilled and knowledgeable user and can be time intensive. VR display of 3D CE MR angiography has been shown to be particularly better than MIP and MPR for the evaluation of renal artery stenoses [38].

Adjunctive MR techniques: "bright blood"

Postcontrast gradient echo imaging

After 3D CE MR angiography, the additional performance of a fat-suppressed T1-weighted fast 2D spoiled gradient echo pulse sequence in an orthogonal plane may be useful for evaluation of the abdominal viscera (Fig. 8) or further evaluation of the aortic wall. This imaging also allows illustration of mural thrombosis and a secondary confirmation of vascular findings. Abnormal enhancement of the vessel wall and perivascular tissues and the parenchyma also can be assessed [19]. A newer 3D fat-suppressed T1-weighted

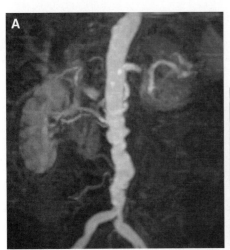
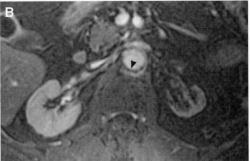

Fig. 8. A 76-year-old woman with severe atherosclerotic disease. (*A*) On 3D CE MR angiography (coronal MIP), the abdominal aorta has an irregular contour consistent with diffuse atherosclerotic plaque. The left renal artery is occluded, and there are two right renal arteries. Further subvolume MIP reconstruction (not shown) showed a severe stenosis of the main right renal artery. (*B*) After 3D CE MR angiography, axial fat-suppressed 2D fast spoiled gradient echo imaging shows a small scarred left kidney consistent with long-term ischemic nephropathy. A thin dark curvilinear band (*arrowhead*) consistent with atherosclerotic plaque also is seen lining the posterior wall of the abdominal aorta.

spoiled gradient echo pulse sequence that uses a radial k-space trajectory (T1 high-resolution isotropic volume examination [THRIVE], Philips Medical Systems) is showing promise for post-contrast imaging (Fig. 9).

Steady-state free precession

As previously mentioned, SSFP pulse sequences can be a valuable tool not only for initial screening of the abdominal vasculature (see Fig. 1), but also as a postcontrast vascular imaging tool. On SSFP, vascular signal is improved by the Gd and remains high 20 minutes after contrast injection [39]. These sequences are highly dependent on T2-to-T1 ratio and may be less helpful for imaging the hepatic vessels because the signal within the hepatobiliary system also is bright. After 3D CE MR angiography, cine SSFP

can be used to confirm the presence of thrombus or an intimal tear. SSFP imaging is particularly sensitive to B_0 inhomogeneity and sensitive to metallic susceptibility artifacts from metallic stents or clips.

Phase-contrast imaging

PC is a flow-based technique that relies on the detection of phase shifts of moving spins for the generation of signal. Although this technique can be performed without the use of Gd-chelate contrast agents, signal is improved on PC acquisitions after Gd has been administered [40]. PC imaging requires the appropriate operator prescription of velocity encoding (VENC) and direction of flow sensitivity. Postcontrast 3D PC MR angiography has been shown to be of particular value as an adjunct to renal 3D CE

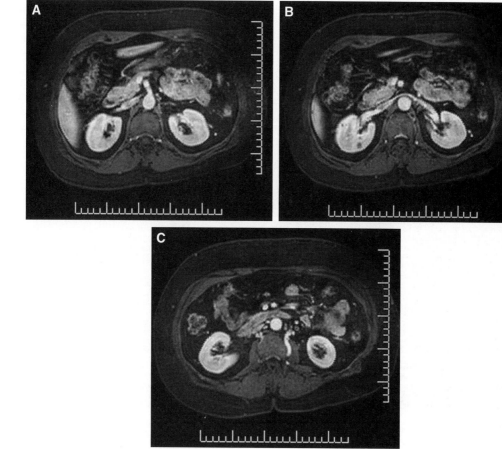

Fig. 9. (*A–C*) Fat-suppressed T1-weighted imaging using a new fast 3D spoiled gradient echo technique that uses a radial k-space trajectory called THRIVE. Shown are select source images (*A–C*, cranial to caudal) from 100 partitions obtained during an 18-second breath hold after 3D CE MR angiography.

MR angiography [41,42] because its sensitivity to phase persists after Gd-chelate contrast administration. On 3D PC MR angiography, turbulent flow through a hemodynamically significant stenosis results in phase dispersion (also called *intravoxel dephasing*) and signal loss; this results in stenosis appearing more severe on 3D PC MR angiography than on initial 3D CE MR angiography [41,42]. PC also can be performed in a 2D cine mode for flow measurement. This technique can be used to confirm stent patency in segments otherwise not visualized on 3D CE MR angiography (Fig. 10).

Adjunctive MR techniques: "black blood"

"Black blood" imaging (eg, spin echo, fast spin echo, double inversion recovery fast spin echo) is a standard part of most abdominal MR angiography examinations [6,43]. Black blood images provide relevant morphologic information about the wall and diameter of the abdominal aorta and its immediate adjacent tissues and should be part of the precontrast imaging protocol. Although 3D CE MR angiography is good for angiographic illustration, this technique provides a "luminogram," and it does not illustrate the wall of the vessels. Intramural hematoma and extramural pathology, both of which can be crucial items of information, may not be displayed on 3D CE MR angiography, and black blood imaging should be included in the abdominal MR

angiography protocol. With the speed of newer black blood imaging techniques, precontrast axial T1-weighted and T2-weighted black blood imaging usually can be included easily into the scan protocol at little expense in terms of time.

MR of selected conditions of the abdominal aorta

Abdominal aortic aneurysm

The protean manifestations of atherosclerosis can be exquisitely shown on MR. One of the most common manifestations of this complex disease process is AAA (see Fig. 4). An AAA is a pathologic, permanent, localized dilation of at least one segment of the normal aorta with a diameter at least 1.5 times the normal expected diameter of the involved segment [44]. AAAs are significantly more common than thoracic aortic aneurysms and often are clinically unsuspected. The incidence of AAA increases abruptly after age 55 in men and age 70 in women [45,46]. The incidence of AAA has increased measurably, from 8.7 per 100,000 person-years in 1951 to 36.5 to 60 per 100,000 person-years in 1971 to 1980 [47]. The increased incidence applies to aneurysms of all sizes. Possible contributing factors to the increase include the aging of the population, increased awareness of the condition and its associated coexisting disease entities, and improved diagnostic techniques [46]. The prevalence of AAAs in people 50 years old and older is at least 3% [48].

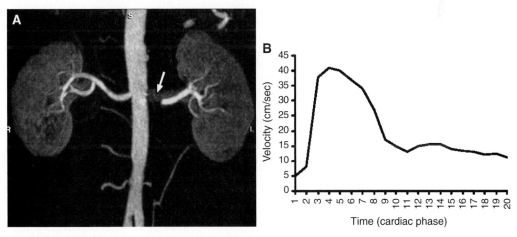

Fig. 10. (*A*) 3D CE MR angiography in a patient with a history of prior stenting for left renal artery stenosis. Coronal MIP from 3D CE MR angiography shows a normal right renal artery and, more importantly, a poorly visualized segment of the left renal artery secondary to significant T2* susceptibility artifact from the stent (*arrow*). Cine phase contrast (images not shown) was performed distal to the stent in a plane perpendicular to the left renal artery. (*B*) Flow quantification using commercially available software showed a normal pulsatile left renal artery flow pattern, which suggests patency of the stent lumen.

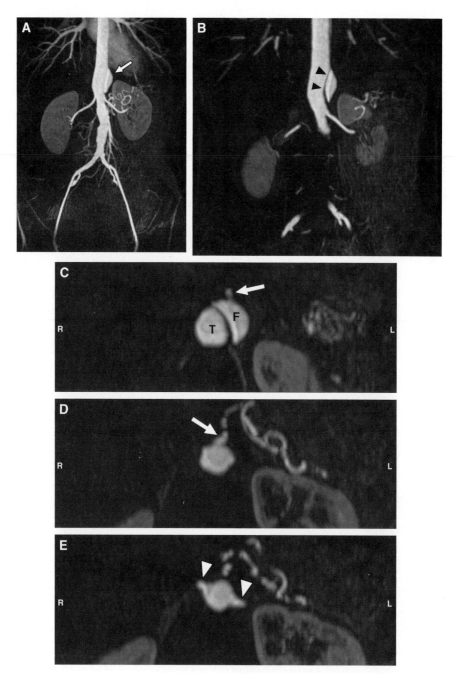

Fig. 11. (*A–F*) Thoracoabdominal aortic dissection on 3D CE MR angiography. (*A*) On coronal MIP, a focal bulge (*arrow*) suggesting an aneurysm is seen in the suprarenal aorta. (*B*) Thinner reconstruction of the 3D data set using subvolume MIP reveals an intimal tear (*arrowheads*) consistent with aortic dissection. (*C*) Axial subvolume MIP at the level of the celiac artery (*arrow*) shows the dissection separating the true lumen (T) from the false lumen (F). The celiac artery (*arrow*) is shown to arise from the false lumen. (*D* and *E*) More distal axial subvolume MIP evaluation of the aorta shows no extension of the dissection and normal origins for the superior mesenteric artery (*arrow* in *D*) and renal arteries (*arrowheads* in *E*). (*F*) VR projection summarizes the aforementioned findings with the celiac artery (*arrowhead*) seen arising from the false lumen (F) and the superior mesenteric artery (*arrow*) slightly displaced but arising from the true lumen.

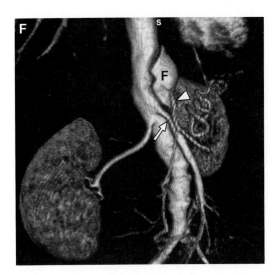

Fig. 11 (*continued*)

The etiology of AAA traditionally has been attributed to atherosclerosis, although it is now evident that multiple factors must be considered as they interact with each other [46]. The morphology of atherosclerotic disease of the abdominal aorta manifests commonly as a fusiform aneurysm. Saccular aneurysms are less common, and stenotic disease of the distal aorta is even rarer (see Fig. 2). The infrarenal aorta is the site most affected by the atherosclerotic process and is the most common site of the development of AAA (see Fig. 1). Suprarenal AAAs are uncommon and tend to arise as a distal extension of a thoracic aneurysm and more commonly are called *thoracoabdominal aneurysms*. AAA and the branch vessel relationships can be well illustrated on 3D CE MR angiography [49–53].

In addition to atherosclerosis, genetic factors and cellular mechanisms, such as the mediation of proteolytic enzymes, play a role in the development of AAA [53–58]. The pathophysiology of AAA also may include an inflammatory component with elevated levels of cytokines and increased numbers of macrophages within the wall of the aneurysm [57,58]. Another important element of the process is the formation of thrombus as a result of decreased blood flow and stagnation in the aneurysmal segment. Because the thrombus and atherosclerotic debris can embolize distally, their presence on MR is important to note. The most significant risk of AAA is rupture [46,59]. In approximately 80% of ruptured AAAs, the blood decompresses into the left retroperitoneum, which can contain the

collection. In the remaining 20% of patients, AAA rupture extravasates directly into the peritoneal cavity, which results in uncontrolled hemorrhage and rapid deterioration of the patient's clinical status. Rarely an aneurysm can rupture into an adjacent venous structure, such as the inferior vena cava, iliac vein, or renal vein.

Aortic dissection

Aortic dissection is the term used to describe the process that begins when blood dissects into the media of the aortic wall through an intimal tear [60,61]. The intimal flap that subsequently develops divides the lumen into a false lumen and a true lumen. On presentation, greater than 90% of patients complain of pain, which can be focal or multicentric and may radiate. Of patients with dissection, 70% have a history of hypertension, and most are receiving treatment with antihypertensives. Twenty percent of patients are in shock on admission.

Although dissection more commonly is associated with the thoracic aorta, it commonly extends into the abdomen aorta (see Fig. 3). The typical appearance of a dissection consists of a posterolateral spiral from the thoracic aorta, which then courses inferiorly, staying to the left side of the aorta as the intimal tear extends. The key branch vessels in the abdomen that are most frequently compromised are the left renal artery and the celiac and superior mesenteric arteries. Occasionally, dissection may be more localized (Fig. 11). 3D CE MR angiography displays the extent of the dissection and involvement of branch vessels with exquisite clarity (see Figs. 3 and 11). At least two delayed phase postcontrast acquisitions are prudent to ensure optimal visualization of the false channel, where blood flow is much slower than in the true lumen [6,9].

Renal artery stenosis

Atherosclerotic disease of the renal arteries accounts for 75% to 84% clinically significant renovascular lesions [62–67]. Atherosclerotic renal artery stenosis (RAS) can be identified commonly with vascular disease affecting other vascular beds. Studies in patients undergoing coronary angiography indicate that 19% to 20% have RAS with greater than 50% narrowing of the renal artery lumen [63–65]. Aortograms obtained in patients with peripheral vascular disease indicate that 30% to 50% of patients have renal

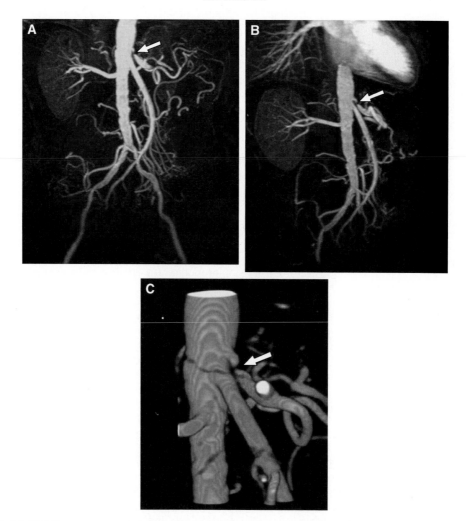

Fig. 12. (*A–C*) Celiac artery stenosis in a patient with diffuse atherosclerosis. (*A* and *B*) 3D CE MR angiography (*A*, coronal MIP; *B*, oblique subvolume MIP) shows a severe proximal celiac artery stenosis (*arrow*). (*C*) VR projection shows the celiac artery stenosis and its relationship to the adjacent superior mesenteric artery.

artery lesions of some degree [66,67]. A high index of clinical suspicion is key to the diagnosis of RAS. Although it is not cost-effective to screen all hypertensive patients for RAS, a thorough review of the medical history and a careful physical examination should be performed to recognize important features suggesting renovascular hypertension [68], including onset of hypertension before age 30 years or after 55 years; malignant or accelerated hypertension; sudden onset of uncontrolled hypertension that previously was well controlled; evidence of diffuse atherosclerosis; epigastric bruit, particularly during diastole; azotemia induced by angiotensin-converting enzyme inhibitor; unexplained azotemia; a unilateral small

kidney; or flash pulmonary edema in the presence of hypertension and normal left ventricular function. 3D CE MR angiography can be a good screening tool for patients with suspected atherosclerotic renovascular hypertension (see Fig. 4) [41,69–72].

Fibromuscular dysplasia

FMD is a relatively uncommon but important cause of renovascular hypertension accounting for approximately 15% to 20% of all cases [73–75]. There are four types of FMD. Medial fibromuscular dysplasia accounts for approximately 70% of all cases of FMD. It occurs most often in

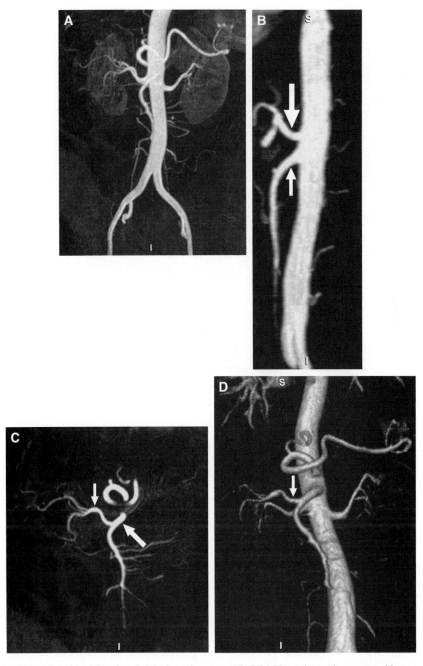

Fig. 13. (*A–D*) Normal variant of replaced right hepatic artery. 3D CE MR angiography can provide a good anatomic roadmap of the abdominal arteries. (*A* and *B*) 3D CE MR angiography (*A*, coronal MIP; *B*, sagittal subvolume MIP) shows the renal arteries, celiac trunk (*large arrow* in *B*) and superior mesenteric artery (*small arrow* in *B*) to arise normally from the aorta and to have normal caliber. (*C*) Further analysis using coronal subvolume MIP shows a normal vascular variant of a replaced right hepatic artery (*small arrow*), arising from the superior mesenteric artery (*large arrow*). (*D*) The replaced right hepatic artery (*arrow*) is particularly well visualized on VR display. The replaced right hepatic artery is not as well visualized on coronal MIP (*A*) because it overlaps the right renal artery and is obscured on MIP.

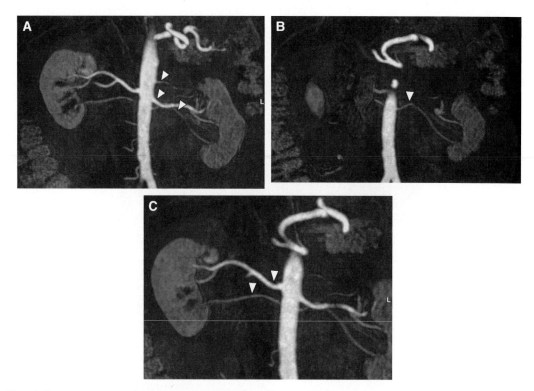

Fig. 14. Supernumerary renal arteries. (*A–C*) Subvolume MIP from 3D CE MR angiography shows the three left renal arteries (*arrowheads* in *A* and *B*) and the two right renal arteries (*arrowheads* in *C*).

women between ages 25 and 50 and is rare in children. FMD primarily affects the distal two thirds of the main renal artery and its major branches. The pathologic process of FMD begins when the internal elastic membrane is lost or thinned, and collagen bands replace the muscle. These bands within the renal artery lead to focal areas of narrowing that often are accompanied by segments of poststenotic dilatation with a resulting classic appearance of the "string of beads" (see Fig. 6). The spatial resolution demands for proper recognition of FMD are high and continue to be a challenge and known pitfall for renal 3D CE MR angiography. The use of adjunctive MR features and tools such as renal flow measurement can improve diagnostic accuracy MR for detection of renovascular hypertension and are discussed elsewhere in this issue by Michaely et al [76].

Mesenteric ischemia

Acute mesenteric ischemia (AMI) is the result of an acute interruption of the blood supply to the small bowel or colon with potentially devastating results. The mortality rate has been reported as greater than 60% in AMI [77]. AMI is usually the result of one of four underlying insults to the mesenteric vasculature: (1) superior mesenteric artery (SMA) embolus, (2) SMA thrombosis, (3) mesenteric venous thrombosis, or (4) nonocclusive mesenteric vasoconstriction. Rarely, aortic dissections also can cause AMI. Typically, these patients are extremely sick with the potential to become rapidly unstable, so MR evaluation should be done in a controlled, well-monitored environment with anesthesia and surgical support if needed [78]. Acute emboli to the SMA are reported as the etiology for approximately 40% to 50% of all cases of AMI [77]. Acute mesenteric arterial thrombosis usually is associated with a preexisting atherosclerotic lesion and tends to occlude typically within the first 2 cm of its origin (in contrast to acute embolic occlusions). Nonocclusive mesenteric ischemia reportedly accounts for approximately 25% of cases of AMI, and the mortality rate can reach 70% [79]. Nonocclusive mesenteric ischemia typically develops during an episode of cardiogenic shock or a state of hypoperfusion, owing to excessive sympathetic activity

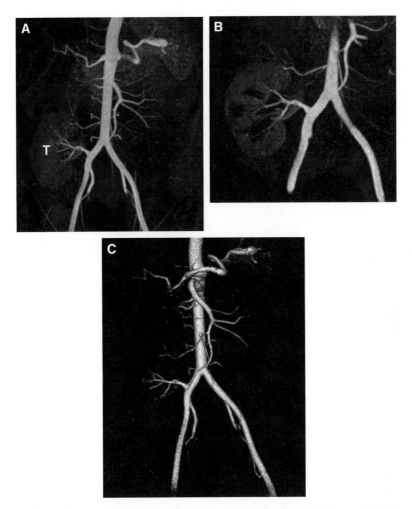

Fig. 15. (*A–C*) Renal transplant surveillance using 3D CE MR angiography. (*A* and *B*) Coronal MIP (*A*) and subvolume MIP (*B*) from 3D CE MR angiography shows the transplanted kidney (T) and its patent transplant artery. The individual segmental branches of the transplant artery also are well seen. (*C*) The transplant artery also is well seen on VR display.

that results in secondary vasoconstriction of the mesenteric arteries. MR usually is requested for evaluation of chronic mesenteric ischemia, which typically is secondary to severe atherosclerotic disease of the abdominal aorta and its branches and is classically characterized by postprandial abdominal pain, weight loss, and anorexia [77]. An autopsy study shows significant stenoses of the mesenteric and celiac arteries in 67% of subjects 80 years old or older [80]. Although atherosclerotic disease of the mesenteric branches is frequent, mesenteric ischemia is relatively uncommon because of the rich collateral circulation associated with the mesenteric vessels. It is

believed that at least two of the three main vessels must be affected either by occlusive or by stenotic disease to produce clinical symptoms, although exceptions to this rule exist. Chronic mesenteric ischemia in the setting of proximal or segmental mesenteric artery stenosis or occlusion in only one affected vessel is rare, but can occur. 3D CE MR angiography also is well suited for the evaluation of patients with celiac (Fig. 12) and mesenteric stenoses [81]. Although 3D CE MR angiography seems to be fairly accurate in the evaluation of stenoses of the celiac artery and SMA, the inferior mesenteric artery at times is difficult to evaluate because of its small diameter.

Periprocedural evaluation

Presurgical roadmapping

3D CE MR angiography is a valuable method for noninvasive roadmapping of abdominal vascular anatomy. Vascular mapping is beneficial for a variety of surgeries, including hepatic resection and transplant planning. With the increased use of less invasive procedures, such as partial nephrectomy, the acquisition of a preprocedural roadmap of pertinent vascular anatomy is sometimes essential. 3D CE MR angiography readily shows normal variants (Fig. 13).

3D CE MR angiography is used by many sites to screen potential renal donors [82–84]. 3D CE MR angiography can provide the crucial information without exposing the potential donor to ionizing radiation or nephrotoxic contrast media. The key to the preoperative evaluation of potential donors is to determine the most suitable kidney for expedient and safe removal [85,86]. 3D CE MR angiography permits the identification of the number of renal arteries, including supernumerary renal arteries (found in 27% of kidneys), and the presence of any early branching arteries, while allowing the detection of previously unsuspected renovascular disease or any parenchymal disease (eg, renal cell carcinoma) that may influence the choice of kidney (Fig. 14) [86]. Renovascular anatomy and anomalies, such as renal ectopia and retroaortic or circumaortic renal veins, also are readily identifiable. Although not all of these anatomic variations or other conditions constitute a contraindication for renal donation, the preoperative identification of these findings may affect the choice of kidney for transplant or may redirect the surgical approach.

Postprocedural surveillance

Renal transplant evaluation

MR commonly is requested for the evaluation of renal transplants. 3D CE MR angiography provides angiographic illustration of the vascular anastomosis (Fig. 15). Stenosis of the transplant artery is the most common vascular complication of renal transplantation, occurring in 1% to 12% of transplanted renal arteries, and is easily treated using percutaneous angioplasty and possibly stent placement [87,88]. Other potential complications include arterial and venous thrombosis, intrarenal arteriovenous fistulas and pseudoaneurysms secondary to transplant biopsy, and potential urinary or vascular leaks. Urologic complications are relatively uncommon, consisting mainly of urinary leaks and urethral obstruction.

Endovascular abdominal aortic aneurysm repair and graft surveillance

3D CE MR angiography also can be used to detect complications of endovascular procedures, such as endoleaks. Endovascular AAA repair is an increasingly common procedure and requires routine imaging surveillance [89,90]. Most investigational clinical trials have required evaluation using contrast-enhanced CT, and MR is not routinely performed in these patients. 3D CE MR angiography also can provide proper illustration of endoleaks, however [91]. The presence or absence of an isolated endoleak does not indicate either failure or success of the procedure, and additional information is required to make an accurate assessment. The goal of postprocedural evaluation should include the following determinations: (1) size of the aneurysm, (2) position of the stent-graft relative to landmarks (renal arteries in the abdomen), (3) evidence of change in position of the endoprosthesis, (4) structural integrity of the device, (5) endoleak, (6) change in characteristics of a known endoleak or a new endoleak.

Summary

MR angiography, especially using 3D CE MR angiography, has evolved rapidly into a robust diagnostic tool with ever-increasing flexibility for tailored applications for illustration of the abdominal aorta and its branches. The abdominal indications for MR angiography continue to expand as technical advances overcome old barriers, such as motion and the time required for a high-quality diagnostic study. 3D CE MR angiography is now standard practice in the noninvasive evaluation of a wide range of clinical situations and has expanded to include multiple applications involving the periprocedural evaluation of patients, giving clinicians the ability to diagnose safely and effectively patients who are not able to tolerate invasive procedures or iodinated contrast material.

References

[1] Koelemay MJ, Lijmer JG, Stoker J, et al. Magnetic resonance angiography for the evaluation of lower extremity arterial disease: a meta-analysis. JAMA 2001;285:1338–45.

[2] Nelemans PJ, Leiner T, de Vet HC, et al. Peripheral arterial disease: meta-analysis of the diagnostic performance of MR angiography. Radiology 2000; 217:105–14.

[3] Yucel EK, Anderson CM, Edelman RR, et al. AHA scientific statement. Magnetic resonance angiography: update on applications for extracranial arteries. Circulation 1999;100:2284–90.

[4] Prince MR, Yucel EK, Kaufman JA, Harrison DC, Geller SC. Dynamic gadolinium-enhanced three-dimensional abdominal MR arteriography. J Magn Reson Imaging 1993;3:877–81.

[5] Prince MR. Gadolinium-enhanced MR aortography. Radiology 1994;191:155–64.

[6] Ho VB, Corse WR. MR angiography of the abdominal aorta and peripheral vessels. Radiol Clin North Am 2003;41:115–44.

[7] Prince MR. Contrast-enhanced MR angiography: theory and optimization. Magn Reson Imaging Clin N Am 1998;6:257–67.

[8] Ho VB, Foo TK, Czum JM, et al. Contrast-enhanced magnetic resonance angiography: technical considerations for optimized clinical implementation. Top Magn Reson Imaging 2001;12:283–99.

[9] Schneider G, Prince MR, Meaney JF, Ho VB, editors. Magnetic resonance angiography: techniques, indications and practical applications. Milan (Italy): Springer-Verlag; 2004.

[10] Kaufman JA, McCarter D, Geller SC, et al. Two-dimensional time-of-flight MR angiography of the lower extremities: artifacts and pitfalls. AJR Am J Roentgenol 1998;171:129–35.

[11] Pereles FS, McCarthy RM, Baskaran V, et al. Thoracic aortic dissection and aneurysm: evaluation with nonenhanced true FISP MR angiography in less than 4 minutes. Radiology 2002;223:270–4.

[12] Marks B, Mitchell DG, Simelaro JP. Breath-holding in healthy and pulmonary-compromised populations: effects of hyperventilation and oxygen inspiration. J Magn Reson Imaging 1997;7:595–7.

[13] Chung T, Krishnamurthy R. Contrast enhanced MR angiography in infants and children. Magn Reson Imaging Clin N Amer 2005, in press.

[14] Trost DW, Zhang HL, Prince MR, et al. Three-dimensional MR angiography in imaging platinum alloy stents. J Magn Reson Imaging 2004;20:975–80.

[15] Weiger M, Pruessmann KP, Kassner A, et al. Contrast-enhanced 3D MRA using SENSE. J Magn Reson Imaging 2000;12:671–7.

[16] van den Brink JS, Watanabe Y, Kuhl CK, et al. Implications of SENSE MR in routine clinical practice. Eur J Radiol 2003;46:3–27.

[17] Maki JH, Wilson GJ, Eubank WB, Hoogeveen RM. Utilizing SENSE to achieve lower station submillimeter isotropic resolution and minimal venous enhancement in peripheral MR angiography. J Magn Reson Imaging 2002;15:484–91.

[18] Chen Q, Quijano CV, Mai VM, et al. On improving temporal and spatial resolution of 3D contrast-enhanced body MR angiography with parallel imaging. Radiology 2004;231:893–9.

[19] Glockner JF. Three-dimensional gadolinium-enhanced MR angiography: applications for abdominal imaging. Radiographics 2001;21:357–70.

[20] Knopp MV, Floemer F, Schoenberg SO, et al. Non-invasive assessment of renal artery stenosis: current concepts and future directions in magnetic resonance angiography. J Comput Assist Tomogr 1999;23:S111–7.

[21] Runge VM. Safety of approved MR contrast media for intravenous injection. J Magn Reson Imaging 2000;12:205–13.

[22] Runge VM, Knopp MV. Off-label use and reimbursement of contrast media in MR. J Magn Reson Imaging 1999;10:489–95.

[23] Kopka L, Vosshenrich R, Rodenwaldt J, Grabbe E. Differences in injection rates on contrast-enhanced breath-hold three-dimensional MR angiography. AJR Am J Roentgenol 1998;170:345–8.

[24] Lee VS, Rofsky NM, Krinsky GA. Single-dose breath-hold gadolinium-enhanced three-dimensional MR angiography of the renal arteries. Radiology 1999;211:69–78.

[25] Boos M, Scheffler K, Haselhorst R, Reese E, Frohlich J, Bongartz GM. Arterial first pass gadolinium-CM dynamics as a function of several intravenous saline flush and Gd volumes. J Magn Reson Imaging 2001;13:568–76.

[26] Earls JP, Rofsky NM, DeCorato DR, Krinsky GA, Weinreb JC. Breath-hold single dose Gd-enhanced three-dimensional MR aortography: usefulness of a timing examination and MR power injector. Radiology 1996;201:705–10.

[27] Willems JL, Roelandt JR, Van de Vel HR, Joossens JV. The circulation time in the aged. Am J Cardiol 1971;27:155–61.

[28] Hany TF, McKinnon GC, Leung DA, Pfammatter T, Debatin JF. Optimization of contrast timing for breath-hold three-dimensional MR angiography. J Magn Reson Imaging 1997;7:551–6.

[29] Foo TKF, Saranathan M, Prince MR, Chenevert TL. Automated detection of bolus arrival and initiation of data acquisition in fast, three-dimensional, gadolinium-enhanced MR angiography. Radiology 1997;203:275–80.

[30] Ho VB, Foo TKF. Optimization of gadolinium-enhanced magnetic resonance angiography using an automated bolus-detection algorithm (MR SmartPrep). Invest Radiol 1998;33:515–23.

[31] Wilman AH, Riederer SJ, King BF, Debbins JP, Rossman PJ, Ehman RL. Fluoroscopically triggered contrast-enhanced three-dimensional MR angiography with elliptical centric view order: application to the renal arteries. Radiology 1997;205:137–46.

[32] Riederer SJ, Fain SB, Kruger DG, Busse RF. Real-time and triggering of 3D contrast-enhanced MR

angiograms using MR fluoroscopy. MAGMA 1999; 8:196–206.

[33] Riederer SJ, Bernstein MA, Breen JF, et al. Three-dimensional contrast-enhanced MR angiography with real-time fluoroscopic triggering: design specifications and technical reliability in 330 patient studies. Radiology 2000;215:584–93.

[34] Korosec FR, Frayne R, Grist TM, Mistretta CA. Time-resolved contrast-enhanced 3D MR angiography. Magn Reson Med 1996;36:345–51.

[35] Finn JP, Baskaran V, Carr JC, et al. Thorax: low-dose contrast-enhanced three-dimensional MR angiography with subsecond temporal resolution—initial results. Radiology 2002;224:896–904.

[36] Maki JH, Prince MR, Londy FL, Chenevert TL. The effects of time varying signal intensity and k-space acquisition order on three-dimensional MR angiography image quality. J Magn Reson Imaging 1996;6:642–51.

[37] Glockner JF. MR angiography image processing and interpretation. Magn Reson Imaging Clin N Am 2005, in press.

[38] Baskaran V, Pereles S, Nemcek AA, et al. Gadolinium-enhanced 3D MR angiography of renal artery stenosis: a pilot comparison of maximum intensity projection, multiplanar reformatting, and 3D volume-rendering postprocessing algorithms. Acad Radiol 2002;9:50–9.

[39] Foo TK, Ho VB, Marcos HB, Hood MN, Choyke PL. MR angiography using steady-state free precession. Magn Reson Med 2002;48:699–706.

[40] Bass JC, Prince MR, Londy FJ, et al. Effect of gadolinium on phase-contrast MR angiography of the renal arteries. AJR Am J Roentgenol 1997;168:261–6.

[41] Prince MR, Schoenberg SO, Ward JS, et al. Hemodynamically significant atherosclerotic renal artery stenosis: MR angiographic features. Radiology 1997;205:128–36.

[42] Hood MN, Ho VB, Corse WR. Three-dimensional phase contrast MR angiography: a useful clinical adjunct to gadolinium-enhanced 3D renal MRA? Milit Med 2002;167:343–9.

[43] Fenlon HM, Yucel EK. Advances in abdominal, aortic, and peripheral contrast-enhanced MR angiography. Magn Reson Imaging Clin N Am 1999;7: 319–36.

[44] Johnston KW, Rutherford RB, Tilson MD, Shah DM, Hollier L, Stanley JC. Suggested standards for reporting on arterial aneurysms. Subcommittee on Reporting Standards for Arterial Aneurysms, Ad Hoc Committee on Reporting Standards, Society for Vascular Surgery and North American Chapter, International Society for Cardiovascular Surgery. J Vasc Surg 1991;13:452–8.

[45] Bengtsson H, Bergqvist D, Sternby NH. Increasing prevalence of abdominal aortic aneurysms: a necropsy study. Eur J Surg 1992;158:19–23.

[46] Isselbacher EM. Diseases of the aorta. In: Braunwald E, Zipes DP, Libby P, editors. Heart disease: a textbook of cardiovascular medicine. 6th edition. Philadelphia: WB Saunders; 2001. p. 1422–50.

[47] Bickerstaff LK, Hollier LH, Van Peenan HJ, Melton LJ 3rd, Pairolero PC, Cherry KJ. Abdominal aortic aneurysms: the changing natural history. J Vasc Surg 1984;1:6–12.

[48] Anidjar S, Kieffer E. Pathogenesis of acquired aneurysms of the abdominal aorta. Ann Vasc Surg 1992;6:298–305.

[49] Prince MR, Narasimham DL, Stanley JC, et al. Breath-hold gadolinium-enhanced MR angiography of the abdominal aorta and its major branches. Radiology 1995;197:785–92.

[50] Kaufman JA, Geller SC, Petersen MJ, et al. MR imaging (including MR angiography) of abdominal aortic aneurysms: comparison with conventional angiography. AJR Am J Roentgenol 1994;163: 203–10.

[51] Laissy JP, Soyer P, Tebboune D, et al. Abdominal aortic aneurysms: assessment with gadolinium-enhanced time-of-flight coronal MR angiography (MRA). Eur J Radiol 1995;20:1–8.

[52] Petersen MJ, Cambria RP, Kaufman JA, et al. Magnetic resonance angiography in the preoperative evaluation of abdominal aortic aneurysms. J Vasc Surg 1995;21:891–8.

[53] Prince MR, Narasimham DL, Stanley JC, et al. Gadolinium-enhanced magnetic resonance angiography of abdominal aortic aneurysms. J Vasc Surg 1995;21:656–69.

[54] Verloes A, Sakalihasan NL, Koulischer L, Limet R. Aneurysms of the abdominal aorta: familial and genetic aspects in three hundred thirteen pedigrees. J Vasc Surg 1995;21:646–55.

[55] Davies MJ. Aortic aneurysm formation: lessons from human studies and experimental models. Circulation 1998;98:193–5.

[56] Reilly JM, Brophy CM, Tilson MD. Characterization of an elastase from aneurysmal aorta which degrades intact aortic elastin. Ann Vasc Surg 1992; 6:499–502.

[57] Anidjar S, Dobrin PB, Eichorst M, Graham GP, Chejfec G. Correlation of inflammatory infiltrate with the enlargement of experimental aortic aneurysms. J Vasc Surg 1992;16:139–47.

[58] Pearce WH, Koch AE. Cellular components and features of immune response in abdominal aortic aneurysms. Ann N Y Acad Sci 1996;800:175–85.

[59] Darling RC. Ruptured arteriosclerotic abdominal aortic aneurysms: a pathologic and clinical study. Am J Surg 1970;119:397–401.

[60] Erbel R. Diseases of the thoracic aorta. Heart 2001; 86:227–34.

[61] Meszaros I, Morocz J, Szlavi J, et al. Epidemiology and clinicopathology of aortic dissection. Chest 2000;117:1271–8.

[62] Hansen KJ. Prevalence of ischemic nephropathy in the atherosclerotic population. Am J Kidney Dis 1994;24:615–21.

[63] Conlon PJ, O'Riordan E, Kalra PA. New insights into the epidemiologic and clinical manifestations of atherosclerotic renovascular disease. Am J Kidney Dis 2000;35:573–87.

[64] Harding MB, Smith LR, Himmelstein SI, et al. Renal artery stenosis: prevalence and associated risk factors in patients undergoing routine cardiac catheterization. J Am Soc Nephrol 1992;2:1608–16.

[65] Rihal CS, Textor SC, Breen JF, et al. Incidental renal artery stenosis among a prospective cohort of hypertensive patients undergoing coronary angiography. Mayo Clin Proc 2002;77:309–16.

[66] Swartbol P, Thorvinger BO, Parsson H, Norgren L. Renal artery stenosis in patients with peripheral vascular disease and its correlation to hypertension: A retrospective study. Int Angiol 1992;11:195–9.

[67] Choudhri AH, Cleland JG, Rowlands PC, Tran TL, McCarty M, al-Kutoubi MA. Unsuspected renal artery stenosis in peripheral vascular disease. BMJ 1990;301:1197–8.

[68] Krijnen P, van Jaarsveld BC, Steyerberg EW, Man in't Veld AJ, Schalekamp MA, Habbema JD. A clinical prediction rule for renal artery stenosis. Ann Intern Med 1998;129:705–11.

[69] Schoenberg SO, Essig M, Bock M, et al. Comprehensive MR evaluation of renovascular disease in five breath holds. J Magn Reson Imaging 1999;10:347–56.

[70] Bakker J, Beek FJ, Beutler JJ, et al. Renal artery stenosis and accessory renal arteries: accuracy of detection and visualization with gadolinium-enhanced breath-hold MR angiography. Radiology 1998;207:497–504.

[71] De Cobelli F, Vanzulli A, Sironi S, et al. Renal artery stenosis: evaluation with breath-hold, three-dimensional, dynamic, gadolinium-enhanced versus three-dimensional, phase contrast MR angiography. Radiology 1997;205:689–95.

[72] Hany TF, Leung DA, Pfammatter T, Debatin JF. Contrast-enhanced magnetic resonance angiography of the renal arteries. Invest Radiol 1998;33:653–69.

[73] Hartman RP, Kawashima A, King BF Jr. Evaluation of renal causes of hypertension. Radiol Clin North Am 2003;41:909–29.

[74] Fenves AZ, Ram CV. Fibromuscular dysplasia of the renal arteries. Curr Hypertens Rep 1999;1(6):546–9.

[75] Kaplan NM. Clinical hypertension. 7th edition. Baltimore: Williams & Wilkins; 1998, p. 306.

[76] Michaely HJ, Schoenberg SO, Ringer JR, et al. MR angiography in patients with renal disease. Magn Reson Imaging Clin N Am 2005, in press.

[77] Hagspiel KD, Angle JF, Spinosa DJ, et al. Mesenteric ischemia: angiography and endovascular interventions. In: Longo W, Peterson GJ, Jacobs DL,

editors. Intestinal ischemia disorders: pathophysiology and management. St. Louis: Quality Medical Publishing; 1999. p. 105–54.

[78] Hagspiel KD, Leung DA, Angle JF, et al. MR angiography of the mesenteric vasculature. Radiol Clin North Am 2002;40:867–86.

[79] Bassiouny HS. Nonocclusive mesenteric ischemia. Surg Clin North Am 1997;77:319–26.

[80] Jarvinen O, Laurikka J, Sisto T, Salenius JP, Tarkka MR. Atherosclerosis of the visceral arteries. Vasa 1995;24:9–14.

[81] Meaney JF, Prince MR, Nostrant TT, Stanley JC. Gadolinium-enhanced MR angiography of visceral arteries in patients with suspected chronic mesenteric ischemia. J Magn Reson Imaging 1997;7:171–6.

[82] Low RN, Martinex AG, Steinberg SM, et al. Potential renal transplant donors: evaluation with gadolinium-enhanced MR angiography and MR urography. Radiology 1998;207:165–72.

[83] Rankin SC, Jan W, Koffman CG. Noninvasive imaging of living related kidney donors: evaluation with CT angiography and gadolinium-enhanced MR angiography. AJR Am J Roentgenol 2001;177:349–55.

[84] Rusnack D, Israel GM. Kidney transplantation: evaluation of donors and recipients. Magn Reson Imaging Clin N Am 2004;12:505–14.

[85] Frick MP, Goldberg ME. Uro- and angiographic findings in a "normal" population: screening of 151 symptom-free potential transplant donors for renal disease. AJR Am J Roentgenol 1980;134:503–5.

[86] Spring DB, Salvatierra O Jr, Palubinskas AJ, Amend WJ Jr, Vincenti FG, Feduska NJ. Results and significance of angiography in potential kidney donors. Radiology 1979;133:45–7.

[87] Surlan M, Popovic P. The role of interventional radiology in management of patients with end-stage renal disease. Eur J Radiol 2003;46:96–114.

[88] Israel GM, Lee VS, Edye M, et al. Comprehensive MR imaging in the preoperative evaluation of living donor candidates for laparoscopic nephrectomy: initial experience. Radiology 2002;225:427–32.

[89] Thurnher S. Imaging of aortic stent-grafts and endoleaks. Radiol Clin North Am 2002;40:799–833.

[90] White GH, Yu W, May J, Chaufour X, Stephen MS. Endoleak as a complication of endoluminal grafting of abdominal aortic aneurysms: classification, incidence, diagnosis, and management. J Endovasc Surg 1997;4:152–68.

[91] Lookstein RA, Goldman J, Pukin L, Marin ML. Time-resolved magnetic resonance angiography as a noninvasive method to characterize endoleaks: initial results compared with conventional angiography. J Vasc Surg 2004;39:27–33.

ELSEVIER
SAUNDERS

Magn Reson Imaging Clin N Am
13 (2005) 91–111

MAGNETIC
RESONANCE
IMAGING CLINICS
of North America

MR Angiography of the Peripheral Arteries

James F.M. Meaney, FRCR*, Niall Sheehy, MRCPI

Department of Diagnostic Imaging, St. James's Hospital, James's Street, Dublin 8, Ireland

Atherosclerosis is virtually ubiquitous in Western societies. Although atherosclerotic narrowing can affect any artery in the body, the greatest burden of disease falls on the lower extremities [1–7]. Patients with peripheral vascular disease (PVD) typically present with one of two distinct clinical syndromes: (1) intermittent claudication, a lifestyle-modifying disease predominantly reflecting proximal vessels (large vessel disease); or (2) if the disease is more severe, limb-threatening ischemia. Most of the latter patients are diabetics in whom severe distal (small vessel) disease is present [1,2,7]. In the United States, the annual burden of arteriosclerotic lower limb disease amounts to approximately 60,000 percutaneous angioplasty procedures and 100,000 amputations [4].

Atherosclerotic lesions have a predilection for branching points and for sites of mechanical stress on the artery. These factors help to explain the consistent clinical syndromes that are encountered in patients with PVD, with localization of lesions at the aortic bifurcation (often with encroachment onto one or both common iliac artery origins), common femoral artery bifurcation, and adductor canal. Predisposing factors are smoking (in almost all patients) and a history of diabetes mellitus. Rates of lower extremity amputation are 15 to 46 times higher in diabetic patients when compared with nondiabetic patients [5]. A large recent surgical review of patients undergoing distal bypass grafting to the pedal arteries recorded a 95% incidence of diabetes mellitus [6,7].

Traditional algorithms for investigating PVD have been influenced by the fact a "road map" could only be acquired by subjecting the patient to invasive catheter angiography, usually performed via a transfemoral approach [8]. Patients with limb-threatening disease require angiographic documentation of the distribution and severity of disease or, in some cases, immediate surgery without preoperative imaging. Nevertheless, because of the limited availability and morbidity [9,10] of catheter angiography, referring physicians traditionally have referred patients with intermittent claudication for catheter angiography only after noninvasive testing (eg, Doppler sonography or plethysmography) has been performed [11]. These noninvasive studies help to determine the severity of disease and are useful for stratifying patients into those with "inflow" (aortoiliac) and "outflow" (femoropopliteal) disease [8].

Because of the widespread and systemic nature of the disorder and the multiplicity of lesions that typically occur, optimal therapeutic strategies can be formulated only when accurate mapping of the peripheral arterial tree has been performed. Because of its noninvasive nature, MR angiography offers substantial benefits to physicians and patients when used as a screening test. Refinements in technique over the last decade, notably, the advent of contrast-enhanced three-dimensional (3D) MR angiography coupled with moving table/bolus chase method, have led to the potential for comprehensive noninvasive evaluation of the vasculature from above the aortic bifurcation to the pedal arch without arterial catheterization, ionizing radiation, or nephrotoxic contrast agents. Although other modalities such as multidetector CT show promise, CT is more invasive than MR angiography and has the drawbacks of ionizing radiation and nephrotoxic contrast agent exposure [12–14].

Relevant anatomy for MR angiography

Knowledge of the peripheral arterial anatomy and its relevant segments is necessary not only for

* Corresponding author.
E-mail address: jmeaney@meaneys.com
(J.F.M. Meaney).

1064-9689/05/$ - see front matter © 2005 Elsevier Inc. All rights reserved.
doi:10.1016/j.mric.2004.12.012

mri.theclinics.com

image interpretation but also for planning of a suitable MR angiography protocol. Most current peripheral protocols use a multistation bolus chase 3D contrast-enhanced (Fig. 1) approach whereby imaging is performed using a series of overlapping coronal 3D volume acquisitions. Recognition of the anatomic landmarks ensures proper placement of the imaging volumes for inclusion of the relevant vascular structures.

The abdominal aorta bifurcates at the L4 level into the common iliac arteries. The common iliac arteries bifurcate into internal iliac and external iliac arteries in front of the sacroiliac joints at the level of L5/S1. The common and external iliac arteries sometimes follow a fairly redundant course within the pelvis owing to the large amount of "dead-space" into which the vessels can elongate as part of the normal aging process; therefore, increasing the imaging volume dimension in the anteroposterior plane is often required to include the vessels. To preserve spatial resolution in the slice direction, one must increase the number of partitions in the volume and the imaging time. Although the internal iliac arteries travel posteriorly for a modest distance, only the origins need to be imaged, minimizing the spatial coverage requirements within the abdomen and pelvis. The external iliac artery continues anteriorly as the common femoral artery (length of 4 to 6 cm only), but there is no identifiable anatomic landmark separating these structures on MR angiography. The common femoral artery divides into the profunda femoris artery, a medium-sized artery arising from the lateral aspect, and the superficial femoral artery, its direct continuation. The first imaging volume of a moving table contrast-enhanced MR angiography or of a single-station contrast-enhanced MR angiography typically encloses all of these arteries in the 3D volume.

The superficial femoral artery passes through the adductor hiatus (not identifiable on MR imaging), approximately at the junction of the upper two thirds and lower third of the femur. Upon entering the adductor canal, the superficial femoral artery gives rise to the medial and lateral genicular branches, which typically enlarge and form collateral channels in patients with severe stenosis or occlusion of the superficial femoral artery, and becomes the popliteal artery. The popliteal artery terminates at its bifurcation into the anterior tibial artery and tibioperoneal trunk. The second imaging volume of a moving table contrast-enhanced MR angiography or of

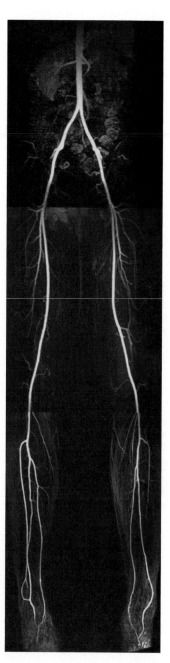

Fig. 1. Three-station moving table contrast-enhanced MR angiography demonstrating normal appearance of the arteries from the level of the renal arteries to the foot in anteroposterior projection. Note the progressive decrease in vessel size from the aorta to foot. This emphasizes the requirement for independent tailoring of the scan parameters at all three locations.

a single-station contrast-enhanced MR angiography typically encloses all of these arteries in the 3D volume, with some overlap with the first volume cranially and the third volume caudally.

Below the knee, the popliteal artery gives rise to the tibioperoneal trunk, its direct continuation at the take-off of the anterior tibial artery (usually, the largest of the infrapopliteal arteries). The tibioperoneal trunk divides into the peroneal (typically, the smallest of the infrapopliteal arteries) and posterior tibial artery. These arteries are collectively known as the "trifurcation" or "run-off" vessels. The pedal arteries are the direct continuation of the anterior and posterior tibial arteries and pass forward onto the foot. The posterior tibial artery continues as the common plantar artery, which then bifurcates into the medial and lateral plantar arteries. The anterior tibial artery becomes the dorsalis pedis artery, which then divides into the medial and lateral tarsal arteries. The deep plantar artery joins the anterior (dorsalis pedis and tarsal arteries) and posterior circulation (the plantar arteries), contributing to an arcade.

For imaging of the third location, the operator may decide between two different scenarios. The first scenario involves imaging the arteries to the level of the ankle joint only. This approach requires a smaller 3D imaging volume with a shorter scan time and is appropriate in patients with intermittent claudication, because distal bypass grafting is generally not required, and depiction of the pedal arch is superfluous. The second scenario mandates a much larger 3D imaging volume extended to include the pedal arteries as well as the arteries of the calf in the imaging volume, which can be performed in the coronal or sagittal plane. This approach of extended spatial coverage is essential in patients with limb-threatening ischemia, because distal bypass grafting is frequently the only alternative to amputation in these cases.

Scope of MR angiography

The goal of MR angiography is to replace x-ray digital subtraction angiography as a diagnostic tool in the majority of patients [15]. For this to occur, MR angiography must be reproducible, readily available, accurate, free from artifacts, and time efficient. Because of poor spatial coverage per unit time, resulting in unacceptably long examination times, and a tendency for overestimation of the severity of stenoses, noncontrast

MR angiography techniques do not offer a valid screening alternative to digital subtraction angiography [16–25]. Nevertheless, these techniques have been widely used for patients with contraindications to conventional arteriography (iodinated contrast material allergy, renal impairment, failed arteriography, and patients in whom arteriography is not possible) and have also been proven to be beneficial for detecting angiographically occult pedal arteries in patients in whom distal bypass procedures are being considered.

The introduction of contrast-enhanced MR angiography techniques [26–30], which deliver a road-mapping capability similar to digital subtraction angiography without the associated risks of iodinated contrast material [13–14] or arterial catheterization [13,14], marked a major juncture in noninvasive imaging of the lower extremity arteries. Because intravascular contrast is generated by artificial lowering of the blood T1 by intravenous injection of paramagnetic contrast material, images are "flow independent." Use of coronal plane image acquisition in addition to fast gradient-echo imaging is possible with substantial time saving. Unlike time-of-flight (TOF) MR angiography, contrast-enhanced MR angiography does not suffer from flow-related artifacts, and the freedom from imaging plane constraints (coronal plane optimal) and the ability to unleash the speed advantage conferred by fast gradient technology enables a rapid acquisition, with acceptable resolution and appropriate coverage of the relevant anatomy.

Notwithstanding the success of contrast-enhanced MR angiography, the spatial coverage provided by a single acquisition (even when acquired in the coronal plane with the maximum permissible field of view [FOV]) is substantially less than the distance from the midabdominal aorta to pedal arch. This limitation has been addressed by a variety of modifications, including multistation MR angiography performed with a separate injection for each acquisition, and moving table contrast-enhanced MR angiography, in which a single injection is used in conjunction with successive acquisitions at consecutive overlapping locations punctuated in time by rapid table movement [30–39]. Nevertheless, because several (usually three) acquisitions are required to image the relevant anatomy in the coronal plane with moving table MR angiography, the bolus "outstrips" data acquisition in many patients, resulting in venous contamination of the third location with obscuration of some relevant arterial segments in some individuals. Despite this and other minor limitations, moving table contrast-enhanced MR angiography offers an ideal or near-ideal method for noninvasive imaging of the peripheral arteries. Because the major limitation is related to inadequate imaging speed in relation to bolus transit times, numerous modifications aimed at improving acquisition speed have been proposed. These modifications include optimized k-space filling strategies [40–42], the use of location-specific tailored acquisitions, a hybrid 2D/3D technique, "time-resolved" and other "key-hole" techniques, parallel imaging, and the use of a "flow-arrest" technique (tourniquets or blood pressure cuff) to slow the onset of venous enhancement.

Is a universal MR angiography study of the peripheral arteries possible?

Noncontrast (predominantly TOF) MR angiography did not supplant digital subtraction angiography as a screening test for evaluating the peripheral arteries because of the long examination times and frequent artifacts. Although many of the limitations of TOF MR angiography were negated initially by contrast-enhanced MR angiography and later by the moving table method, which extended the spatial coverage to include all of the relevant anatomy, the inability to acquire data with sufficiently high spatial resolution (required to grade stenoses accurately in small arteries) and sufficiently high temporal resolution (required to eliminate venous enhancement) meant than some examinations were suboptimal. As a result, MR angiography has not yet universally supplanted digital subtraction angiography, and an approach tailored to the clinical indication (intermittent claudication versus limb-threatening ischemia) and thus to a specific region of interest (aorta to trifurcation or infrapopliteal arteries, corresponding to the previously mentioned two clinical scenarios) has been favored by many.

A comprehensive examination that covers all of the relevant anatomy from the midabdominal aorta to pedal arch with sufficiently high resolution to grade stenoses accurately in all relevant arteries without confounding venous enhancement now seems possible in virtually all patients using a combination of recently described approaches. If achievable, this "universal" MR angiography addressing all of the relevant disease regardless of whether patients have intermittent claudication or

tissue loss would probably supplant digital subtraction angiography in virtually all patients. To emphasize how this might be achieved, all available technologies are discussed briefly in the following sections to highlight their strengths and limitations.

Summary of MR angiography methodologies

Time-of-flight MR angiography

For TOF MR angiography, one must consider the effect of radiofrequency pulses on stationary tissues and flowing blood separately.

Stationary tissues

The stationary (background tissues) and moving spins both experience radiofrequency pulses, but the resultant signal emanating from each is different. Background tissues (ie, predominantly muscle and fat) become partially saturated after each radiofrequency pulse. In TOF MR angiography, the incomplete recovery of transverse magnetization results in saturation (decreased signal) of these tissues, because the short repetition times (TR) of 20 to 50 ms are shorter than the T1 of most tissues, apart from fat, methemoglobin and gadolinium (Gd)-chelate contrast agent. Although all stationary tissues are partly saturated, tissues with shorter T1s (eg, fat) appear brighter than tissues with a longer T1 (eg, muscle and cerebrospinal fluid).

Flowing blood

For moving spins, the situation is different in TOF MR angiography. Because the radiofrequency pulses are applied to the imaging slice only (typically, 2 to 4 mm thick for 2D TOF imaging), blood outside this imaging slice does not receive any radiofrequency pulses and is fully relaxed. Upon entering the imaging slice, the fully magnetized blood displaces the partially saturated blood (the basis of the term "inflow" effect). If the flowing spins remain within the imaging slice during readout, they will generate a relatively high signal intensity compared with background tissues. As blood becomes progressively saturated as it traverses the imaging slice by successive radiofrequency pulses, for the generation of optimum intravascular signal there is an interdependence of slice thickness TR and flip angle (larger flip angles result in greater degrees of saturation). In areas of very fast and turbulent flow, there may be signal loss. This loss is occasionally manifested beyond severe stenoses (and may be particularly marked in patients with severe aortic coarctation) as a jet effect. Minimizing the echo time (TE) is advantageous for TOF MR angiography, although, in practice, TEs longer than the minimum possible must be accepted owing to the requirement to use flow compensation (gradient motion nulling [GMN]). To further reduce fat signal (because of its short T1), an out-of-phase TE is optimal (the shortest out-of-phase TE consistent with the use of GMN is 6.9 ms at 1.5 T).

Phase-contrast MR angiography

Phase-related signal loss occurs because the phase of the signal is directly related to the velocity of motion in a particular direction along one of the imaging gradients. The slice-select and frequency-encoding gradients actually consist of a pair of gradients (ie, they are bipolar gradients) applied in opposite directions; therefore, for static tissues, the effect of each gradient on the phase of the hydrogen protons is zero (the sum of each opposed gradient). For protons moving in the direction of the applied gradient, the position of a proton will change between the first and second (opposed) gradient pulse so that the effect of each pulse on the phase of the proton is not the same. As a result, moving protons acquire a net phase shift (proportional to velocity) relative to stationary tissues.

Contrast-enhanced MR angiography

The technique of contrast-enhanced MR angiography relies on the intravenous injection of a paramagnetic Gd-chelate contrast agent in conjunction with a heavily T1-weighted gradient-echo acquisition for the generation of intravascular signal (Fig. 2). Since the first description by Prince [26,27], this technique has revolutionized noninvasive vascular imaging of all territories. By synchronizing peak arterial enhancement with contrast-defining central k-space lines, images with unrivalled contrast-to-noise ratio (CNR) are generated [27,40–42]. Because the technique relies on T1 shortening and not on inherent properties of flow, images can be acquired in the coronal plane. For this same reason, short examination times can be achieved giving a 5- to 10-fold speed-up factor (TRs of 2 to 5 ms compared with >30 ms for TOF MR angiography) (see Tables 1 and 2 for a comparison with TOF MR angiography). A further advantage can be gained

by optimizing k-space filling strategies to the arterial bolus. Nevertheless, because current scanners have a spatial coverage limitation (generate images over a maximum FOV of 45 to 50 cm only—less than the distance from the abdominal aorta to pedal arch), and because the temporal resolution offered by commercially available scanners is insufficient to capture the arterial phase at all imaging locations of a three- (or four-) station peripheral MR angiographic study in some patients, several different techniques for contrast-enhanced MR angiography have evolved (see Table 2 for scan parameters).

Contrast-enhanced MR angiography of the peripheral vasculature: variations in approach

Three approaches are used: (1) single-station contrast-enhanced MR angiography, (2) multi-station multi-injection contrast-enhanced MR angiography, and (3) multistation contrast-enhanced MR angiography with a single injection and a moving table. Hybrid approaches employ 3D contrast-enhanced MR angiography in association with another approach (TOF MR angiography or 2D MR–digital subtraction angiography for the third location).

Single-station MR angiography of the peripheral arteries

With this approach, the relevant lesion is predicted from clinical or imaging (eg, duplex) criteria, and a single FOV is evaluated only [28,29,37–39]. Nevertheless, anatomic prediction of the location of occlusive lesions is difficult, and multiple lesions, many of which lie outside a single FOV, occur in the majority of patients. Although it has been shown to be efficacious, this approach is mostly used for evaluating parts of the peripheral vasculature that have been missed by arteriography, especially the pedal arteries in patients in whom distal bypass grafting is an option. The approach also has an essential role in imaging patients with aortic or bilateral iliac occlusion where catheter arteriography is not possible (Fig. 3).

Multistation multi-injection MR angiography of the peripheral arteries

Single-station MR angiography is performed at each of two or three consecutive locations, with a separate injection for each location [43]. Although proven in clinical practice, this technique

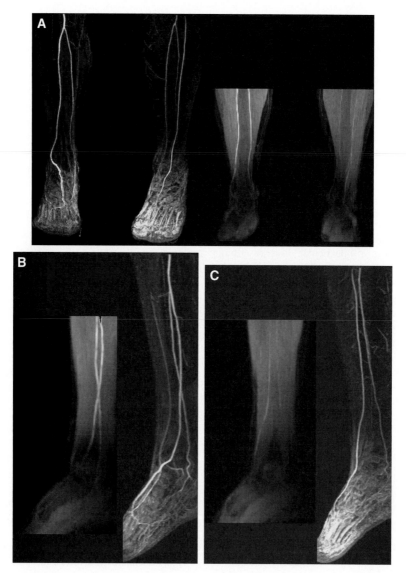

Fig. 2. Comparison of single-station contrast-enhanced MR angiography (left) and TOF MR angiography (right). (*A*) Frontal MIP demonstrates clear visualization of the anterior and posterior tibial arteries on the right and all three arteries on the left on the contrast-enhanced MR angiography and a normal patent dorsalis pedis artery on each side. The images were acquired at isotropic spatial resolution (1 mm³) in a time of 65 seconds. The TOF MR angiography took 5 minutes to obtain at lower resolution (3 mm³) and gives an inferior image quality. Although two infrapopliteal arteries are visualized on both sides, the dorsalis pedis is not visualized on either side. (*B,C*) Comparison of contrast-enhanced MR angiography and TOF MR angiography (lateral MIPs) demonstrates a patent dorsalis pedis artery and patent pedal arch on both sides (*B*, right side; *C*, left side).

is now rarely employed, due to refinements in the moving-table approach.

Moving table contrast-enhanced MR angiography of the peripheral arteries

It is possible to image the arteries of the entire lower half of the body during a single

contrast injection by acquiring three coronally oriented overlapping FOVs while rapidly moving the patient from one location to the next between scans. This approach has evolved from one with "fixed" imaging parameters (ie, identical parameters for all locations) to one with highly adaptable imaging parameters tailored to

Table 1
Comparison of TOF and contrast-enhanced MR angiography techniques

Parameter	TOF	Contrast-enhanced single-station MR angiography	Contrast-enhanced multi-injection multistation MR angiography	Moving table (single injection)
Acquisition time per slice	Long, secondary to use of relatively long TR (>35 ms)	Short, as shortest TR available can be used	Short, as shortest TR available can be used	Short, as shortest TR available can be used
Spatial coverage per unit time	Poor (mandatory use of the axial scan plane)	Excellent Can use coronal plane (greatest anatomic coverage for any FOV and slice thickness combination)	Excellent Can use coronal plane (greatest anatomic coverage for any FOV and slice thickness combination)	Excellent
Extended spatial coverage per unit time	Poor (the axial scan plane gives worst anatomic coverage of all imaging planes)	NA	Good; however, repositioning of table and need for subsequent localizer and mask images introduces inefficiency	Best of all Overlapping coronal acquisitions with minimum time between scans owing to rapid table movement
Artifacts	Flow related, with overestimation of degree of stenosis secondary to turbulent dephasing	Minimal, provided images are synchronized with the arterial peak of contrast enhancement	As per single-station MR angiography, with propensity for some venous enhancement in the second but also especially the third location	Propensity for venous enhancement in the third location

Abbreviation: NA, not applicable.

Table 2
Parameters for TOF and contrast-enhanced MR angiography

Parameter	TOF	Single-station contrast-enhanced MR angiography	Moving table
Sequence	GRE with GMN	Spoiled GRE	Spoiled GRE
TR	>35 ms	<6 ms	<6 ms
TE	7 ms	<2 ms (or out-of-phase = 2.3 ms at 1.5 T)	<2 ms (or out-of-phase = 2.3 ms at 1.5 T)
Flip angle	>45	30–60	30–60
Bandwidth	Optimized	Trade-off: low BW = more SNR but longer scan time; high BW = shorter scan time but lower SNR	Trade-off: low BW = more SNR but longer scan time; high BW = shorter scan time but lower SNR
Scan matrix	256×192	512×192	512×192–512
Matrix size	8 mm^3	1–6 mm^3	6, 4, 1–2 mm^3
k-space filling	Linear	Centric	Centric
Bolus timing	NA	Fluoroscopy or test bolus	Fluoroscopy or test bolus
Subtraction	No	Yes	Yes
Contrast dose	NA	10–20 mL (0.5 M)	20–40 mL (0.5 M)
Injection rate	NA	Monophasic	Monophasic/multiphasic

Abbreviations: GRE, gradient-recalled echo; GMN, gradient motion nulling; NA, not applicable.

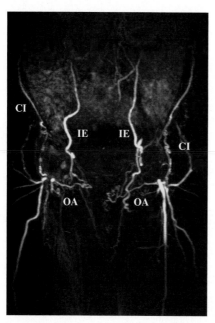

Fig. 3. Single-station contrast-enhanced MR angiography of the aortoiliac arteries demonstrates absence of the aorta and iliac arteries. There is marked collateral formation involving the inferior epigastric (IE), circumflex iliac (CI), and obturator artery (OA) on both sides. In such patients, MR angiography is invaluable, because performance of catheter angiography requires the use of a transfemoral approach. Additionally, because many of the collaterals arise above catheter placement (within the lower thoracic aorta), visualization of the arteries beyond the aortic occlusion is often markedly suboptimal with digital subtraction angiography.

each individual FOV. The requirements are as follows:

Automated table movement (a "floating" table)
A reliable method for reproducible repositioning of the table between pre- and postcontrast images
A robust method for synchronizing the first acquisition with contrast arrival [44–47]
"Flexible" imaging parameters (in-plane resolution, 3D scan volume, and k-space filling optimized individually for each location) [36]

Venous enhancement in the infrapopliteal circulation: the temporal versus spatial resolution trade-off

An inverse relationship exists between temporal and spatial resolution for contrast-enhanced MR angiography, that is, the higher the spatial resolution, the lower the temporal resolution (longer scan time) and vice versa. Prince et al [48] reported that, on average, the contrast material takes only 5 seconds to travel from the common femoral artery to popliteal artery and an additional 7 seconds to reach the ankle arteries (Fig. 4). This rapid transit of contrast material down the leg arteries most likely accounts for the difficulties with bolus timing in bolus chase MR angiography, because the motion of the MR table top and the imaging time are not fast enough to keep up with bolus passage in an average patient. Although the acquisition time for three successive acquisitions with current hardware capability is substantially greater than the transit time from the abdominal aorta to ankle artery, the arterial phase can be prolonged for contrast-enhanced MR angiography simply by using a longer injection time tailored to the duration of the three acquisitions. Although the arterial phase is dictated by the duration of the injection, the arteriovenous window is somewhat unpredictable, and venous enhancement occurs in the third location when central k-space data acquisition, delayed as a result of the finite time required to image the first two locations, coincides with contrast being present in the veins. Careful optimization of peripheral moving table contrast-enhanced MR angiography reduces the likelihood of venous enhancement as follows:

Scan timing: Aortoiliac imaging is commenced as soon as contrast arrives in the region of interest (eg, timing bolus/bolus detection) to ensure that there is no "knock-on" delay for leg imaging [44–47].

Contrast infusion rate and mask subtraction: The infusion is tailored to the duration of the first two scans plus two table movements plus the acquisition time for the central lines of k-space for the third location (the first few seconds only). The reduced injection rate may help to minimize venous enhancement [41,42]. Despite a lower infusion rate, subtraction of a precontrast mask essentially eliminates fat signal from the postcontrast image and gives a dramatically improved image quality [49].

Tailored scan parameters for each region of interest: As the arteries progressively decrease in size from the aorta to foot, it is advantageous to prescribe independent volumes at all three locations (Fig. 5), with the highest resolution reserved for the legs.

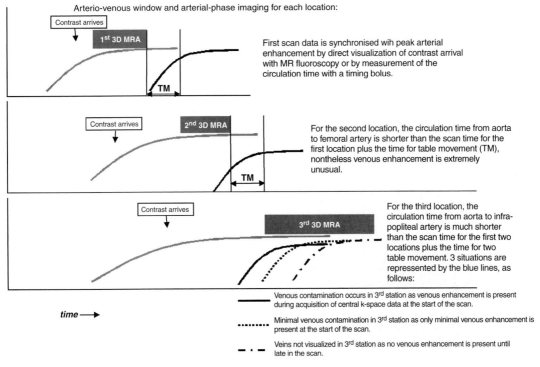

Fig. 4. Time course and risk of venous enhancement in the legs. Methods for reducing the incidence of venous enhancement include ensuring little or no redundancy in positioning the 3D imaging volumes, the use of satisfactory rather than highest possible resolution, and the use of tourniquets to slow the onset of venous enhancement. (*Modified from* Meaney JFM. MR angiography of the peripheral arteries: lower extremities. In: Schneider G, Prince MR, Meaney JFM, et al, editors. Magnetic resonance angiography: techniques, indications and applications. New York: Springer; 2005. p. 278; with permission.)

Isotropic voxel imaging is sacrificed in favor of shorter scan times.

Optimized k-space filling strategies: Although "centric" k-space data acquisition reduces the likelihood of venous enhancement at all locations, it also facilitates higher-resolution imaging of the (smaller) leg arteries by allowing the acquisition of resolution-defining peripheral k-space mapping to continue regardless of venous enhancement [40,42]. Nevertheless, slightly longer imaging (plus table motion) times would be acceptable if the centers of k-space were aligned such that the first acquisition collected the center of k-space toward the end of acquisition, whereas the last acquisition collected the center of k-space toward the beginning of acquisition (Fig. 6). This strategy would have the effect of "left-shifting" the entire acquisition, because scan data could be initiated for the first location before contrast arrival within the aorta (eg, once contrast was present within the left atrium) and would also allow use of a shorter bolus with improved T1 shortening for the same injected volume of contrast agent [35].

Enhancements to moving table contrast-enhanced MR angiography

Despite using a highly optimized approach for moving table contrast-enhanced MR angiography, most "failures" are secondary to venous enhancement in the third (calf) station and reflect the limitation of acquisition speed compared with circulation times. Because of this limitation, numerous novel approaches have been implemented to improve the temporal resolution.

Time-resolved imaging

Time-resolved imaging can be performed with a 2D approach [50], a hybrid 2D/3D approach

[51,52], or a 3D (time-resolved acquisition imaging of contrast kinetics [TRICKS]) approach [53].

Two-dimensional approach

The technique of 2D contrast-enhanced MR angiography is referred to as "MR–digital subtraction angiography" to highlight the similarities with conventional catheter arteriography [50]. For both techniques, projection images are acquired during the visualization of bolus passage through the region of interest. However, 3D imaging offers

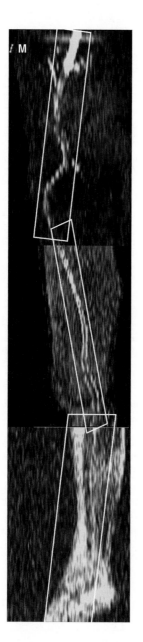

advantages, including the ability to reconstruct multiple projections, eliminating the requirement for imaging in multiple planes with separate injections, as is used for catheter arteriography. Because the large amount of dead space within the pelvis allows vessel tortuosity with resultant overlap on AP views, 2D imaging is not advocated for the first location. As the arteries of the thighs and legs course between muscle groups, there is no dead space that can facilitate arterial tortuosity with increasing age; hence, 2D imaging is appropriate for these locations. 2D images offer much shorter scan times compared with 3D images. 2D images (with a slice thickness appropriate to the anatomy, typically 6 to 8 cm) with complex subtraction and high in-plane spatial resolution can be achieved in less than 3 seconds [53,54].

Hybrid three-dimensional (aortoiliac and femoropopliteal) and two-dimensional (infrapopliteal) imaging

The speed advantage of 2D imaging can be exploited as part of a hybrid technique that uses 3D acquisitions for the aortoiliac location, 2D acquisitions for the thighs, and 2D or 3D acquisitions for the legs and feet [50–52]. The rationale for this approach is that 2D imaging reduces the overall time before central k-space data are collected for the third location. Alternatively, 2D imaging of the infrapopliteal arteries can be performed before a moving table approach of the first two locations [51,52].

Fig. 5. Appropriate positioning of the 3D imaging volumes with respect to the localizer. The MIP images from the (low resolution) TOF localizer delineate the arteries sufficiently well to facilitate placement of the 3D volumes. On the third location localizer, the small arteries of the leg and foot are hardly visualized at all. Nevertheless, by ensuring that the cephalad part of the imaging volume encloses the popliteal artery and by placing the posterior aspect of the 3D volume just posterior to the medial malleolus (visible on the axial localizer images), all of the relevant arteries will be included. For the third location, either a large imaging volume (to include the pedal arch, as shown here) or a smaller imaging volume (shorter acquisition time) can be used to image the arteries to the level of the ankle joint only. This approach is appropriate in patients with intermittent claudication who have a proximal pattern of disease but not in patients with tissue loss owing to the critical importance of the pedal arteries in this group.

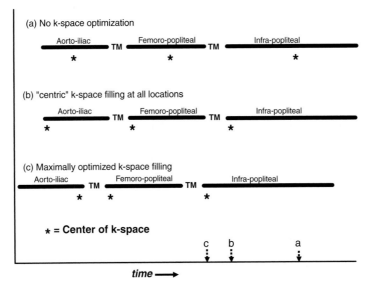

Fig. 6. k-Space schema demonstrating the benefit of optimization of k-space filling strategies for each location. (*A*) Graph demonstrates "linear" k-space filling at all three locations. With this method, the time interval between the collection of central k-space data (denoted by *) is significantly longer than for the other two methods, and the time at which central k-space data are completed for the third location is significantly later (denoted by "a" on the time axis). (*B*) Using "centric" phase encoding at all three locations, the interval between the k-space centers for all three acquisitions is shorter; additionally, the time at which the central lines of k-space for the last acquisition are completed (denoted by "b" on the time axis) occurs earlier. (*C*) By moving the center of k-space to the middle or end of the acquisition for the first location only, the interval between the k-space centers becomes even shorter; completion of central k-space data acquisition for the last station occurs even earlier, assuming that "triggering" at the first location was performed before the onset of enhancement within the aorta.

"Segmented" k-space approach

Two separate approaches that exploit the unique nature of the k-space domain wherein central k-space data govern image contrast and peripheral k-space data govern spatial resolution have been implemented.

Three-dimensional time-resolved acquisition imaging of contrast kinetics. A different approach to contrast-enhanced MR angiography involves acquiring multiple 3D volumes during the passage of the contrast agent bolus by using a time-resolved acquisition. With time-resolved acquisition imaging of contrast kinetics (TRICKS), repeated sampling of the critical central k-space views is combined with temporal interpolation to produce a series of time-resolved 3D images [53]. Time-resolved acquisitions such as TRICKS obviate timing tests and a separate acquisition of precontrast images for mask-mode subtraction. TRICKS imaging is particularly useful in patients with markedly asymmetric flow.

"Shoot 'n' scoot." To keep up with the rapid transit of the contrast bolus and to reduce the interval between contrast arrival in the aorta and the initiation of imaging for the third location, Foo et al [54] have successfully demonstrated the feasibility of acquiring central k-space data only during the first arterial pass of the contrast material bolus for the first two locations for moving table peripheral MR angiography of the lower extremities [54] (Fig. 7). A full k-space data set is acquired for the third location. After completion of the data scan for the third location, the table moves back to the second and then first locations where the higher spatial frequency k-space data are filled in during recirculation of the contrast material. When the initial k-space acquisition constitutes at least 34% of the total acquisition, the 3D shoot 'n' scoot images do not exhibit noticeable artifacts despite the discontinuity in amplitude and phase between the central k-space core and the higher spatial frequencies. Although promising, this technique of shoot 'n' scoot is not yet commercially available.

Parallel imaging

Parallel imaging has a major impact on peripheral moving table contrast-enhanced MR

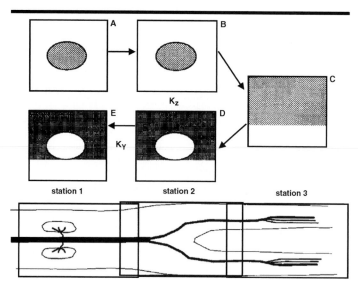

Fig. 7. Shoot 'n' scoot (SNS) segmented volume approach. Diagram shows k-space segmentation and acquisition sequence for three-station peripheral run-off MR angiography by using 3D SNS. As in all experiments, a partial Fourier acquisition (0.5 signal acquired) is used. For the first two stations, only the central core k_y and k_z data are acquired during the first pass. Data acquisition for the third station (tibioperoneal arteries) is not segmented. The remaining k-space views for stations 1 and 2 are completed at the end of the study. The shaded areas indicate portions of k-space data in k_y and k_z acquired in the order of A, B, C, D, and E, with the diagonal-striped regions acquired during the first pass and the black regions acquired during the subsequent pass. Note that for station 1, data are acquired in reverse elliptic centric order, with the center of k-space placed at the end of the initial acquisition, whereas those for stations 2 and 3 are with normal elliptic centric order (center of k-space at the start of acquisition). (Courtesy of Drs. V.B. Ho and T. Foo.)

angiography. It offers substantial savings in time (a factor of two or more) that can be used to increase resolution or decrease time (or a combination of both) [55,56]. If implemented in moving table MR angiography for the first or second locations, imaging times can be reduced to levels that virtually eliminate the risk of venous enhancement within the third location.

This approach gives increased acquisition speed by using multiple phase-array coils with known sensitivities. The scan time is typically reduced by at least a factor of two, although higher sensitivity encoding (SENSE) factors may be used to give greater time reductions. There is a penalty in the signal-to-noise ratio (SNR) proportional to the square root of the time reduction (ie, halving the scan time gives an SNR penalty of $\sqrt{1/2} = 30\%$ penalty). For any SENSE factor, all of the savings can be exploited in the interest of more rapid imaging, the resolution can be doubled for any scan time, or a combination of the two can be used. SENSE is particularly attractive for the peripheral vasculature, where most of the time reduction can be invested in more rapid

imaging for the first two locations, with use of much higher resolution for the legs.

Tourniquets to slow down the circulation

Until recently, most efforts to reduce venous enhancement have focused on increasing the speed of acquisition. Nevertheless, a simpler method is to increase the amount of time available for imaging the arterial phase by delaying the egress of contrast agent into the veins. Several investigators have reported that compression of the thigh by means of a tourniquet or an inflatable cuff is an effective method for reducing venous enhancement within the legs that can be implemented without costly hardware or software upgrades [57,58]. It is ideally suited for and facilitates high spatial resolution imaging of the lower extremity arterial system using a moving table approach with a single injection of contrast material. This approach is a modification of the timed arterial compression technique used for upper extremity imaging; however, the supra-arterial pressures (eg, 200 mm Hg) employed to "freeze" the circulation once contrast has filled the arteries of interest in the upper extremity would almost certainly not be tolerated by patients with already compromised arterial blood supply. In the lower extremity, researchers have employed thigh cuff inflation of 40, 50, and 60 mm Hg in three independent studies, with a successful reduction in venous enhancement rates without impairing arterial blood flow to the pedal arch. Zhang et al have demonstrated that unilateral thigh compression during time-resolved MR angiography with elastic tourniquets increases contrast travel time

from the common femoral artery to the popliteal artery by 62%, whereas subsystolic (60 mm Hg) inflation of thigh blood pressure cuffs slows travel time by 94% [57] (Fig. 8). The improved sharing of the contrast bolus between stations may result in better correlation of peak arterial enhancement with the center of k-space and correspondingly improved SNR.

Although the mechanism of action remains unproven, it has been hypothesized that improved venous suppression occurs owing to engorgement of veins with blood before the injection of

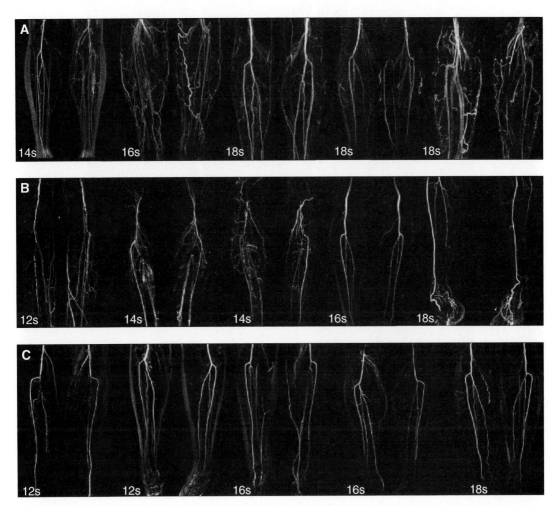

Fig. 8. Role of thigh compression in reducing venous enhancement. Comparison of tourniquet and blood pressure cuff compression. Calf stations of 3D bolus chase MR angiography in patients with fast rate of flow (contrast travel time to popliteal artery trifurcation <20 s). (*A*) On time-resolved 2D projection MR angiograms obtained without thigh compression, all patients show some venous contamination. (*B,C*) Time-resolved 2D projection MR angiograms were obtained with thigh compression applied by tourniquets (*B*) and blood pressure cuffs (*C*). Note that the least soft tissue enhancement and venous contamination occur with subsystolic thigh compression applied by blood pressure cuffs. (Courtesy of Drs. H.L. Zhang and M. Prince.)

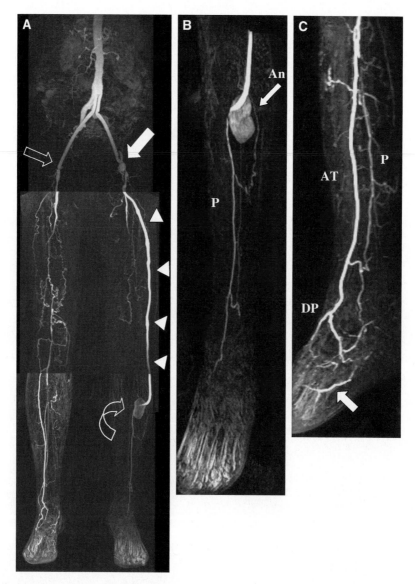

Fig. 9. (*A*) Three-station moving table MR angiography demonstrates a patent aortobifemoral graft. There is a mild stenosis at the distal anastomosis on the right (*open arrow*) and a small left-sided anastomotic pseudoaneurysm within the left groin (*solid arrow*). There is also a patent left femoropopliteal graft (*arrowheads*). Note the relatively large anastomotic popliteal pseudoaneurysm (*curved arrow*). (*B*) Lateral MIP of the left infrapopliteal arteries demonstrated the pseudoaneurysm (An) arising eccentrically at the anastomosis and a single patent infrapopliteal (peroneal) artery. The dorsalis pedis artery is occluded. (*C*) On the right side, a patent dorsalis pedis artery (DP) arises from the anterior tibial artery (AT). The posterior tibial artery is occluded; however, the peroneal artery (P) is patent. The lateral plantar artery (*arrow*) reconstitutes via the pedal arch.

gadolinium so that when the contrast material eventually arrives in peripheral veins, it is rapidly diluted. This effect would explain why the improvement in perceived image quality occurs despite the fact that the effect on travel time is so minor. To avoid misregistration artifact, the cuff must be inflated before acquisition of the localizer images. Zhang and Prince have suggested that standard lower extremity blood pressure cuffs can be used; however, several dual cuffs that provide bilateral venous compression are currently being developed.

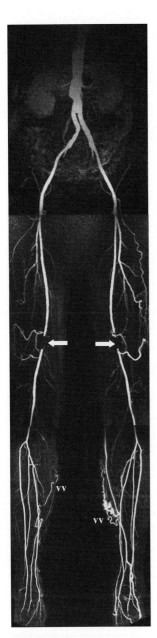

Fig. 10. Three-station moving table contrast-enhanced MR angiography in a patient who previously underwent aortobifemoral bypass grafting. There is a short-segment occlusion of the distal superficial femoral artery at the level of the adductor canal on both sides (*arrows*). Mild bilateral superficial venous enhancement (VV) does not interfere with the diagnosis.

Receiver coils

A dedicated peripheral MR angiography coil gives optimal results (the coil typically extends from the pelvis to foot arteries). Alternatively, a "moving" coil can be used that remains in the magnet bore, as the patient is moved between locations [59]. An acceptable option is to use the integral body coil for signal transmission/reception for the first and second locations, and a flexible phase-array coil for evaluation of the legs (where the arteries are smallest). Although the integral body coil was initially used for moving table peripheral MR angiography with excellent results, it is no longer recommended owing to higher clinical expectations and refinements in technique that accept multichannel coils.

Contrast agents

Initially it was presumed that all 0.5 M contrast agents had a similar profile for contrast-enhanced MR angiography, but it is now known that this is not true. Nonetheless, all currently available extracellular contrast agents have shown high degrees of accuracy when compared with catheter angiography, and all are adequate for contrast-enhanced MR angiography. Some studies have suggested an advantage for Gd-BOPTA (Multihance) for peripheral MR angiography when compared with other 0.5 M contrast agents, possibly because of its weak protein binding and superior relaxivity. Knopp et al [60] demonstrated that the SNR and contrast-to-noise ratio (CNR) at nine vessel segments from the distal abdominal aorta to the lower leg were significantly greater after the injection of Gd-BOPTA (0.1 mmol/kg) compared with Gd-DTPA (Magnevist, Schering, Germany) at the same dose and injection rate, with the greatest benefit for Gd-BOPTA in the smaller more distal vessels of the lower leg. Other investigators have reported improved performance of Gd-BOPTA when compared with Gd-DOTA [61]. More recently, Gadovist (Schering, Germany), which is formulated at 1.0 M, has become available in the European market [62,63]. The higher "strength" undoubtedly offers an improved SNR and CNR for any contrast dose, and this agent has also been validated for peripheral contrast-enhanced MR angiography [62,63].

Postprocessing

Although a surface-shaded display and video "angioscopy" (fly-through) are available, the

Table 3
Accuracy of 2D TOF MR angiography for significant (>50%) stenosis or occlusion by territory, aortoiliac arteries

Study	Year	No. of patients	No. of segments	Sensitivity	Specificity
Baumgartner	1993	15	15	82	100
Glickerman	1996	23	161	89	98
Snidow	1996	42	68	100	23
Quinn	1993	30	118	94	91
Yucel	1993	25	93	93	83
Poon	1997	15	90	100	86

Modified from Meaney JFM. MR angiography of the peripheral arteries: lower extremities. In: Schneider G, Prince MR, Meaney JFM, et al, editors. Magnetic resonance angiography: techniques, indications and applications. New York: Springer; 2004; with permission.

Table 4
Femoropopliteal arteries

Study	Year	No. of patients	No. of segments	Sensitivity	Specificity
Baumgartner	1993	15	26	88	100
Glickerman	1996	23	324	88	98
Snidow	1996	42	170	92	82
Yucel	1993	25	82	93	92

Modified from Meaney JFM. MR angiography of the peripheral arteries: lower extremities. In: Schneider G, Prince MR, Meaney JFM, et al, editors. Magnetic resonance angiography: techniques, indications and applications. New York: Springer; 2004; with permission.

Table 5
Infrapopliteal arteries

Study	Year	No. of patients	No. of segments	Sensitivity	Specificity
Glickerman	1996	23	384	86	91
Snidow	1996	42	88	92	91
McDermott	1995	24	216	89	91

Modified from Meaney JFM. MR angiography of the peripheral arteries: lower extremities. In: Schneider G, Prince MR, Meaney JFM, et al, editors. Magnetic resonance angiography: techniques, indications and applications. New York: Springer; 2005; with permission.

Table 6
Accuracy of 3D contrast-enhanced MR angiography for significant (>50%) stenosis or occlusion

Study	Year	No. of patients	No. of segments	Sensitivity	Specificity
Ho	1997	28	242	92	93
Yamashita	1998	20	140	96	83
Meaney	1999	20	620	85	93
Ruehm	2001	61	1739	92	98
Rofsky	2000	15	150	97	96

Modified from Meaney JFM. MR angiography of the peripheral arteries: lower extremities. In: Schneider G, Prince MR, Meaney JFM, et al, editors. Magnetic resonance angiography: techniques, indications and applications. New York: Springer; 2005; with permission.

Table 7
Pedal digital subtraction angiography versus MR angiography for treatment planning

Study	Year	Technique	No. of patients	Results
Baum	1995	2D TOF	155	MR angiography >> digital subtraction angiography Odds of demonstrating patent vessel 1.6 times greater on MR angiography vs digital subtraction angiography
Kreitner	2000	3D contrast-enhanced MR angiography	24	18% of segments identified by MR angiography only No segments visualized by digital subtraction angiography were missed by MR angiography
Dorweiler	2002	3D contrast-enhanced MR angiography	15	Angiographically occult vessels detected by MR angiography with subsequent successful grafting
Hoffmann	2002	3D contrast-enhanced MR angiography	37	MR angiography superior to digital subtraction angiography for showing suitable graft recipient and demonstrated more patent segments

Modified from Maki JH. Pedal MR angiography. In: Schneider G, Prince MR, Meaney JFM, et al, editors. Magnetic resonance angiography: techniques, indications and applications. New York: Springer; 2005; with permission.

maximum intensity projection (MIP) gives a satisfactory overview of the affected arteries and is the format closest to image display for conventional arteriography [64]. The following approach may be used (see Figs. 9 and 10 for clinical examples):

- All data sets should be interrogated using multiplanar reformatting, whole volume and subvolume MIP, to demonstrate the arterial tree optimally.
- For the pelvis, at least three projections should be generated, corresponding to standard angiographic projections.
- For the thighs, frontal MIPs corresponding to standard angiographic projections should be generated.
- For the legs, frontal MIPs corresponding to standard angiographic projections should be generated in addition to a lateral view of the foot when the pedal arteries are visualized.

Summary of clinical results

The impressive accuracy of TOF MR angiography, contrast-enhanced MR angiography, and moving table MR angiography along with their impact on decision making is summarized in Tables 3 to 8. The accuracy of MR angiography

has been underpinned by several meta-analyses, the results of which are summarized in Table 8 [65–67].

Future developments

Currently, the most widespread method for evaluating the entire run-off arteries relies on the acquisition of three static acquisitions in rapid succession with three coronal-oriented overlapping acquisitions. Researchers have recently devised a method for data acquisition using continuous table motion [68]. This acquisition is achieved by differential sampling of 3D k-space during continuous motion of the patient table. Although in its infancy, this technique offers promise for the future as another novel and potentially useful method for peripheral MR angiography. Resolution can be tailored to the progressively smaller arteries by filling in more k-space views as imaging progresses more distally. Potentially, the table speed can be matched to bolus passage, reducing or eliminating venous enhancement within the lower locations. Newer contrast agents, including "blood-pool" agents, may offer significant advantages over existing agents [69–71]. Continuous refinements in pulse sequence methodology and the potential for functional assessment in the future offer further

Table 8
Summary of meta-analysis results for peripheral MR angiography

Study	Technique	No. of studies	No. of patients	Sensitivity (%)	Specificity (%)	DOR[a]
Nelemans [65]	2D TOF	13	344	64–100	68–96	1.0
	3D contrast-enhanced MR angiography	10	253	92–100	91–99	7.46
Koelemay [67]	2D TOF	18	474	69–100	73–97	1.0
	3D contrast-enhanced MR angiography		482	85–97	83–98	2.8
Visser & Hunink [66]	3D contrast-enhanced MR angiography	9	216	97.5	96.2	—
	Duplex ultrasound	18	1059	87.6	94.7	—

[a] The diagnostic odds ratio (DOR) is a measure of the discriminative power of a diagnostic test. It is the ratio of the odds of a positive test result among diseased patients to the odds of a positive test result among nondiseased persons.

Modified from Meaney JFM. MR angiography of the peripheral arteries: lower extremities. In: Schneider G, Prince MR, Meaney JFM, et al, editors. Magnetic resonance angiography: techniques, indications and applications. New York: Springer; 2005; with permission.

promise for improved peripheral MR angiography techniques.

The universal MR angiography study: are we there yet?

An evolution has occurred from cumbersome and not widely accepted noncontrast MR angiography to single-location contrast-enhanced MR angiography to extended FOV imaging with a moving table approach for peripheral artery evaluation. The goal of a highly optimized study with spatial resolution adequate for each location without venous enhancement now seems possible. A carefully tailored three-station moving table MR angiography performed on a scanner equipped with fast gradient technology in association with parallel imaging at the first two (and preferably all three) locations with bolus detection, optimized k-space filling strategies, and thigh compression to delay the onset of venous enhancement will deliver high spatial resolution images free from venous contamination in virtually all patients. The authors believe that this approach will address all of the relevant questions, regardless of symptomatology, and offer the clinician an attractive alternative to invasive testing in all patients who can undergo MR imaging.

References

[1] Fowkes FG, Housley E, Cawood EH, et al. Edinburgh Artery Study: prevalence of asymptomatic and symptomatic peripheral arterial disease in the general population. Int J Epidemiol 1991;20:384–92.

[2] Voyt NT, Wolfson SK, Kuller LH. Lower extremity arterial disease and the ageing process: a review. J Clin Epidemiol 1992;45:529–42.

[3] Dormandy JA, Rutherford RB. Management of peripheral arterial disease (PAD). TASC Working Group. Trans Atlantic Inter-Society Concensus (TASC). J Vasc Surg 2000;31:S192–274.

[4] Jenkins GD, Stanson AW, Toomey BJ, et al. Limb salvage after successful pedal bypass grafting is associated with improved long-term survival. J Vasc Surg 2001;33:6–16.

[5] Armstrong D, Lavery L. Diabetic foot ulcers: prevention, diagnosis and classification. Am Fam Physician 1998;57(6):1325–78.

[6] Pomposelli FJ, Marcaccio E, Gibbons G, et al. Dorsalis pedis arterial bypass: durable limb salvage for foot ischemia in patients with diabetes mellitus. J Vasc Surg 1995;21(3):375–84.

[7] Pomposelli F, Kansal N, Hamdan A, et al. A decade of experience with dorsalis pedis artery bypass: analysis of outcome in more than 1000 cases. J Vasc Surg 2003;37(2):307–15.

[8] Bron KM. Femoral arteriography. In: Abrams HL, editor. Abrams angiography: vascular and interventional radiology. Boston: Little, Brown; 1983. p. 1835–76.

[9] Waugh JR, Sacharias N. Arteriographic complications in the DSA era. Radiology 1992;182:243–6.

[10] Reidy JF, Ludman C. Technical note: safety of outpatient arteriography using 3F catheters. Br J Radiol 1996;66:1048–52.

[11] Wilson YG, George JK, Wilkins DC, et al. Duplex assessment of run-off before femorocrural reconstruction. Br J Surg 1997;84:1360–3.

[12] Ota H, Takase K, Igarashi K, et al. MDCT compared with digital subtraction angiography for

assessment of lower extremity arterial occlusive disease: importance of reviewing cross-sectional images. AJR Am J Roentgenol 2004;182(1):201–9.

[13] Tepel M, van Der Giet M, Schwarzfeld C, et al. Prevention of radiographic contrast agent induced reductions in renal function by acetylcysteine. N Engl J Med 2000;343:180–4.

[14] Conlon PJ, O'Riordan E, Kaldra PA. New insights into the epidemiological and clinical manifestations of atherosclerotic renovascular disease. Am J Kidney Dis 2000;35:573–87.

[15] Brillet PY, Vayssairat M, Tassart M, et al. Gadolinium-enhanced MR angiography as first-line preoperative imaging in high-risk patients with lower limb ischemia. J Vasc Interv Radiol 2003;14(9 Pt 1): 1139–45.

[16] Owen RS, Carpenter JP, Baum RA, et al. Magnetic resonance imaging of angiographically occult runoff vessels in peripheral arterial occlusive disease. N Engl J Med 1992;326:157–8.

[17] Baumgartner I, Maier SE, Koch M, et al. Magnetresonanzarteriographie Duplexsonographie und konventionelle Arteriographie zur Beurteilung der peripheren arteriellen Vers-chlusskrankheit. Rofo Fortschr Geb Rontgenstr Neuen Bildgeb Verfahr 1993;159:167–73.

[18] Quinn SF, Demlow TA, Hallin RW, et al. Femoral MR angiography versus conventional angiography: preliminary results. Radiology 1993;189:181–4.

[19] Yucel EK, Kaufman JA, Geller SC, et al. Atherosclerotic occlusive disease of the lower extremity: prospective evaluation with two-dimensional time-of-flight MR angiography. Radiology 1993;187: 635–41.

[20] Glickerman DJ, Obregon RG, Schmiedl UP, et al. Cardiac-gated MR angiography of the entire lower extremity: a prospective comparison with conventional angiography. AJR Am J Roentgenol 1996; 167:445–51.

[21] Baum R, Rutter C, Sunshine J, et al. Multicenter trial to evaluate vascular magnetic resonance angiography of the lower extremity: American College of Radiology Rapid Technology Assessment Group. JAMA 1995;274(11):875–80.

[22] McDermott VG, Meakem TJ, Carpenter JP, et al. Magnetic resonance angiography of the distal lower extremity. Clin Radiol 1995;50:741–6.

[23] Carpenter JP, Golden MA, Barker CF, et al. The fate of bypass grafts to angiographically occult runoff vessels detected by magnetic resonance angiography. J Vasc Surg 1996;23:483–9.

[24] Cortell ED, Kaufmann JA, Geller SC, et al. MR angiography of tibial run-off vessels: imaging with the head coil compared with conventional arteriography. AJR Am J Roentgenol 1996;167:147–51.

[25] Ho KY, de Haan MW, Oei TK, et al. MR angiography of the iliac and upper femoral arteries using four different inflow techniques. AJR Am J Roentgenol 1997;169:45–53.

[26] Prince MR. Gadolinium-enhanced MR aortography. Radiology 1994;191(1):155–64.

[27] Prince MR, Narasimham DL, Stanley JC, et al. Breath-hold gadolinium-enhanced MR angiography of the abdominal aorta and its major branches. Radiology 1995;197(3):785–92.

[28] Snidow JJ, Johnson MS, Harris VJ, et al. Three-dimensional gadolinium-enhanced MR angiography for aorto-iliac inflow assessment plus renal artery screening in a single breath hold. Radiology 1996;198:725–9.

[29] Poon E, Yucel EK, Pagan-Marin H, et al. Iliac artery stenosis measurements: comparison of two-dimensional time-of-flight and three-dimensional dynamic gadolinium-enhanced MR angiography. AJR Am J Roentgenol 1997;169:1139–44.

[30] Ho KY, Leiner T, de Haan MW, et al. Peripheral vascular tree stenoses: evaluation with moving-bed infusion-tracking MR angiography. Radiology 1998;206:683–92.

[31] Meaney JFM, Ridgway JP, Chakraverty S, et al. Stepping-table gadolinium-enhanced digital subtraction MR angiography of the aorta and lower extremity arteries: preliminary experience. Radiology 1999;211:59–67.

[32] Yamashita Y, Mitsuzaki K, Ogata I, et al. Three-dimensional high resolution dynamic contrast-enhanced MR angiography of the pelvis and lower extremities with use of a phased array coil and subtraction. J Magn Reson Imaging 1998;8:1066–72.

[33] Sueyoshi E, Sakamoro I, Matsuoko Y, et al. Aortoiliac and lower extremity arteries: comparison of three-dimensional dynamic contrast-enhanced subtraction MR angiography and conventional angiography. Radiology 1999;210:683–8.

[34] Ruehm SG, Hany TF, Pfammater T, et al. Pelvic and lower extremity arterial imaging: diagnostic performance of three-dimensional contrast-enhanced MR angiography. AJR Am J Roentgenol 2000;174: 1127–35.

[35] Ho VB, Choyke PL, Foo TK, et al. Automated bolus chase peripheral MR angiography: initial practical experiences and future directions of this work-in-progress. J Magn Reson Imaging 1999;10:376–88.

[36] Leiner T, Ho KYJAM, Nelemans PJ, et al. Three-dimensional contrast-enhanced moving-bed infusion-tracking (MoBI-Track) peripheral MR angiography with flexible choice of imaging parameters for each field of view. J Magn Reson Imaging 2000; 11:368–77.

[37] Kreitner KF, Kalden P, Neufang A, et al. Diabetes and peripheral arterial occlusive disease: prospective comparison of contrast-enhanced three-dimensional MR angiography with conventional digital subtraction angiography. AJR Am J Roentgenol 2000;174: 171–9.

[38] Hofmann W, Forstner R, Kofler B, et al. Pedal artery imaging—a comparison of selective digital subtraction angiography, contrast enhanced magnetic

resonance angiography and duplex ultrasound. Eur J Vasc Endovasc Surg 2002;24(4):287–92.

[39] Dorweiler B, Neufang A, Kreitner K, et al. Magnetic resonance angiography unmasks reliable target vessels for pedal bypass grafting in patients with diabetes mellitus. J Vasc Surg 2002;35(4):766–72.

[40] Mezrich R. A perspective on k-space. Radiology 1995;195:297–315.

[41] Kopka L, Vosshenrich R, Rodenwaldt J, et al. Differences in injection rates on contrast-enhanced breath-hold three-dimensional MR angiography. AJR Am J Roentgenol 1998;170(2):345–8.

[42] Maki J. The effect of time-varying intravascular signal intensity and k-space acquisition order on three-dimensional MR angiographic image quality. J Magn Reson Imaging 1997;6:642–51.

[43] Rofsky NM, Johnson G, Edelman MA, et al. Peripheral vascular disease evaluated with reduced-dose gadolinium-enhanced MR angiography. Radiology 1997;205:163–9.

[44] Earls JP, Rofsky NM, DeCorato DR, et al. Breath-hold single-dose gadolinium-enhanced three-dimensional MR aortography: usefulness of a timing examination and MR power injector. Radiology 1996;201:705–10.

[45] Prince MR, Chenevert TL, Foo TK, et al. Contrast-enhanced abdominal MR angiography: optimization of imaging delay time by automating the detection of contrast material arrival in the aorta. Radiology 1997;203:109–14.

[46] Meaney JFM, Fowler RC, Saysell M, et al. Visualisation of bolus arrival for 3D contrast enhanced renal MRA: use of large field of view dynamic single slice 2-D fluoroscopic acquisition with complex subtraction, real-time reconstruction and real-time display (BolusTrak) [abstract]. In: Proceedings of the Radiological Society of North America. Berkeley (CA): ISMRM; 1999. p. 271.

[47] Riederer SJ, Bernstein MA, Breen JF, et al. Three-dimensional contrast-enhanced MR angiography with real-time fluoroscopic triggering: design specifications and technical reliability in 330 patient studies. Radiology 2000;215:584–93.

[48] Prince MR, Chabra SG, Watts R, et al. Contrast material travel times in patients undergoing peripheral MR angiography. Radiology 2002;224(1):55–61.

[49] Ho KY, de Haan MW, Kessels AG, et al. Peripheral vascular tree stenoses: detection with subtracted and nonsubtracted MR angiography. Radiology 1998;206:673–81.

[50] Lee HM, Wang Y, Sostman HD, et al. Distal lower extremity arteries: evaluation with two-dimensional MR digital subtraction angiography. Radiology 1998;207:505–12.

[51] Maki JH, Ephron JH, Glickerman DJ, et al. Moving table Gd-enhanced MR angiography of the lower extremities: a combination 3D and 2D technique—preliminary results [abstract]. In: Proceedings of the Eighth Scientific Meeting and Exhibition of the International Society for Magnetic Resonance in Medicine. Berkeley (CA): ISMRM; 2000. p. 1810.

[52] Wang Y, Winchester PA, Khilnani NM, et al. Contrast-enhanced peripheral MR angiography from abdominal aorta to the pedal arteries: combined dynamic two-dimensional and bolus-chase three-dimensional acquisition. Invest Radiol 2001; 36:170–7.

[53] Swan JS, Carroll TJ, Kennell TW, et al. Time-resolved three-dimensional contrast-enhanced MR angiography of the peripheral vessels. Radiology 2002;225(1):43–52.

[54] Foo TK, Ho VB, Hood MN, et al. High-spatial-resolution multistation MR imaging of lower-extremity peripheral vasculature with segmented volume acquisition: feasibility study. Radiology 2001;219(3):835–41.

[55] Weiger M, Pruessmann KP, Kassner A, et al. Contrast-enhanced 3D MRA using SENSE. J Magn Reson Imaging 2000;12:671–7.

[56] Maki JH, Wilson GJ, Eubank WB. 3D Gd-enhanced moving table peripheral MR angiography using multi-station SENSE to include the pedal vasculature [abstract]. In: Programs and Abstracts of the International Society of Magnetic Resonance in Medicine, ISMRM, Annual Meeting. Berkeley (CA): ISMRM; 2002. p. 1743.

[57] Zhang HL, Ho BY, Chao M, et al. Decreased venous contamination on 3D gadolinium-enhanced bolus chase peripheral MR angiography using thigh compression. AJR Am J Roentgenol 2004;4:1041–7.

[58] Vogt FM, Ajaj W, Hunold P, et al. Venous compression at high-spatial resolution three-dimensional MR angiography of peripheral arteries. Radiology 2004;233:913–20.

[59] Goyen M, Ruehm SG, Barkhausen J, et al. Improved multi-station peripheral MR angiography with a dedicated vascular coil. J Magn Reson Imaging 2001;13:475–80.

[60] Knopp MV, Giesel FL, von Tengg-Kobligk H, et al. Contrast-enhanced MR angiography of the run-off vasculature: intraindividual comparison of gadobenate dimeglumine with gadopentetate dimeglumine. J Magn Reson Imaging 2003;17:694–702.

[61] Wyttenbach R, Gianella S, Alerci M, et al. Prospective blinded evaluation of Gd-DOTA versus Gd-BOPTA–enhanced peripheral MR angiography, as compared with digital subtraction angiography. Radiology 2003;227:261–9.

[62] Hentsch A, Aschauer MA, Balzer JO, et al. Gadobutrol-enhanced moving-table magnetic resonance angiography in patients with peripheral vascular disease: a prospective, multi-centre blinded comparison with digital subtraction angiography. Eur Radiol 2003;13(9):2103–14.

[63] Gregor M, Tombach B, Hentsch A, et al. Peripheral run-off CE MRA with a 1.0 molar gadolinium

chelate (Gadovist) with intra-arterial DSA comparison. Acad Radiol 2002;9(Suppl 2):S398–400.

[64] Hany TF, Schmidt M, Davis CP, et al. Diagnostic impact of four post-processing techniques in evaluating contrast-enhanced three-dimensional MR angiography. AJR Am J Roentgenol 1998;170:907–12.

[65] Nelemans PJ, Leiner T, de Vet HCW, et al. Peripheral arterial disease: meta-analysis of the diagnostic performance of MR angiography. Radiology 2000; 217:105–14.

[66] Visser K, Hunick MG. Peripheral arterial disease: gadolinium-enhanced MR angiography versus color-guided duplex US—a meta-analysis. Radiology 2000;216:67–77.

[67] Koelemay MJ, Lijmer JG, Stoker J, et al. Magnetic resonance angiography for the evaluation of lower extremity arterial disease: a meta-analysis. JAMA 2001;285:1338–45.

[68] Kruger DG, Riederer SJ, Grimm RC, et al. Continuously moving table data acquisition method for long FOV contrast-enhanced MRA and whole-body MRI. Magn Reson Med 2002;47(2): 224–31.

[69] Knopp MV, von Tengg-Kobligk H, Froemer F, et al. Contrast agents for MRA: future directions. J Magn Reson Imaging 1999;10:314–6.

[70] Perreault P, Edelman MA, Baum RA, et al. MR angiography with gadofosveset trisodium for peripheral vascular disease: phase II trial. Radiology 2003;229:811–20.

[71] Leon M, Mohler E. Results of a dose-ranging diagnostic trial of magnetic resonance angiography with MS-325, a blood pool contrast agent, for the detection of vascular occlusive disease in the aortoiliac region. J Am Coll Cardiol 2002;368[A]: 1140–51.

ELSEVIER
SAUNDERS

Magn Reson Imaging Clin N Am
13 (2005) 113–129

MAGNETIC
RESONANCE
IMAGING CLINICS
of North America

MR Venography

Florian M. Vogt, MD*, Christoph U. Herborn, MD,
Mathias Goyen, MD

*Department of Diagnostic and Interventional Radiology, University Hospital Essen,
Hufelandstrasse 55, 45122 Essen, Germany*

Background

In the industrialized world, venous thromboembolic (VTE) disease has an incidence of one to two cases per 1000 people of the general population and is a major cause of morbidity and mortality. More than 50% of VTE manifestations relate to deep vein thrombosis (DVT) of the lower extremities. The probability of subsequent pulmonary embolism increases with the extent of DVT to more proximal veins, which is related to the severity of the initiating prothrombic stimulus and to the duration of the stimulus [1]. Early and extensive diagnosis of thromboembolic disease would allow immediate and effective patient management, thereby preventing severe complications. Various imaging methods have been used for diagnosing DVT, including X-ray venography, which is still considered the reference standard [2]. Because of its invasiveness, the use of iodinated contrast media, and its limited diagnostic value for the pelvic veins, alternative techniques such as duplex sonography have gained more acceptance [3,4]. Although duplex sonography offers the advantages such as low costs, wide clinical availability, and lack of invasiveness, its accuracy depends on a variety of factors, and it has been reported to be less sensitive for the detection of DVT in more distal vessels [5–7]. Furthermore, most patients have multisegmental thrombosis at multiple locations at the time of diagnosis, and duplex sonography cannot provide an explicit overview of the entire venous pathology.

Reflecting the rapid developments in hardware and software, helical multidetector CT has become the main noninvasive imaging modality in many institutions to evaluate patients with suspected VTE disease. New protocols combine CT venography of the pelvis and lower extremities with CT pulmonary angiography to evaluate two vascular regions in a single examination [8,9]. The need to use considerable doses of ionizing radiation and to administer high doses of potentially nephrotoxic iodinated contrast agents for combined protocols are the main drawbacks of this modality.

MR venography has been reported to be an accurate method for assessing the venous system for many years [10–14]. With the development of new and faster sequences and the implementation of well-tolerated MR contrast agents, high-quality imaging of even small, deep veins in the calf and superficial as well as perforating veins became possible. This technique lacks ionizing radiation, and the contrast agents have better safety profiles than the CT compounds. Thus, MR is increasingly applied for diagnosis of venous thromboembolic disease.

This article describes existing MR techniques for the assessment of the venous system and summarizes the clinical experience. It also discusses new applications that are likely to increase the use of MR venography in clinical practice.

Techniques for MR venography

In principle, two MR venography techniques can be differentiated: those that do not use contrast enhancement and three-dimensional (3-D) contrast-enhanced MR venography.

---

* Corresponding author.

E-mail address: florian.vogt@uni-essen.de (F.M. Vogt).

1064-9689/05/$ - see front matter © 2005 Elsevier Inc. All rights reserved.
doi:10.1016/j.mric.2004.12.004

mri.theclinics.com

Non–contrast-enhanced techniques

Non-enhanced flow-dependent MR techniques

Conventional time-of-flight (TOF) and phase-contrast (PC) techniques use flow effects to isolate vessels from surrounding tissue without requiring the injection of a paramagnetic contrast agent. Both techniques have been applied successfully in clinical practice and can be considered accurate methods with good sensitivities and specificities for the assessment of the venous system [11,13]. These techniques, however, have shown to be less accurate in the depiction of small, deep or superficial veins because of the very slow flow [15]. PC techniques can be adapted to a slow flow at the expense of increased sensitivity to global motion artifacts as the acquisition time increases. Furthermore, known limitations, including susceptibility effects, pulsation artifacts, in-plane saturation effects, and spin dephasing, coupled with lengthy acquisition times have restricted the use of both techniques to specific indications in clinical practice.

Time-of-flight MR venography

Commonly, TOF MR angiographic techniques are based on spoiled gradient recall echo (GRE) sequences that rely on the inflow of blood alone to create vascular signal. The signal from stationary tissue within the imaging volume is suppressed by the application of multiple radio frequency (rf) pulses. When short repetition time (TR) values are chosen, the longitudinal magnetization of the tissue does not have sufficient time to redevelop, resulting in very low signal [16]. Flowing spins in the vessels, however, are consistently refreshed

and therefore appear bright in the MR experiment [17,18]. This inflow enhancement is maximized when blood receives only one rf pulse before flowing out of the imaging plane; the technique becomes less effective when longer vessel sections lie within the imaged volume and receive multiple excitations. The intravascular signal intensity may then be reduced to the signal intensity of surrounding tissue, and differentiation may be more difficult. The intraluminal brightness further depends on TR, echo time (TE), and flip angle. Using longer TR leads to an increased number of relaxed spins entering the imaging plane.

TE should be short. A TE of 8 milliseconds (on a 1.5-T MR scanner) is recommended to diphase the signal from water and fat, respectively, and thereby reduce the signal of stationary fat.

A low flip-angle is important to minimize in-plane flow saturation. Very small flip angles, however, result in noisy images, whereas large flip angles might saturate the venous signal. The optimal flip angle depends on the orientation of the slice to the axis of the vessels. For imaging longitudinal flow (ie, in-plane flow), an angle between 20° to 25° should be used. For through-plane flow, a flip angle of 45° is considered optimal.

Because with TOF MR angiography both arterial and venous vessels appear bright, a flow presaturation band is mandatory in the upstream direction of arterial flow, eliminating inflow enhancement by nulling inflowing arterial spins.

TOF images are frequently acquired as a series of two-dimensional (2-D) sections separated by thin gaps. The large coverage areas and the ability to detect small vessels with slow flow make 2-D TOF an ideal candidate for venous imaging (Fig. 1).

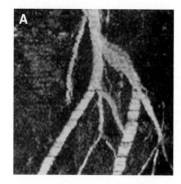
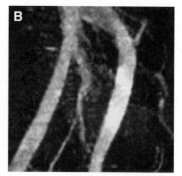

Fig. 1. TOF MR venography of pelvic veins. MIP images were rendered from 2-D data sets, which were acquired in transverse orientation. (*A*) Normal deep venous system of the inferior vena cava, internal and external iliac veins, and inferior mesenteric vein without evidence of DVT. (*B*) Venogram fails to depict the internal iliac vein on the left side because of venous thrombosis.

3-D TOF sequences offer contiguous imaging but have a compromised field-of-view and in-plane spatial resolution and prolonged imaging times.

Phase-contrast MR venography

PC MR venography is based on the observation that spins moving through a magnetic field gradient have different phases (phase shift) when compared with static spins. For PC imaging, two interleaved views are acquired over successive TRs. There is only one difference between the two views: the second view has an added bipolar gradient along one direction (bipolar gradient → (+) Area = (−) Area) [19]. This bipolar gradient affects only moving spins that acquire a different phase dependent on their specific flow characteristics. The phase difference between two successively acquired images is thus limited to phase shifts from moving spins, and a true velocity map is provided. The measured phase difference in individual pixels with flow is directly related to the flow velocity along the direction of the first moment change, which is referred to as the "velocity-encoded direction" and may be along the x-, y-, or z-axis. By definition, flow is bright if it flows from right to left (in the x-plane), anterior to posterior (in the y-plane), or superior to inferior (in the z-plane). Flow in the opposite direction is depicted as black. The technique is unique in that it gives a direct velocity map, and the voxel signal intensity values are proportional to the actual flow velocity in a particular direction. The flow sensitivity can be adjusted. The velocity-encoding value helps to determine the largest measurable velocity. The velocity-encoding value should be chosen to exceed the maximum expected velocity by about 25%. A velocity-encoding value of approximately 20 cm/sec has been suggested for MR venography. PC imaging also has been used for the assessment of the portal venous system [20] because it permits direct quantitative characterization of flow dynamics over time [21]. The time-consuming examinations and motion artifacts have kept this technique from wide clinical use in MR venography.

Nonenhanced flow-independent sequences

Rather than using flow effects to isolate vessels from surrounding structures, flow-independent venography exploits differences in T1, T2, and chemical shift in blood [22–24]. The high intravascular signal intensity of blood comes from its relatively long T2 value, which varies from approximately 60 to 220 milliseconds depending on the physiologically relevant range of oxygen

saturation [25,26]. For fast spin echo (FSE) sequences with a long tau (time between 180° refocusing pulses), the T2 of blood is substantially longer than that of other tissues. Thus heavily T2-weighted FSE sequences (rapid acquisition relaxation enhancement [RARE], turbo spin echo [TSE]) have been used, especially for MR venography of lower extremities and vessels with slow flow. In these applications, they provide good delineation of the vascular anatomy in relatively short acquisition times [27].

The aforementioned techniques use multiple phase-encoded spin echoes; instead of collecting one Fourier line per TR, multiple rf refocusing pulses are used to create additional spin echoes. Those spin echoes are phase encoded and sorted into the same k-space matrix of the excited slice. Usually TR is extended in comparison to conventional spin-echo imaging to achieve better contrast, and usually the matrix size is increased to improve spatial resolution. Both actions eliminate the consequences of reduced signal contribution of Fourier lines acquired with late echoes. Because the objectives for MR venography are to eliminate signal from arterial blood flow, fat, and muscle and to enhance the venous blood signal, these sequences must be optimized further by adapting parameters like TE, tau 180, inversion pulses, bandwidth, and flow compensation [27,28]. Oxygen saturation usually is between 60% and 75% for venous blood, and the measured T2 decreases from 220 milliseconds for arterial blood to about 60 milliseconds for venous blood. Thus a short TE (<100 milliseconds) and a long tau 180 increase the difference in signal between arterial and venous blood. Suppression of muscle tissue can be provided by sufficiently long TE (>60 milliseconds), whereas fat can be nulled using an inversion pulse in a short-T1 inversion recovery preparation. Venous flow velocities can be minimized further by using a tourniquet to reduce flow artifacts.

Because of their lack of flow dependence and their increased resolution, these imaging techniques can depict very small branches. Because of the high number of depicted veins, however, maximum-intensity projections (MIPs) are not considered helpful. Furthermore, venous vessels with higher flow rates are not clearly depicted by such techniques.

This disadvantage can be overcome by recently developed steady-state free-precession (SSFP) gradient echo sequences (eg, True fast imaging with steady precision, fast imaging employing steady state acquisition, balanced fast field echo), which are characterized by balanced gradients in all three directions, ensuring maximum recovery of the transverse magnetization. At the end of the TR, the transverse magnetization is refocused, and the next excitation can be started without further preparation. The main advantage of this sequence is the high signal intensity of fluids. The resulting high contrast delineates vessels as bright structures and at the same time displays all other morphology. The image contrast is determined by favorable T2*/T1 properties that are nearly independent of blood flow [29]; thus flow-artifacts can be totally suppressed if constant venous flow is present. The venous blood stream of the upper extremity veins, the vena cava, and the pelvis veins can be visualized without motion artifacts in conjunction with high spatial resolution (Fig. 2). Recently developed multislice steady-state sequences are capable of covering the entire thoracic or abdominal veins, even in the axial plane, within short acquisition times.

For optimal vessel imaging, short TRs are mandatory to avoid T2* effects but are restricted to the most powerful gradient systems. Short TRs and TEs reduce susceptibility artifacts and lead to extremely short data acquisition times. Further echo sharing can be used to improve temporal resolution [30]. A disadvantage in SSFP imaging is patient-induced inhomogeneities of the magnetic field. Therefore, local shim volumes should be used to eliminate such effects. In cardiac MR imaging there is increasing interest in assessing global and regional ventricular dimensions and cardiac functions with SSFP. These pulse sequences, however, have not become established as the modality of choice for vessel imaging because the inherent high signal intensity of both fluids and fat limits the application of postprocessing algorithms (eg, MIPs or multiplanar reformats). Furthermore, both arteries and veins are displayed with bright signal [31]. Nevertheless, the high spatial resolution and the ability to examine large regions without the use of a contrast agent might make fast SSFP MR venography the technique of choice for excluding venous thrombosis in pregnant patients or in patients with other contraindications to contrast media. Thrombus and slow-flowing blood can be differentiated easily.

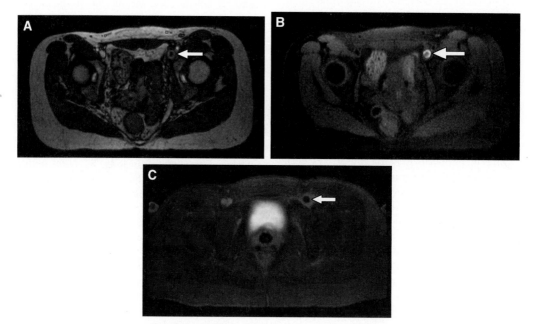

Fig. 2. A 37-year-old woman with a hypercoagulated state and clinical signs of DVT in the left leg. (*A*) A non–contrast-enhanced steady-state free-precision image demonstrates hypointense thrombus material in the left common femoral vein (*arrow*), whereas the right common femoral vein is of normal (bright) signal intensity. (*B*) A non–contrast-enhanced black-blood T2-weighted image correlates well with Fig. 2A. Note the bright signal around the thrombus caused by slow flow (ie, persistence of spins within the imaging slice). The right common femoral vein, however, appears dark, as would be expected in a patent vessel where blood washout is brisk. (*C*) High-spatial-resolution contrast-enhanced VIBE image demonstrates a dark filling defect (*arrow*), confirming the DVT.

Three-dimensional contrast-enhanced MR venography techniques

Gadolinium contrast-enhanced 3-D MR venography combines the intravenous bolus application of a non-nephrotoxic contrast agent, gadolinium chelate, with the acquisition of a 3-D data set, thereby raising the vessel-to-background contrast-to-noise ratio and eliminating flow artifacts [32]. Hence, the signal intensity of blood is no longer flow dependent. The flow-induced artifacts seen with noncontrast TOF or PC MR angiographic techniques therefore are largely eliminated, and images can be collected in the plane coinciding with the course of the vessels of interest. This technique allows coronal coverage of large vascular territories in very short imaging times.

3-D contrast-enhanced MR venography can be performed using an indirect or direct approach. With the indirect approach, the veins are imaged during the contrast-equilibrium phase following the injection of a paramagnetic contrast agent, gadolinium chelate, into an antecubital vein [14,33]. To compensate for considerable dilution as the contrast bolus passes through the lungs, the arterial system, and the capillary bed, indirect MR venography requires large doses of contrast agent. To avoid significant redistribution of the contrast

agent in the extracellular fluid compartment, timing of the acquisition relative to the administration of the contrast agent is crucial. Dynamic gadolinium-enhanced 3-D MR venography, based on the use of very short repetition (<2 milliseconds) and echo times (<1 millisecond), permits the acquisition of consecutive 3-D data sets in less than 30 seconds [34]. This method obviates the need for timing the contrast bolus and has been shown to display the central veins reliably. The indirect approach does not require cannulation of the vein in the effected extremity. For a better contrast-to-noise ratio, images obtained during the venous phase can be subtracted from those acquired in the arterial phase [33]. Subtraction is of less use in the chest and abdomen because of potential spatial misregistration artifacts caused by respiratory motion.

Direct MR venography, like conventional venography, uses a continuous infusion of a diluted dose of gadolinium chelate but is performed proximal or "upstream" to the target venous system [35,36]. Lower or upper extremity MR venography requires injection on the side of the affected extremity. To avoid T2-shortening effects, the contrast medium should be diluted with saline in a ratio of 1:20. The 3-D data sets are collected during injection of the contrast agent (Fig. 3). Imaging should start following the injection of the

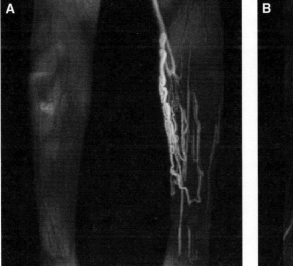
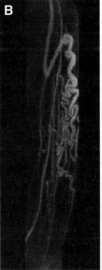

Fig. 3. A 64-year-old patient with varicosity of the left lower limb. Direct MR venography was performed after injection of contrast agent in the distal lower limb vein. An MIP image of the calf demonstrates an extensive varicosity. (*A*) Frontal-projection MIP image. (*B*) 30° rotated oblique MIP image.

first 50 to 60 mL of diluted contrast agent. Repeated acquisitions can be performed to assess functional obstructions of veins.

Although less contrast agent is required with this method, contrast-to-noise ratios are higher than with the indirect approach. First-pass imaging, however, requires a venous access site at the clinically symptomatic limb and does not allow complete evaluation of the chest veins, even after bilateral peripheral infusion [37].

Technical considerations of pulse sequences

The pulse-sequence design for contrast-enhanced MR venography is based on a 3-D Fourier transform GRE sequence with rapid rf pulsing. To achieve maximal T1 weighting, spoiled sequences should be employed. TR and TE should be as short as possible. Flip angles between 30° and 40° provide adequate suppression of the surrounding tissues and render excellent image quality for imaging venous vessels. The partition dimensions (ie, partition thickness, matrix size, field of view) should be prescribed to achieve the smallest possible voxel size to allow sufficient spatial coverage of the target vessel [38]. Conventional sequential phase ordering in which the center k-space views are collected in the middle of the imaging period allows more time for displaying venous collaterals in the presence of venous occlusion.

Recently, 3-D GRE with uniform fat saturation has been introduced for multiphase imaging of adequate anatomic coverage [39,40]. The volumetric interpolated breath-hold examination (VIBE) technique combines angiographic capacities with detailed imaging of the surrounding tissue. The technique uses a symmetric echo in the read direction, partial in-plane Fourier sampling in the phase-encoding direction, and asymmetric echo sampling and interpolation (zero-filling) along the partition direction. An interpolated matrix size with maximum in-plane pixel resolution can be reached within one breath-hold. Partial volume effects are minimized, thereby providing nearly isotropic resolution. Thus, VIBE examinations offer images in any plane from the data sets obtained during arterial and venous phase. Postcontrast images can be reconstructed by using MIP algorithms, thereby incorporating the advantages of contrast-enhanced 3-D MR venography. Use of surface coils for signal reception leads to improved signal-to-noise ratio.

Image analysis

The high contrast between gadolinium-containing luminal (bright) and extraluminal (dark) spins and the true 3-D nature of the acquired data sets provide the basis for a variety of postprocessing algorithms. Analysis should never be limited to MIPs or surface-shaded display. The three-dimensionality inherent in the technique can be exploited fully only if the data are viewed interactively on a workstation using multiplanar reformations.

Direct thrombus imaging

Visualization and evaluation of thrombus in veins can be achieved either by noncontrast or contrast techniques. The noncontrast techniques rely on changes in T1 of thrombus and visualize thrombus against a suppressed dark background [41]. During the process of thrombus formation, the reduction in T1 time of the clot reflects the presence of methemoglobin [42]. High signal intensity occurs initially on T1-weighted images and is present at the margins of the thrombus, extending toward the center over time. In addition, the accumulation of hemoglobin degradation products in macrophages, which have been shown to invade the margin of thrombi in large numbers during thrombus organization, explains the progressive loss of signal intensity observed in the periphery of thrombi on T2-weighted images [43,44]. Thus, changes in clot signal intensity over time may allow estimation of the age of thrombus.

To increase the contrast of clot versus blood further, an inversion recovery pulse can be implemented to null the signal of unclotted blood. Because the signal intensity of the thrombus increases while the contrast between thrombus and blood decreases, however, no exact diagnosis is possible when unclotted blood cannot be nulled completely. Suppression of background signal on T1-weighted data sets can be optimized by selective rf excitation of water molecules, thereby reducing fat signal.

With gadolinium-enhanced MR venography, detection of thrombus is based on the depiction of a dark intraluminal defect. The timing of the 3-D acquisitions needs to be planned so that the acquisition of the k-space coincides with the venous phase of the contrast bolus. Because clinically available extracellular paramagnetic gadolinium chelate contrast agents diffuse rapidly into the interstitial spaces, venous signal intensity rapidly decreases, mandating the use of high doses of contrast agent. Furthermore, delayed filling of collateral or superficial veins, especially in the presence of post-thrombotic changes, is often depicted insufficiently, and the decreases in signal intensity in the late equilibrium phases makes correct diagnosis even more difficult. This dilemma might be overcome by several new paramagnetic, intravascular, gadolinium-based agents that have recently become available and are currently undergoing preclinical and clinical testing [45–48]. These contrast agents either have a macromolecular structure that prevents leakage from the intravascular bed or bind to albumin when injected. These characteristics confine the agents to the intravascular compartment for an extended time, resulting in a high vascular signal-to-noise ratio during equilibrium-phase imaging. The longer vascular half-life of such blood-pool contrast agents might permit imaging of additional vascular sites, such as the pulmonary arteries, that do not require arterial-phase imaging. The T1 relaxation of these blood-pool agents also tends to be several-fold higher than that of gadolinium chelate. Therefore, the blood-pool agents can be used at doses that are several times lower than needed with gadolinium chelate. The higher equivalent-injection rate produces a more highly concentrated bolus, thereby improving arterial-phase imaging as well. Improving both the arterial-phase and equilibrium-phase images should make the final pure venogram superior [49]. First clinical trials have shown these agents offer significantly improved diagnostic conspicuity and contrast in ilio-caval venous opacification when compared with conventional extracellular contrast agents [50].

Ultrasmall superparamagnetic iron oxide (USPIO) preparations also can be used as positive contrast agents in T1-weighted imaging. These suspensions have a high T1 relaxation and a long plasma half-life, making them well suited for MR venography in equilibrium phases. Recently published studies revealed prolonged and improved visualization of the peripheral venous vasculature, particularly of the inferior vena cava and internal iliac veins after intravenous injection of USPIO [50]. MR venography seemed to offer substantive improvements over conventional venography and color Doppler ultrasound [47]. Sensitivities and specificities were lower for the evaluation of vessels below the knee, however [48].

One of the major drawbacks of contrast-enhanced MR venography with intravascular contrast agents is the need for postprocessing. Because the compounds are present in arteries as well as in veins, arterial vessels must be distinguished from venous vessels to yield selective venous angiograms. Without dedicated separation, vessels may be obscured on MIP images. Single-slice viewing can overcome these problems, but this technique is time consuming. Various postprocessing methods for removing arterial signal from venous images have been proposed. New approaches, such as double subtraction or factor analysis of dynamic studies, should have a considerable impact, especially in imaging the vessels below the knee, but still are under evaluation [41,51].

USPIO particles may be expected to accumulate in thrombi and thus affect their signal intensity on MR images [52]. Age-related changes in signal caused by the organizational stage of a thrombus were found on T1-weighted images in an animal model. Hyperintensity of thrombus material increased significantly after administration of a USPIO contrast agent in 3-, 5-, and 7-day-old thrombi, but not at a thrombus age of 1 or 9 days [44,53]. The assessment of thrombus age might be offer important clinical information on whether a thrombus will respond to therapy.

Superior vena cava and upper extremities

Thrombosis of systemic chest veins, commonly presenting as superior vena cava syndrome, is an important cause of morbidity in patients with malignancies, hematologic diseases, or long-term indwelling catheters. This syndrome is characterized by cyanosis and swelling of the head, neck, and arm in combination with the distension of veins on the neck and trunk. Prompt diagnosis and adequate therapy must be provided to restore patency of the veins. The role of imaging is to demonstrate the presence of venous thrombosis, its site and extent, and possible causes.

Thrombo-occlusive disease of the chest veins, including the axillary, subclavian, and innominate veins and the superior vena cava has been evaluated accurately by MR imaging using 2-D TOF methods. In a study by Finn et al [54] with 30 patients, 2-D TOF MR venographic results of the thoracic veins were completely corroborated in 19 of 22 cases (86%), and MR findings were predictive of successful venous catheterization in 11 patients. Hartnell et al [55] reported agreement between 2-D TOF MR venography and conventional venographic findings in cases in which conventional venographic correlation was available.

These techniques have the advantage of not requiring contrast material, but, because data acquisition is required in variable planes with the scan plane perpendicular to the venous vessels, they are limited by long examination times and potentially misleading artifacts [54,56]. To overcome these limitations, recent reports have proposed the use of gadolinium-enhanced 3-D body MR venography [14].

Initially, direct MR venography of the superior vena cava was performed using an injection of diluted contrast media to avoid the T2-shortening effects of a compact bolus [35,36,56,57]. Thornton et al [57] obtained breath-hold 3-D spoiled GRE images during first pass as well as in delayed arteriovenous-phase images after manual injection of a gadolinium chelate contrast agent for imaging of central veins. They reported high sensitivities and specificities. For bilateral evaluation of the axillary, subclavian, and brachiocephalic veins and the assessment of the superior vena cava,

simultaneous injections of the right and left upper extremities should be performed. Before contrast administration, tourniquets can be placed around upper arms to assure adequate filling of the deep venous systems. Bilateral injection of 50 to 60 mL of diluted contrast agent by two operators must be coordinated so that the injections of the first syringes are completed at approximately the same time. The acquisition of the imaging data should be performed during injections of the second syringes. First-pass imaging requires a venous access site at the clinically symptomatic limb (or in both arms for bilateral injection) and does not allow complete evaluation of the chest veins, even with bilateral injection, because unenhanced blood flow in the internal jugular veins may lead to flow-related artifacts.

With the indirect approach, the veins are imaged during the contrast-equilibrium phase following the injection of gadolinium chelate contrast agent (Figs. 4, 5). The necessary venous

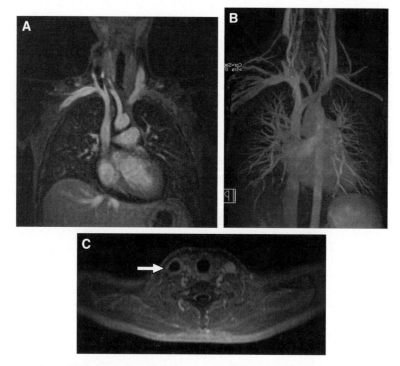

Fig. 4. 3-D contrast-enhanced indirect venography of a 37-year-old man after removal of a central venous catheter in the right internal jugular vein. The patient was referred to assess the veins in the upper extremities to exclude venous thrombosis. (*A*) Contrast-enhanced source image of a 3-D data set acquired in the venous phase shows contrast filling a defect in the right internal jugular vein. (*B*) In an MIP image, there is a partial lack of display of the right internal jugular vein, and some collateral vessels in the supraclavicular region are visualized. (*C*) High-spatial-resolution 3-D VIBE image, acquired in a transverse orientation, displays the widened and clotted right internal jugular vein (*arrow*) with rimlike enhancement of the vessel wall.

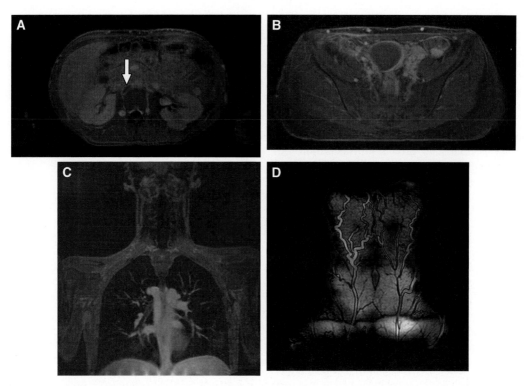

Fig. 5. A 34-year-old woman with complete occlusion of the inferior vena cava and a distinct net of superficial collateral veins at the chest and abdominal wall. A MR study was performed to evaluate vessel status for optimal therapeutic stratification. (*A*) Contiguous 3-D VIBE image data sets of abdomen and pelvis confirmed complete occlusion of the inferior vena cava (*arrow*) from the right atrium down to bifurcation. (*B*) Contrast-enhanced 3-D VIBE images of the pelvis revealed convolution of parauterine and paraovarian veins that drain into superficial veins of the abdominal wall. (*C*) Coronary images showed dilated azygos and hemiazygos veins draining into the superior vena cava. (*D*) High-spatial-resolution non–contrast-enhanced 3-D TrueFISP images demonstrate multiple superficial veins that drain into the superior vena cava.

access can be established anywhere in the body. This approach is especially useful for imaging the chest veins in patients in whom bilateral venous access in the forearms is problematic or when information concerning both arterial and venous vessels is needed. Shinde et al [33] reported the feasibility of this approach in patients who need evaluation of central veins or for placement of a hemodialysis graft. For better a contrast-to-noise ratio, images obtained in the venous phase were subtracted from those acquired in the arterial phase.

Kroencke et al [58] extrapolated the mean time of maximum contrast enhancement of the thoracic veins and chose a time delay of 15 seconds between the acquisition of the arterial and venous phase. Thereby they ensured that patients could breathe before the diagnostic image set was

acquired during suspended respiration at end-inspiration in the phase of maximal venous contrast enhancement. This approach obviated the need for multiple acquisitions after administration of contrast agent. In a prospective study of 16 patients with clinically suspected thromboembolic disease of the chest, MR venography detected thrombus in all patients, and the complete extent of disease could be determined in 15 of 16 patients. Moreover, MR venography provided additional information in 38% when compared with color-coded duplex sonography, digital subtraction angiography, and CT.

The introduction of dynamic gadolinium-enhanced 3-D MR venography, based on the use of very short TR and TE, respectively, permit the acquisition of up to six 3-D data sets in less than 24 seconds [34]. This method obviates the need for timing the contrast bolus and has been shown to be reliable for the display of central veins. This type of dynamic imaging allows the assessment of thoracic veins in different arm positions. MR venograms were of diagnostic quality for all 14 included patients and compared well with duplex sonography.

Another approach toward MR venography of upper chest veins is high-resolution SSFP imaging. This technique promises visualization of thrombus with high contrast relative to the surrounding blood pool without requiring the administration of contrast agents. So far investigations of the technique in patients with DVT and suspected pulmonary embolism have been promising [31]. To the authors' knowledge, no studies have yet investigated the value of SSFP imaging for the assessment of the chest veins including cardiac-triggering and multislice options. The authors' initial experience has been promising, however.

Inferior vena cava and lower extremities

Indications for MR venography of the inferior vena cava include the assessment of extrinsic or intrinsic caval obstruction, congenital anatomic variations, and display of venous anatomy before operation or intervention. Thrombosis of the pelvic veins or the inferior vena cava leads to the development of multiple collateral vessels. In patients with unilateral iliac thrombosis, blood may drain to the contralateral side through a wide variety of collaterals including the sacral, rectal, vesical, uterine, or prostatic plexus. Complete thrombosis of the inferior vena cava leads to drainage of blood into abdominal epigastric veins and through thoracic epigastric veins into the superior vena cava. Most DVTs, however, originate in the deep venous system of the lower extremities.

Both TOF and PC MR angiography depict anatomic variations of the inferior vena cava and pelvic and upper extremity veins (eg, duplications, anomalous course of the left renal vein) and have been established as a reliable means for detecting DVT of pelvic and upper extremity veins [12,59,60]. In pelvic imaging for the evaluation of DVT, MR venography offers advantages over sonography and conventional venography. In a study conducted by Spritzer et al [61], the frequency of isolated DVT detected with MR venography was higher than that reported in previous studies using sonography or conventional ascending venography. Carpenter [11] reported a sensitivity of 100% and a specificity of 96% for the evaluation of DVT from the inferior vena cava to the popliteal vein comparing 2-D TOF MR venography and conventional venography. Evans et al [13] demonstrated a sensitivity of 87% and specificity of 97% for MR venography in detecting infrapopliteal DVT. Lengthy acquisition times have limited the use of the unenhanced techniques mainly to the pelvis, however. Because in-plane flow saturation prevents reliable depiction of perforating veins that run in the horizontal plane, and because of the inherent lack of sensitivity to slow or retrograde flow, TOF MR angiography has not been employed for assessing varicose veins or post-thrombotic changes.

Heavily T2-weighted FSE sequences (eg, RARE, TSE) exploit the intrinsic MR properties of blood and have shown excellent depiction of extremity veins with slow flow, providing good depiction of the venous anatomy in the calf in relatively short acquisition times. Bluemke et al [27] reported using this technique to depict lower extremity veins with relatively high resolution. Gallix et al [28] optimized flow-independent techniques for the depiction of peripheral veins in volunteers. The feasibility of this technique was shown in six patients. DVT findings diagnosed by duplex sonography were also seen on MR venography. Other potential applications of this technique include evaluation of vascular malformations, venous stasis, and varicosities. The recently introduced SSFP technique demonstrated clear thrombus visualization with high contrast to the surrounding blood pool even in calf veins. No contrast media was needed. Diagnosis was achieved within an acquisition time of 10 minutes and was proved by conventional venography, CT, or sonography [31].

If peripheral high-resolution MR venography is required, direct MR venography with injection of diluted contrast agent into a foot vein can be performed, regardless of the underlying flow characteristics and orientation of the vessel. Ruehm et al [62] demonstrated that this technique is suited for the accurate display of deep and superficial venous morphology, post-thrombotic changes, and varicosities affecting the lower extremity. Several limitations have been reported, however, including the need to obtain peripheral venous access and to apply multiple tourniquets to an extremity that may be swollen. In the pelvic veins, dilution from draining venous tributaries can cause a reduction of the very bright signal. To display the pelvic veins and inferior vena cava with direct MR venography, it is useful to use a slightly less-diluted contrast agent (eg, 1:10). To achieve a superior contrast-to-noise ratio, which translates into better image quality and a detailed depiction of the more peripheral venous anatomy, a dedicated vascular coil should be used.

Indirect gadolinium-enhanced MR venography is another means of visualizing the inferior vena cava and the iliac, femoral, and distal extremity veins. Recently published studies have demonstrated that gadolinium-enhanced MR venography provides excellent assessment of inferior vena cava and iliac veins and is equivalent to or even better than conventional venography in delineating DVT [14,58,63,64]. Furthermore, diagnostic conspicuity and contrast were improved significantly using intravascular contrast agents compared with conventional extracellular contrast agents [50].

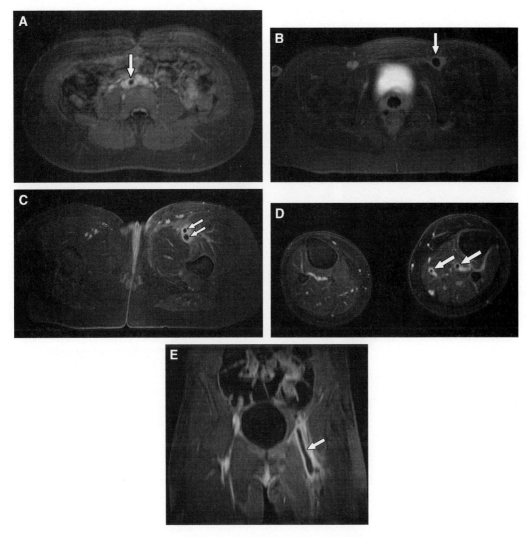

Fig. 6. An 18-year-old woman suffering from a swollen left leg and pain at rest was referred for the evaluation of DVT (*arrows*). Multistation high-spatial-resolution contrast-enhanced 3-D data sets of the entire legs were acquired by combining the continuous moving table technique and surface coils in the equilibrium phase after injection of a single dose of contrast agent. (*A–D*) Images show the thrombosed inferior vena cava, common femoral vein, superficial and deep femoral vein, and clotted fibular and posterior tibial veins. (*E*) Coronal reformatted MR image of the pelvis shows extent of thrombus (*arrow*) in the left superficial femoral vein.

Although it has been reported that subtraction techniques for indirect MR venography add little diagnostic value for the assessment of thromboembolism and that contrast enhancement of arterial vessel segments did not cause difficulties in detecting thrombotic material in the veins [58], the generation of pure MR venograms reduces image interpretation and reporting time. In a recent study, a double-subtraction algorithm, in which two early and two late measurements were used, was evaluated. Images of higher venous signal intensity were obtained with the double-subtraction algorithm than with a single-subtraction algorithm. This technique was called "venous-enhanced subtracted peak arterial MR venography". It created a pure 3-D MR venogram without the need to cannulate a dorsal foot vein [41].

Little is known about the accuracy of indirect visualization of the deep veins in lower extremities. Kluge et al [63] and Aschauer et al [47] have shown good correlation compared with conventional venography in evaluation of DVT in the calf. Larsson et al [48], however, reported sensitivity and specificity values merely in the range of 21% to 58% for vessels below the knee, although they used intravascular contrast agents. Further studies are needed. High-resolution 3-D VIBE imaging seems to offer new opportunities (Fig. 6). The combination of the continuous moving table technique and surface coils will allow high-resolution MR venography in the equilibrium phase, even of the whole body, using a single-dose injection of contrast agent.

A major advantage of MR angiography over alternative diagnostic strategies for investigation

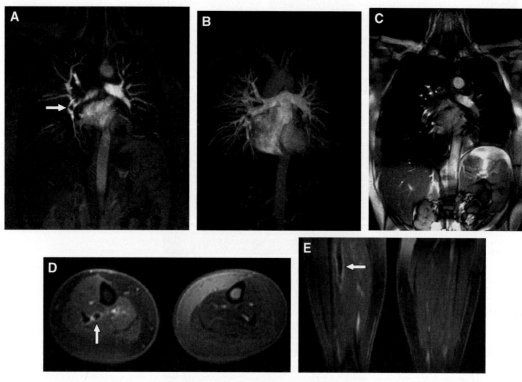

Fig. 7. A 43-year-old man with dyspnea and a swollen right lower limb was referred to exclude pulmonary embolism A MR angiogram of the pulmonary vasculature was complemented by a MR venogram of the pelvic and femoral veins in one session. (*A*) Coronal image from a MR pulmonary angiogram shows a filling defect consistent with an embolus in the right main pulmonary artery extending into the right lower lobe artery (*arrow*). (*B*) A MIP MR venogram of the same data set. (*C*) A real-time TrueFISP data set in corresponding coronal views also depicts the thrombus material. This data set was acquired before the injection of contrast agent. (*D*) Following the MR angiogram of the pulmonary arteries, indirect high-spatial-resolution venography of the peripheral veins from the pelvis to the lower limbs was performed. Thrombus material in the veins of the right lower limb could be visualized (*arrow*). (*E*) Coronal reformatted MR image of the lower leg shows the extent of the thrombus (*arrow*) in the right fibularis vein.

of patients with suspected thromboembolic disease relates to the fact that MR venography of the pelvic and femoral veins may be complemented by MR angiography of the pulmonary vasculature. Recently, some investigators have combined CT pulmonary angiography with venous-phase imaging of the lower extremity and pelvic veins, revealing excellent correlation with sonography and the discovery of clinically important, unsuspected DVT [8,9]. Nevertheless, the feasibility of combined MR protocols (Fig. 7) has still to be determined.

Ultrafast 3-D data acquisitions in conjunction with fast table repositioning permits rapid chase of the contrast bolus through several vascular territories, even extending to whole-body MR angiography [65]. In the near future whole-body indirect MR venography with a single-dose injection of contrast agent is likely to become available and provide high spatial resolution in the equilibrium phase.

Venous malformations

Congenital vascular malformations may present as isolated, small, circumscribed lesions or as complex vascular masses affecting the venous, arterial, or lymphatic system [66,67]. They differ in structural and topographic appearance and develop as a result of unknown genetic and environmental influences on the primitive vascular system in early embryonic life [68]. Subclassification of peripheral congenital vascular malformations remained poorly structured because of the heterogeneous morphologic and functional characteristics of the malformations. Generally, they are classified into slow-flow malformations (capillary, venous, lymphatic, capillary-venous, or capillary-lymphatic-venous malformations) and high-flow malformations (arterio-venous fistulas or arteriovenous malformations).

Venous malformations are the most common vascular malformations and involve the head and neck in about 40% of affected persons and the extremities and trunk in 40% and 20%, respectively [10]. Treatment depends on the local extent of the malformation. Optimal therapeutic stratification requires a comprehensive evaluation of feeding and draining vessels and of adjacent structures. MR imaging has become established as an attractive method to evaluate venous malformations by displaying their extent and their morphologic and functional characteristics (Fig. 8) [69–72]. The standard protocol should include T1-weighted,

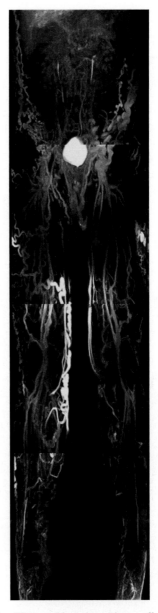

Fig. 8. An 18-year-old male patient suffering from Küppel-Trenauny syndrome. The coronal contrast-enhanced 3-D MR venogram (MIP) visualizes excessive varicosities with venous return mainly through superficial collaterals. Pelvic suprapubic and retroperitoneal collaterals can be seen as well.

T2-weighted, and dynamic contrast-enhanced and late-phase equilibrium fat-saturated T1-weighted sequences. Heavily T2-weighted sequences are highly accurate in delineating vascular malformations. Because of the inherent signal characteristics of this technique, the fluid-filled vascular structures are extremely bright, whereas the surrounding tissues are totally dark. A gradient-echo T2*-weighted sequence can be helpful for detecting hemorrhage or thrombosis. The use of a contrast medium allows venous and arterial malformations to be differentiated from those with lymphatic involvement. Time-resolved contrast-enhanced 3-D MR angiography allows analysis of the different phases and thus permits evaluation of the speed and intensities of blood flow over time (Fig. 9) [73].

Summary

MR venography has successfully shown its potential to evaluate DVT, central venous pathology, and anatomic variants such as venous malformations with high accuracy and has become a supplementary imaging technique to conventional venography, duplex sonography, and CT. Technical limitations, high cost, limited availability, and logical constraints still prevent widespread clinical use, however. As MR

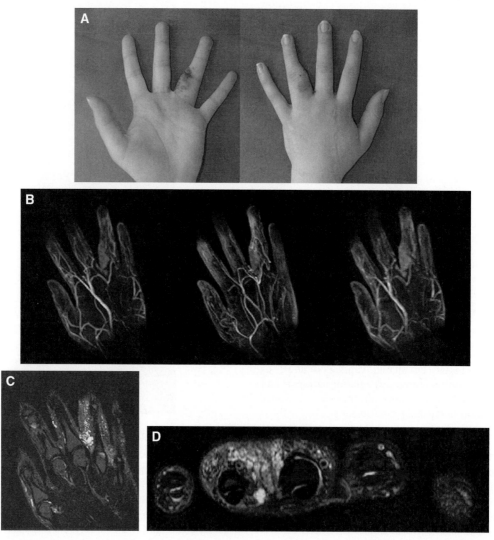

Fig. 9. A 17-year-old female patient with a venous vascular malformation in the fourth digit of the left hand. (*A*) Photographs of the palm and dorsum of the left hand show the ectatic veins and dermal changes in the affected finger. (*B*) Time-resolved MR imaging of the vascular malformation. Early-, venous-, and late-phase PC-enhanced MR angiograms show vascular enhancement patterns of venous vascular malformation. Coronal (*C*) and transverse (*D*) short-tau inversion recovery images reveal that the surrounding subcutaneous and muscular tissues are involved.

technology further improves and becomes more readily available, the role of MR venography in evaluating thromboembolic disease will probably expand. New contrast agents are likely to further improve the technique.

References

[1] Kearon C. Natural history of venous thromboembolism. Semin Vasc Med 2001;1:27–38.

[2] Benenati JF, Becker GJ, Mail JT, et al. Digital subtraction venography in central venous obstruction. AJR Am J Roentgenol 1986;147:685–8.

[3] Lensing AW, Levi MM, Buller HR, et al. Diagnosis of deep-vein thrombosis using an objective Doppler method. Ann Intern Med 1990;113:9–13.

[4] Bettmann MA, Robbins A, Braun SD, et al. Contrast venography of the leg: diagnostic efficacy, tolerance, and complication rates with ionic and nonionic contrast media. Radiology 1987;165:113–6.

[5] Baxter GM. The role of ultrasound in deep venous thrombosis. Clin Radiol 1997;52:1–3.

[6] Turkstra F, Kuijer PM, van Beek EJ, et al. Diagnostic utility of ultrasonography of leg veins in patients suspected of having pulmonary embolism. Ann Intern Med 1997;126:775–81.

[7] Wells PS, Lensing AW, Davidson BL, et al. Accuracy of ultrasound for the diagnosis of deep venous thrombosis in asymptomatic patients after orthopedic surgery. A meta-analysis. Ann Intern Med 1995;122:47–53.

[8] Katz DS, Loud PA, Bruce D, et al. Combined CT venography and pulmonary angiography: a comprehensive review. Radiographics 2002; 22 Spec No:S3–19; discussion S20–14.

[9] Loud PA, Katz DS, Klippenstein DL, et al. Combined CT venography and pulmonary angiography in suspected thromboembolic disease: diagnostic accuracy for deep venous evaluation. AJR Am J Roentgenol 2000;174:61–5.

[10] Butty S, Hagspiel KD, Leung DA, et al. Body MR venography. Radiol Clin North Am 2002;40:899–919.

[11] Carpenter JP, Holland GA, Baum RA, et al. Magnetic resonance venography for the detection of deep venous thrombosis: comparison with contrast venography and duplex Doppler ultrasonography. J Vasc Surg 1993;18:734–41.

[12] Erdman WA, Weinreb JC, Cohen JM, et al. Venous thrombosis: clinical and experimental MR imaging. Radiology 1986;161:233–8.

[13] Evans AJ, Sostman HD, Knelson MH, et al. 1992 ARRS Executive Council Award. Detection of deep venous thrombosis: prospective comparison of MR imaging with contrast venography. AJR Am J Roentgenol 1993;161:131–9.

[14] Lebowitz JA, Rofsky NM, Krinsky GA, et al. Gadolinium-enhanced body MR venography with subtraction technique. AJR Am J Roentgenol 1997;169:755–8.

[15] Holtz DJ, Debatin JF, McKinnon GC, et al. MR venography of the calf: value of flow-enhanced time-of-flight echoplanar imaging. AJR Am J Roentgenol 1996;166:663–8.

[16] Lenz GW, Haacke EM, Masaryk TJ, et al. In-plane vascular imaging: pulse sequence design and strategy. Radiology 1988;166:875–82.

[17] Bradley WG Jr, Waluch V. Blood flow: magnetic resonance imaging. Radiology 1985;154:443–50.

[18] Dumoulin CL, Hart HR Jr. Magnetic resonance angiography. Radiology 1986;161:717–20.

[19] Constantinesco A, Mallet JJ, Bonmartin A, et al. Spatial or flow velocity phase encoding gradients in NMR imaging. Magn Reson Imaging 1984;2:335–40.

[20] Edelman RR, Zhao B, Liu C, et al. MR angiography and dynamic flow evaluation of the portal venous system [see comments]. AJR Am J Roentgenol 1989;153:755–60.

[21] Pelc NJ, Herfkens RJ, Shimakawa A, et al. Phase contrast cine magnetic resonance imaging. Magn Reson Q 1991;7:229–54.

[22] Wright GA, Nishimura DG, Macovski A. Flow-independent magnetic resonance projection angiography. Magn Reson Med 1991;17:126–40.

[23] Brittain JH, Olcott EW, Szuba A, et al. Three-dimensional flow-independent peripheral angiography. Magn Reson Med 1997;38:343–54.

[24] Gronas R, Kalman PG, Kucey DS, et al. Flow-independent angiography for peripheral vascular disease: initial in-vivo results. J Magn Reson Imaging 1997;7:637–43.

[25] Wright GA, Hu BS, Macovski A. 1991 I.I Rabi Award. Estimating oxygen saturation of blood in vivo with MR imaging at 1.5 T. J Magn Reson Imaging 1991;1:275–83.

[26] Li KC, Wright GA, Pelc LR, et al. Oxygen saturation of blood in the superior mesenteric vein: in vivo verification of MR imaging measurements in a canine model. Work in progress. Radiology 1995;194:321–5.

[27] Bluemke DA, Wolf RL, Tani I, et al. Extremity veins: evaluation with fast-spin-echo MR venography. Radiology 1997;204:562–5.

[28] Gallix BP, Achard-Lichere C, Dauzat M, et al. Flow-independent magnetic resonance venography of the calf. J Magn Reson Imaging 2003;17:421–6.

[29] Plein S, Bloomer TN, Ridgway JP, et al. Steady-state free precession magnetic resonance imaging of the heart: comparison with segmented k-space gradient-echo imaging. J Magn Reson Imaging 2001;14:230–6.

[30] Barkhausen J, Goyen M, Ruhm SG, et al. Assessment of ventricular function with single breath-hold real-time steady-state free precession cine MR imaging. AJR Am J Roentgenol 2002;178:731–5.

[31] Spuentrup E, Buecker A, Stuber M, et al. MR-venography using high resolution True-FISP. Rofo 2001;173:686–90.

[32] Prince MR. Gadolinium-enhanced MR aortography. Radiology 1994;191:155–64.

[33] Shinde TS, Lee VS, Rofsky NM, et al. Three-dimensional gadolinium-enhanced MR venographic evaluation of patency of central veins in the thorax: initial experience. Radiology 1999;213:555–60.

[34] Goyen M, Barkhausen J, Kuehl H, et al. [Contrast-enhanced 3D MR venography of central thoracic veins: preliminary experience]. Rofo 2001;173: 356–61 [in German].

[35] Ruehm S, Zimny K, Debatin J. Direct contrast-enhanced 3D MR venography. Eur Radiol 2001; 11:102–12.

[36] Ruehm SG, Wiesner W, Debatin JF. Pelvic and lower extremity veins: contrast-enhanced three-dimensional MR venography with a dedicated vascular coil-initial experience. Radiology 2000;215: 421–7.

[37] Broglia L, Ambrogi G, Rossi M, et al. Upper limb deep venous thrombosis: evaluation with contrast-enhanced MR venography. In: Proceedings of the 12th European Congress of Radiology. Vienna (Austria); Springer-Verlag: 2000. p. 300.

[38] Prince MR. Contrast-enhanced MR angiography: theory and optimization. Magn Reson Imaging Clin N Am 1998;6:257–67.

[39] Rofsky NM, Lee VS, Laub G, et al. Abdominal MR imaging with a volumetric interpolated breath-hold examination. Radiology 1999;212:876–84.

[40] Biederer J, Liess C, Charalambous N, et al. Volumetric interpolated contrast-enhanced MRA for the diagnosis of pulmonary embolism in an ex vivo system. J Magn Reson Imaging 2004;19: 428–37.

[41] Fraser DG, Moody AR, Morgan PS, et al. Diagnosis of lower-limb deep venous thrombosis: a prospective blinded study of magnetic resonance direct thrombus imaging. Ann Intern Med 2002;136: 89–98.

[42] Moody AR, Pollock JG, O'Connor AR, et al. Lower-limb deep venous thrombosis: direct MR imaging of the thrombus. Radiology 1998;209:349–55.

[43] Francis CW, Totterman S. Magnetic resonance imaging of deep vein thrombi correlates with response to thrombolytic therapy. Thromb Haemost 1995;73: 386–91.

[44] Schmitz SA, Winterhalter S, Schiffler S, et al. USPIO-enhanced direct MR imaging of thrombus: preclinical evaluation in rabbits. Radiology 2001; 221:237–43.

[45] Chambon C, Clement O, Le Blanche A, et al. Superparamagnetic iron oxides as positive MR contrast agents: in vitro and in vivo evidence. Magn Reson Imaging 1993;11:509–19.

[46] Mayo-Smith WW, Saini S, Slater G, et al. MR contrast material for vascular enhancement: value of superparamagnetic iron oxide. AJR Am J Roentgenol 1996;166:73–7.

[47] Aschauer M, Deutschmann HA, Stollberger R, et al. Value of a blood pool contrast agent in MR venography of the lower extremities and pelvis: preliminary results in 12 patients. Magn Reson Med 2003; 50:993–1002.

[48] Larsson EM, Sunden P, Olsson CG, et al. MR venography using an intravascular contrast agent: results from a multicenter phase 2 study of dosage. AJR Am J Roentgenol 2003;180:227–32.

[49] Prince MR, Sostman HD. MR venography: unsung and underutilized. Radiology 2003;226:630–2.

[50] Sharafuddin MJ, Stolpen AH, Dang YM, et al. Comparison of MS-325- and gadodiamide-enhanced MR venography of iliocaval veins. J Vasc Interv Radiol 2002;13:1021–7.

[51] Martel AL, Fraser D, Delay GS, et al. Separating arterial and venous components from 3D dynamic contrast-enhanced MRI studies using factor analysis. Magn Reson Med 2003;49:928–33.

[52] Weissleder R, Elizondo G, Wittenberg J, et al. Ultrasmall superparamagnetic iron oxide: characterization of a new class of contrast agents for MR imaging. Radiology 1990;175:489–93.

[53] Schmitz SA, Winterhalter S, Schiffler S, et al. USPIO-enhanced direct thrombus MRI. Acad Radiol 2002;9(Suppl 2):S339–40.

[54] Finn JP, Zisk JH, Edelman RR, et al. Central venous occlusion: MR angiography. Radiology 1993;187: 245–51.

[55] Hartnell GG, Hughes LA, Finn JP, et al. Magnetic resonance angiography of the central chest veins. A new gold standard? Chest 1995;107:1053–7.

[56] Li W, David V, Kaplan R, et al. Three-dimensional low dose gadolinium-enhanced peripheral MR venography. J Magn Reson Imaging 1998;8:630–3.

[57] Thornton MJ, Ryan R, Varghese JC, et al. A three-dimensional gadolinium-enhanced MR venography technique for imaging central veins. AJR Am J Roentgenol 1999;173:999–1003.

[58] Kroencke TJ, Taupitz M, Arnold R, et al. Three-dimensional gadolinium-enhanced magnetic resonance venography in suspected thrombo-occlusive disease of the central chest veins. Chest 2001;120: 1570–6.

[59] Lanzer P, Gross GM, Keller FS, et al. Sequential 2D inflow venography: initial clinical observations. Magn Reson Med 1991;19:470–6.

[60] Spritzer CE, Sostman HD, Wilkes DC, et al. Deep venous thrombosis: experience with gradient-echo MR imaging in 66 patients. Radiology 1990;177: 235–41.

[61] Spritzer CE, Arata MA, Freed KS. Isolated pelvic deep venous thrombosis: relative frequency as detected with MR imaging. Radiology 2001;219:521–5.

[62] Ruehm SG, Wiesner W, Debatin JF. Pelvic and lower extremity veins: contrast-enhanced three-dimensional MR venography with a dedicated vas-

cular coil-initial experience. Radiology 2000;215: 421–7.

[63] Kluge A, Rominger M, Schonburg M, et al. [Indirect MR venography: contrast medium protocols, post-processing and combination in diagnosing pulmonary emboli with MRI]. Rofo 2004;176:976–84 [in German].

[64] Fraser DG, Moody AR, Davidson IR, et al. Deep venous thrombosis: diagnosis by using venous enhanced subtracted peak arterial MR venography versus conventional venography. Radiology 2003; 226:812–20.

[65] Goyen M, Quick HH, Debatin JF, et al. Whole-body three-dimensional MR angiography with a rolling table platform: initial clinical experience. Radiology 2002;224:270–7.

[66] Breugem CC, van Der Horst CM, Hennekam RC. Progress toward understanding vascular malformations. Plast Reconstr Surg 2001;107:1509–23.

[67] Szilagyi DE, Smith RF, Elliott JP, et al. Congenital arteriovenous anomalies of the limbs. Arch Surg 1976;111:423–9.

[68] Mulliken JB, Glowacki J. Classification of pediatric vascular lesions. Plast Reconstr Surg 1982;70:120–1.

[69] Cohen JM, Weinreb JC, Redman HC. Arteriovenous malformations of the extremities: MR imaging. Radiology 1986;158:475–9.

[70] Meyer JS, Hoffer FA, Barnes PD, et al. Biological classification of soft-tissue vascular anomalies: MR correlation. AJR Am J Roentgenol 1991;157: 559–64.

[71] Huch Boni RA, Brunner U, Bollinger A, et al. Management of congenital angiodysplasia of the lower limb: magnetic resonance imaging and angiography versus conventional angiography. Br J Radiol 1995; 68:1308–15.

[72] Baker LL, Dillon WP, Hieshima GB, et al. Hemangiomas and vascular malformations of the head and neck: MR characterization. AJNR Am J Neuroradiol 1993;14:307–14.

[73] Herborn CU, Goyen M, Lauenstein TC, et al. Comprehensive time-resolved MRI of peripheral vascular malformations. AJR Am J Roentgenol 2003; 181:729–35.

ELSEVIER
SAUNDERS

Magn Reson Imaging Clin N Am
13 (2005) 131–151

MAGNETIC
RESONANCE
IMAGING CLINICS
of North America

MR Angiography in Patients with Renal Disease

Henrik J. Michaely, MD*, Stefan O. Schoenberg, MD,
Johannes R. Rieger, MD, Maximilian F. Reiser, MD

*Department of Clinical Radiology, University Hospitals, Ludwig Maximilians University-Munich,
Grosshadern Marchioninistrasse 15, Munich 81377, Germany*

Three-dimensional contrast-enhanced (3-D CE) MR angiographic examinations of the renal arteries have been widely used in clinical practice since their introduction approximately 10 years ago [1–3]. The previously used MR angiographic techniques, time-of-flight MR angiography [4] and phase-contrast (PC) MR angiography [5], have major limitations for imaging the abdominal vessels. Today, almost every scanner in use meets the hardware requirements for 3-D CE MR angiography. A complete examination can be performed easily in 20 minutes and yields high-resolution, high-contrast images of the abdominal arteries. 3-D CE MR angiography has become a widely accepted imaging technique, especially in patients with suspected renal artery disease. In this application, it has some key advantages over its alternatives, standard X-ray angiography and CT angiography. 3-D CE MR angiography does not expose the patient to ionizing radiation and therefore was proposed and has been used as screening technique [6–9]. In properly screened patient populations, few if any serious risks are associated with 3-D CE MR angiography, whereas conventional X-ray angiography carries a minimal risk of distal embolization and arterial wall dissection. Furthermore, both X-ray angiography and CT angiography require the use of iodine-based contrast agents, which are potentially nephrotoxic. This additional concern is significant, particularly in patients with impaired renal function, who are the very individuals likely to require renal artery evaluation [10–13]. The gadolinium chelate contrast agents used in

3-D CE MR angiography, however, are safe even in patients with renal insufficiency [14]. The 3-D volumetric nature of 3-D CE MR angiography allows easy reformatting and the exact depiction of complicated vessel anatomy, such as renal transplant arteries. In addition, 3-D CE MR angiography can be extended easily into a comprehensive renal examination with added MR-flow and MR-perfusion measurements.

These capabilities and advantages have made 3-D CE MR angiography the mainstay of vascular MR studies. The clinical indications for renal MR angiography examinations are growing rapidly.

So far, the main indication for 3-D CE MR angiography of the renal arteries has been renovascular disease, especially atherosclerotic renal artery stenosis (RAS). Atherosclerotic RAS can be found in 90% of patients with RAS; fibromuscular dysplasia (FMD) accounts for the remaining 10% of cases [15–18]. RAS is characterized by impaired renal blood flow and reactive hypertension resulting from renin release and the activation of the lipoxygenase pathway [19,20]. RAS is a rare entity with a prevalence of approximately 4% [21]. The prevalence of atherosclerotic RAS increases with age, however, and in patients with hypertension, diabetes mellitus, or coronary artery disease the prevalence of RAS can reach 47% [15,22–25]. If not detected and treated correctly, RAS leads to ischemic nephropathy and end-stage renal disease [16]. RAS is estimated to account for 10% to 40% of end-stage renal disease in patients without identified primary renal disease [26].

Recent indications for 3-D CE MR angiography include the surveillance of dialysis grafts [27–30] and the assessment of renal transplants using a combination of morphologic sequences, MR angiography, and functional sequences [31–34].

---

* Corresponding author.
E-mail address: henrik.michaely@med.uni-muenchen.de (H.J. Michaely).

1064-9689/05/$ - see front matter © 2005 Elsevier Inc. All rights reserved.
doi:10.1016/j.mric.2004.12.007

These functional sequences include MR perfusion measurements based on spin-labeling techniques [35–37], CE techniques [38–44], PC MR-flow measurements [45–47], and blood oxygen level–dependent techniques [48–51]. With functional imaging, new perspectives for renal MR imaging arise, such as the detection of isolated parenchymal disease, the detection of acute renal failure, and the assessment of split renal function [52,53].

Imaging techniques

Technical considerations

The clinical requirement for high-resolution 3-D CE MR angiography has driven the hardware development in the past years, with a focus on the improvement of the gradient systems. The gradient systems in current scanners, with a gradient strength of 45 mT/m and slew rate of 200 mT/m/s, allow repetition times of about 3 milliseconds and thus the imaging of an entire high-resolution 3-D dataset within one breath-hold period. 3-D CE MR angiography typically is performed using a spoiled gradient echo (GRE) sequence acquiring the entire 3-D data set in 20 to 30 seconds. To decrease scanning times, partial Fourier and asymmetric echo techniques are commonly used. Typically, a spatial resolution of $1.5 \times 1.5 \times 1.5$ mm^3 is achieved. This spatial resolution, however, is still significantly inferior to that of digital subtraction angiography by a factor of three to five. Therefore, a different approach to improve the spatial resolution of the 3-D CE MR angiography has been introduced: new data sampling and reconstruction methods such as parallel imaging. Parallel-imaging techniques require multichannel MR scanners with multiple receiver coils used simultaneously to undersample the data. With a given number of phase-encoding steps, the acquisition time can be reduced by an acceleration factor, or the spatial resolution can be increased by an acceleration factor. The current standard 1.5-T MR systems typically allow acceleration factors of two to four. All vendors offer parallel-imaging options for their scanners marketed as ASSET (General Electric, Milwaukee, Wisconsin), iPAT (Siemens Medical Systems, Erlangen, Germany) or SENSE (Philips Medical Systems, Best, The Netherlands). With parallel-imaging techniques, only a given part of the data defined by the acceleration factor is acquired, and the undersampled images must be unfolded. Two techniques and their derivates are used to reconstruct the undersampled data: simultaneous acquisition of spatial harmonics (SMASH) [54,55] and sensitivity encoding (SENSE) [56,57]. SENSE uses a prescan to acquire the coil sensitivity profiles before the actual scan. With these profiles, the aliased image is reconstructed in the image domain. SMASH relies on the ability to approximate low-order harmonics of the desired field of view (FOV) by linear combination of sensitivity functions in the k-space. Both techniques can be combined with conventional techniques, such as fractional echo or partial Fourier approaches. With parallel imaging, however, the signal-to-noise-ratio (S/N) is inversely proportional to the square root of the acceleration factor times a geometry factor, g. The geometry factor g depends on the receiver coil arrangement. Therefore, dedicated coils with multiple receiver elements with optimized geometry should be used for parallel imaging. Using an acceleration factor of two or three on a high-field-strength MR system equipped with high performance gradients, the authors acquire a 3-D CE MR angiography with a submillimeter isotropic resolution of 0.9 mm^3 within a single breath-hold. Fig. 1 shows a patient without RAS. The scanner allows acceleration factors to be selected in the phase-encoding direction and parallel imaging in three gradient directions. Therefore, an acceleration factor of 12 is theoretically possible. These higher acceleration factors will certainly be exploited in the future, when higher field strengths offset the possible S/N

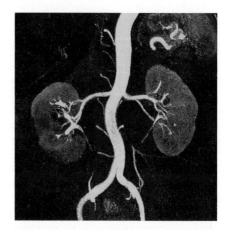

Fig. 1. MIP view of a 3-D CE MR angiography (resolution, 0.9 mm^3; iPAT factor, 3; acquisition time, 21 seconds) (Magnetom Avanto, Siemens) in a 49-year-old patient with suspected renal artery stenosis. The renal arteries are patent and can be followed into the periphery. There is already excretion of contrast agent resulting from the previous perfusion measurement.

drop. Today, to compensate for the S/N loss associated with parallel imaging, the 1-molar contrast agent gadobutrol (Gadovist; Schering AG, Berlin, Germany) or higher-relaxivity contrast agents such as Gd-BOPTA (Multihance; Bracco SpA, Milan, Italy), with a dose of 0.1 to 0.15 mmol/kg body weight, can be used. Gadobutrol has already been approved in Europe for MR angiography and has the additional advantage of a better-defined bolus and hence better arterial contrast.

Renal anatomy

Every renal MR examination needs to include pulse sequences that deliver detailed anatomic information about the kidneys and the perinephric tissue. These sequences typically consist of T2-weighted (T2W) imaging in a transverse orientation and T1-weighted (T1W) imaging before and after contrast administration in a second orientation, preferably coronal. Postcontrast T1W images may add additional information if performed with spectral fat saturation. Anatomic imaging must enable the determination of the kidney size, the visual assessment of the renal parenchyma, the detection of focal renal lesions, such as cysts, renal cell carcinomas, or angiomyolipomas, and yield information about perinephric masses or lymph nodes. Standard T1W GRE pulse sequences and T2W turbo spin echo pulse sequences used for other abdominal applications can be used to detect these lesions. To correct for respiratory-induced motion, respiratory gating with navigator correction should be used.

MR angiography

3-D CE MR angiography is performed using fast 3-D GRE sequences. For correct depiction of the arteries, the sequence parameters and the administration of contrast agent need to be planned carefully. Because the voxel size and image contrast ultimately determine the diagnostic value of the study, it is essential to find the best compromise between high S/N and high spatial resolution within the patient's breath-hold time. The FOV should be kept as small as possible to allow high resolution but should be large enough to avoid aliasing. Typically, a FOV of 350 mm is suitable. A slab thickness of approximately 80 mm should be chosen to contain entire abdominal aorta and its main branches. A native 3-D MR angiography can be obtained first and may be used for subtraction. At Ludwig Maximilians University, which has Siemens MR scanners, a spoiled 3-D fast

low angle shot sequence with generalized autocalibrating partially parallel acquisitions (GRAPPA) and an integrated parallel acquisition technique factor of two is used with the following parameters: TR = 3.79 milliseconds, TE = 1.39 milliseconds, FOV read = 400 mm, FOV phase = 87%, slices per slab = 80, slice thickness = 0.9 mm, frequency-encoding steps = 512, flip angle = 25°, bandwidth = 50 Hz/pixel. These parameters yield a voxel size of $1.0 \times 0.9 \times 1.0$ mm^3. Three phases of the MR angiography should be acquired: the arterial phase, the venous phase about 20 seconds after the arterial scan, and a delayed phase. For high S/N and minimal venous contamination, exact synchronization of the acquisition of the k-space center, the area of greatest image contrast, with the peak of the contrast agent bolus is crucial. If the acquisition starts before the arrival of the contrast agent bolus, the desired arteries are not seen. If the center of k-space is obtained during the actual arrival of the bolus, when gadolinium concentration is rapidly increasing, ringing artifacts occur. If the acquisition is too late, venous enhancement may obscure arteries and significantly impair the diagnostic value of the study.

There are several methods to ensure proper timing for 3-D CE MR angiography. The authors use a test-bolus of 2 mL of contrast agent followed by a 30-mL saline flush to determine the correct acquisition timing. Automatic or semiautomatic MR-fluoroscopy approaches, such as CareBolus (Siemens), SmartPrep (General Electric) or BolusTrak (Philips), can be used instead. If venous contamination is feared or a high-flow fistula is suspected, the k-space can also be filled using an elliptic centric phase ordering [58]. In an elliptic centric k-space acquisition, the k-space is filled from the center to the periphery using an elliptical or spiral trajectory. The combination of elliptic centric k-space acquisition with MR fluoroscopy can be advantageous, because the central k-space is filled first, when the arrival of the contrast agent bolus is detected. The resulting image has purely arterial contrast because the venous enhancement takes place when the periphery of the k-space is read out. The contrast agent is administered through an antecubital vein using an 18-gauge or 20-gauge needle at a flow rate of 2 mL/second followed by a 30-mL saline flush at the same flow rate. The typical dose of a traditional extracellular gadolinium chelate contrast agent (0.5-molar) is 0.2 mmol/kg, which corresponds to a 30- to 40-mL bolus, depending on patient weight.

Another way to obtain a renal MR angiography without the need for bolus-timing techniques is to use time-resolved MR angiography techniques, such as multiphasic MR angiography [59], or undersampled techniques, such as time-resolved imaging of contrast kinetics (TRICKS) [60], which show enable dynamic visualization transit of the contrast agent. TRICKS undersamples the k-space periphery and relatively oversamples the center of k-space, so the changing contrast information is updated more often than the unchanging detail information. The peripheral k-space data are shared among the individual image sets. Although these dynamic techniques may be valuable for the detection of delayed flow (eg, in dissecting aneurysms or hemodynamically significant RAS), they suffer from relatively poor spatial resolution compared with standard 3-D CE MR angiography. As a rule of thumb, the voxel size of dynamic studies is twice the voxel size of a current state-of-the-art 3-D CE MR angiography. Dynamic imaging techniques may become more practical with higher-field-strength scanners that will allow acceptable spatial resolution.

A relatively new technique for renal MR angiography is to use steady-state free-precession sequences with cardiac and respiratory gating with multiple averages. The first published results report on the use of slice-selective inversion pulses to null the background signal [61,62]. The inherently high vessel contrast obviates the need for contrast agent and avoids the possible errors associated with the bolus timing. Other interesting aspects of this approach are the use of both respiratory and cardiac gating (ie, double gating) and the multiple averages that allow assessment the more distal parts of the renal arteries in healthy volunteers. The visualized part of the vasculature, however, is limited to a relatively small FOV comprising only the renal arteries. Whether this technique will gain acceptance remains to be seen.

Flow measurements

Cine MR using PC has been used to measure flow for at least 10 years [63–65]. Cine PC can be used for the assessment of hemodynamic significance in cases of RAS [45,66,67] and is commonly used as an adjunct to the 3-D CE MR angiography. Some authors have correlated flow parameters with kidney volume to determine the renal volume index to predict the therapeutic success of revascularization [68]. Cine PC flow measurements are based on the principle that spins moving along a gradient experience a phase shift that is proportional to their flow velocity. Retrospective or prospective cardiac gating is used to acquire flow data over the entire cardiac cycle. Cine PC flow measurements yield quantitative flow parameters, such as mean flow velocity, maximum flow velocity, mean temporal flow, and time to peak velocity. In addition, a Doppler-like flow profile can be performed to evaluate the blood flow qualitatively. The temporal resolution of the pulse sequence must not fall below 30 milliseconds to track the pulse-wave correctly and completely. Typical imaging parameters include a 256×256 matrix and a total acquisition time of 3 to 4 minutes, depending on the patient's heart rate. The velocity-encoding value (VENC) should be adjusted carefully to avoid phase aliasing, which occurs if the VENC is set too low (ie, below the peak velocity). Ideally the VENC should be set at or, preferably, just above the peak velocity of the blood flow being measured. In most patients, a VENC of 75 cm/s is appropriate for renal artery evaluation, but in cases of chronic heart failure or other low cardiac output, a lower VENC should be considered. The cine PC flow measurements need to be positioned exactly perpendicular to the vessel axis, with the vessel in the isocenter of the slice plane. This positioning can be performed quite easily on the maximum intensity projections (MIP) derived from the 3-D CE MR angiography. The imaging slice must not be positioned in a stenosis but rather 1 cm distal of the stenosis. If the imaging slice is positioned too close to or even in a stenosis, turbulent flow may generate incorrect results because of aliasing or intravoxel dephasing [69]. In scanners with high gradient strengths, eddy currents may occur and may hamper the flow measurements, making the results unrealistically low. Therefore, a thorough correction for background phase is important to achieve correct results.

To shorten the long acquisition times of the flow measurements, segmented echoplanar imaging (EPI) techniques have been proposed that allow data acquisition within a single breath-hold [70,71]. Even though segmented EPI techniques provide high temporal and spatial resolution, they have not been widely accepted because of the ghosting artifacts. In addition, dedicated ECG-gating systems are necessary to avoid the interference encountered during cardiac gating.

A recent approach to speed up dynamic MR measurements, including flow measurements, is k-t-broad use linear acquisition speed-up technique (BLAST) [72]. In k-t-BLAST, the spatiotemporal correlations in k-space are exploited. After a training phase, spatio-temporal filtering of data acquisition is applied in dynamic imaging. K-t-BLAST does not lead to a loss in S/N and can be performed with only a single receiver coil. Acceleration up to a factor of eight can be reached. K-t-BLAST can be combined with parallel imaging as well. Flow measurements with high temporal and spatial resolution can be obtained in 50 seconds with k-t-BLAST. The resulting quantitative and qualitative results correlate well with standard cine PC flow measurements [73].

Perfusion measurements

Although flow measurements display the flow in the large feeding vessels, perfusion measurements aim at demonstrating the capillary blood flow in the renal parenchyma and especially in the highly vascularized renal cortex. There are numerous rationales for performing perfusion measurements: first, to assess the impact of renal artery stenosis on the relevant renal parenchymal blood flow; second, to assist MR angiography in case of segmental RAS or in case of in-stent restenosis, both of which can be difficult to appreciate in the MR angiography; and third, to establish the diagnosis of parenchymal disease or impaired renal function in the absence of renovascular disease.

Currently there are two main approaches to renal perfusion measurements: arterial spin–labeling (ASL) techniques, which use blood as endogenous contrast agent, and CE techniques that are based on the imaging dynamics of gadolinium contrast agent. ASL techniques are attractive in that they are noninvasive and do not require the administration of contrast agents [74]. Different techniques have been proposed in the literature, but only animal studies or volunteer studies have been performed [36,75–77]. The main disadvantages that impede broad clinical application are the inherent low S/N and the susceptibility for artifacts. Most ASL techniques, such as flow-sensitive alternating inversion recovery (FAIR), measure the signal from arterial blood at a fixed inversion delay after magnetic labeling. Because no image information is sampled during this delay, FAIR measurements are inefficient and time consuming. To avoid this problem a Look-Locker acquisition has been proposed to sample not one but a series of images after each labeling pulse [78]. This technique also overcomes the limitation of ASL sequence in yielding only a single perfusion-weighted slice without the temporal perfusion information and thereby offers the possibility of absolute quantification. A true fast imaging with steady state precession readout for ASL sequences has been proposed recently to increase the S/N and to decrease the susceptibility for artifacts [35]. Even though these techniques are promising, and possible applications such as renal transplant surveillance are in sight, no clinical breakthrough has been achieved so far.

Unlike ASL techniques, CE MR perfusion techniques do not suffer from S/N limitations. The first renal perfusion studies were reported in 1989 [39]. Since then, the technique has evolved, but CE perfusion measurements are not yet widely applied clinically. The basic principle of CE MR perfusion is to administer a bolus of contrast agent and to visualize the arrival of the bolus by using dynamic imaging of the kidneys with a temporal resolution as high as possible. Only intravascular contrast agents allow a pure perfusion imaging; extracellular contrast agents always show some filtration. $T2^*$weighted GRE sequences use intravascular ultrasmall superparamagnetic iron oxide contrast agents such as SHU 555 C (Sehering AG) or NC 100150 (GE Health Care, Little Chalfont, United Kingdom). T1W turbo fast low angle shot (TurboFLASH) sequences use standard gadolinium chelate contrast agents, such as Gd-DTPA or Magnevist (Sehering AG), or macromolecular gadolinium chelates, such as gadomelitol or Vistarem (Guerbet, Paris, France).

Plotting the signal intensity of a user-defined region of interest over the kidney or the renal cortex yields a signal-intensity versus time (SIVT) curve. Fitting the first pass of the SIVT curves with a gamma variate fit delivers semiquantitative parameters such as mean transit time (MTT), time to maximum signal intensity (Tmax), the maximum upslope steepness (MUS), and the maximum signal intensity [79]. To obtain absolute quantitative perfusion parameters, the renal SIVT curves must be deconvoluted with the input function that is in the best case the SIVT curve of the renal artery. For practical reasons, the SIVT curve of the aorta is commonly chosen instead. The need for deconvolution, a complicated mathematical process, is probably the main obstacle to the widespread use of these techniques. Deconvolution can be calculated more easily with intravascular contrast agents such as MS-325 (Epix Pharmaceuticals, Boston, Massachusetts) or NC100150, which do not leave the vessel bed immediately [80–82]. At Ludwig Maximilians University, perfusion measurements are performed using a saturation-recovery

TurboFLASH sequence with a high temporal resolution of four slices per second. For saturation recovery, a series of three 90° pulses in a phase angle of 90° is applied, minimizing inflow effects and providing good signal linearity. The four slices assure good coverage of the renal parenchyma. The total acquisition time is 5 minutes to cover the first pass as well as the filtration of the contrast agent. With this technique, MTT, MUS, and Tmax showed significant differences between healthy kidneys and those with significant RAS. These findings demonstrate that renal blood flow is maintained until the threshold of the autoregulation capacity is crossed. Normally, the autoregulation fails in stenoses of more than 75% of vessel diameter [66].

MR renography

In contrast to perfusion measurements that focus on the (regional) parenchymal blood flow, MR renography aims at assessing the split renal function and the glomerular filtration rate (GFR) according to the method used in renal scintigraphy. MR renography depends on the administration and excretion of an extracellular contrast agent. Extracellular contrast agents such as Gd-DTPA or Gd-DOTA behave at the glomerulus like ^{99m}Tc-DTPA, the tracer used in renal scintigraphy. In contrast, ^{99}Tc-MAG3 is excreted by the tubules to a high degree. Therefore, ^{99}Tc-MAG3 scintigraphy reflects the active tubular excretion in addition to the GFR. Gadolinium chelate contrast agents are freely filtered at the glomerulus without tubular reabsorption or excretion [83]. Thus, their clearance is equivalent to the GFR [84–86]. Based on this property of extracellular contrast agents, Niendorf et al [85] developed a technique that measures the signal intensity in the renal artery and the renal vein and converts it into the gadolinium concentration of the renal artery and the renal vein. Because the lower signal intensity in the renal vein results from the filtration of the gadolinium, the GFR can be calculated from the concentrations of gadolinium and the patient's hematocrit [85]. A larger series reporting on this technique has not been published so far. More recent publications proposed the use of a steady-state free-precession technique [87] using 0.1 mmol/kg Gd-DTPA or a volume-interpolated breath-hold examination sequence for MR renography with a 2-mL Gd-DTPA bolus and temporal resolution of 3 seconds per 3-D data set [88]. From these data, SIVT curves over the kidney, the renal

cortex, and the medulla are obtained. Gates' [89] scintigraphic method allows the calculation of split renal function and GFR using the generated SIVT curves [41,90]. Captopril was used in some studies to increase specificity [87,88]. All these techniques showed good correlation with scintigraphy results. Captopril is an angiotensin I–converting enzyme inhibitor that reduces the arterial blood pressure. Captopril's mechanism of action is vasodilatation of the efferent vessel of the glomerula and thus reduces the transglomerular filtration pressure. In cases of RAS with impaired renal blood flow, the reduced transglomerular filtration pressure leads to a drop in GFR. Systematic studies that compare MR renography with scintigraphy are lacking, however, and none of these MR techniques is used regularly in clinical practice.

Applications

General remarks

Most renal MR angiography examinations are performed in patients with hypertension and with a clinical suspicion for RAS. A general diagnostic evaluation, including kidney size, length, assessment of the cortico-medullar differentiation, and the number of renal arteries, needs to be done as the first step of the examination. A normal kidney measures 12.5 cm in women and 13 cm in men in longest dimension and should have a smooth surface and reniform shape. Unilateral small kidneys can result from vascular disease, infarction, pyelonephritis, or ureteral obstruction, whereas bilateral small kidneys can arise from longstanding hypertension, late-stage amyloidosis, and hereditary nephropathies. Enlarged kidneys occur in the setting of renal vein thrombosis (RVT), cellular infiltration such as lymphoma or acute nephritis, glomerulonephritis, and early-stage amyloidosis.

The cortico-medullary differentiation (CMD) and the medullar pyramids can be seen on traditional noncontrast MR images. The renal cortex should be hypointense in T2W images and hyperintense in T1W images in relation to the medulla because of the higher water content of the medulla. On fat-suppressed T1W images, CMD may vanish in patients with a serum creatinine level greater than 3.5 mg/dL or with a serum creatinine level greater than 10.0 mg/dL. In these instances, CMD may not be seen even in CE scans [91]. Traditional T1W and T2W images are helpful in detecting renal congenital abnormalities of the kidneys such as horseshoe kidneys, renal agenesis, renal polycystic disease, and renal hypoplasia or dysplasia. Thorough attention must also be paid to the perirenal structures, especially the adrenal glands.

When analyzing data from 3-D CE MR angiography, one must rememberthat 17% to 24% of the kidneys are supplied by an accessory renal artery [92,93]. Accessory renal arteries are aberrant branches, usually originating directly from the aorta and serving only a small portion of the kidney. In rare cases they can also originate from other arteries. They often are longer and narrower than regular renal arteries, with a lower perfusion pressure and higher vascular resistance [92]. It is important to identify all renal vessels and, if possible, to measure the blood flow in all of them. Several studies have reported accuracies between 80% and 100% in detecting accessory renal arteries [94,95]. A recent multicenter trial reported MR angiography and digital subtraction angiography were in complete agreement in assessing the number of accessory renal arteries in only 82% of the cases (median range, 80% to 88% for seven readers) [96]. The frequency with which the number of accessory arteries was overestimated was similar for MR angiography and digital subtraction angiography. Good results have already been reported for the correct identification of the absolute number and the location of supernumerary vessels in kidney donors being evaluated before transplantation [97]. The significance of accessory RAS remains controversial, however. It is known that a high-grade stenosis of an accessory artery can trigger renin release, but the necessity for intervention is being questioned because of the small vessel caliber and the resulting risk of occlusion. Recent studies showed that the prevalence of accessory renal arteries was not increased in patients with hypertension [98]. Moreover, hemodynamically significant accessory RAS was found only in 1.5% of all patients with RAS, raising questions about the role of renal stenoses in the pathogenesis of renal hypertension [93].

Atherosclerotic renal artery stenosis

Up to 90% of RAS are caused by atherosclerotic vessel disease [16]. Because of the progressive nature of this disease [15,99,100], which can lead to ESRD [101], and the possibility of medical or interventional therapy [16,102], it is important to detect and grade atherosclerotic RAS correctly. Most patients with RAS are in or beyond their fifth decade and usually also suffer from other manifestations of atherosclerotic disease and hypertension,

such as coronary artery disease, peripheral artery disease, and diabetes. Atherosclerotic disease also affects the abdominal aorta and the other main branches that need to be incorporated in the analysis. In the renal artery, atherosclerosis usually leads to ostial stenoses or, rarely, to focal dissections. Distal RAS is rarely seen in atherosclerosis; if present, it affects the branching sites. Bilateral RAS occurs in 32% to 78% of the patients [103]. In cases of high-grade stenosis, collateral vessel webs through capsular and perforating arteries can be seen occasionally. Most stenoses show poststenotic dilatation, and they often are marked by eccentric position [104]. These stenoses may be underestimated, depending on the angle of vessel projection used in the analysis. The authors therefore strongly recommend obtaining reformats perpendicular to the vessel axis at the site of stenosis and distal to the stenosis. These means can measure the stenosis diameter, a measurement that is more robust than the typically used in-plane measurement [105]. For the grading of stenoses, the North American Symptomatic Cartoid Endarterectomy Trial criteria should be used. Correlations of area stenosis with intravascular ultrasound showed good results. When there is uncertainty regarding the hemodynamic relevance or the grade of a RAS, MR flow and perfusion measurements are necessary. MR flow measurements show a distinct loss of the early systolic peak with normal flow values in the case of low- to intermediate-grade RAS. In case of hemodynamically significant stenosis, the blood flow decreases significantly, and the flow profile becomes flattened. MR perfusion measurements show delayed arrival of contrast in the affected renal parenchyma with an elevated mean transit time and lowered MUS. Fig. 2 shows the comprehensive work-up in a patient with bilateral RAS including MR angiography, flow measurements, and MR perfusion measurements.

The literature reports excellent sensitivities and specificities for 3-D CE MR angiography for the detection of renal artery stenosis. Table 1 presents the results of all studies that included 50 or more patients. The recently presented Renal artery Diagnostic Imaging Study in Hypertension shows drastically poorer results, on the order of 60% to 70% for the correct grading of RAS by both CT angiography and MR angiography. This finding emphasizes the importance in grading stenoses of using cross-sectional reformats and flow or perfusion measurements to verify the findings [106]. In addition, it is common to find no or only a low-grade RAS with pathologic perfusion parameters

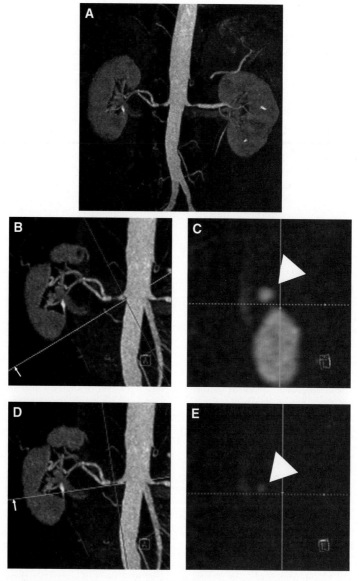

Fig. 2. (*A*) MIP view of a patient with bilateral high-grade atherosclerotic RAS. (*B–E*) To assess the real area of the stenosis, cross-sectional views of the right renal artery were obtained proximal to the stenosis (*B, C*) and in the stenosis (*D, E*). The perpendicular cut vessel is pointed out by an arrowhead (*C, E*). (*F*) The perfusion measurement in the same patient shows an inhomogeneous and slowed arrival of the contrast agent in the renal cortex. (*G*) For further evaluation, a SIVT curve was plotted that shows the patient's perfusion (*dashed line*) and the perfusion of a person without RAS (*solid line*) for comparison. The semiquantitative assessment yielded an elevated mean transit time of 30 seconds in this patient versus a mean transit time of 14 seconds in the healthy person. (*H*) The phase-contrast flow measurement shows a markedly decreased maximum flow velocity (*dashed line*) compared with the healthy person (*solid line*).

in a patient with hypertension. Biopsies of these kidneys often reveal parenchymal disease such as nephrosclerosis secondary to the hypertension. Therefore, MR perfusion measurements can help establish the diagnosis of parenchymal disease in the absence of RAS, as shown in Fig. 3 [79].

Imaging of associated disease

Atherosclerotic RAS is only one manifestation of systemic atherosclerotic disease. In patients undergoing cardiac catheterization, RAS prevalences of 39% were found, with 14.3% being high-

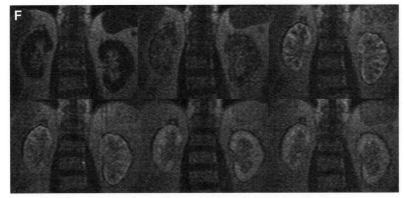

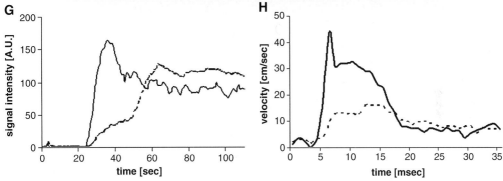

Fig. 2 (*continued*)

grade stenoses [107]. Also in patients with lower extremity occlusive disease or with aortic aneurysms, a RAS prevalence of 39% was reported [24]. Coronary artery disease, myocardial infarction, increased carotid intimal medial thickness, increased internal carotid artery stenosis, and major ECG abnormalities are significantly more common in patients with renovascular disease [108]. In Fig. 4, MR angiographic studies show associated disease in a patient with RAS and coronary artery disease. In addition, a substantially higher morbidity and mortality has been found in patients with RAS undergoing stent therapy. This relationship is amplified further in the presence of renal insufficiency [109].

Fibromuscular dysplasia

FMD is a less common cause of RAS, accounting for less than 10% of cases [16]. The most common type of FMD type, medial fibroplasia, is characterized by the classical string-of-beads appearance of the affected vessel. The "beads" in this type of FMD, which mainly affects middle-aged women, are usually larger than the vessel diameter and can appear aneurysmal, whereas in

Table 1

Sensitivity and specificity of 3D CE MRA studies enrolling more than 50 individuals in the evaluation of renal arteries disease

Authors	Year	n	Sensitivity (%)*	Specificity (%)*	Degree of stenosis (%)
Holland et al [132]	1996	63	100	100	>50
De Cobelli et al [133]	1997	55	100	97	>50
Hany et al [134]	1998	103	93	90	NA
Leung et al [135]	1999	60	90	86	>60
Thornton et al [8]	1999	62	88	98	>50
Shetty et al [136]	2000	51	96	92	NA

* Compared with conventional angiography.

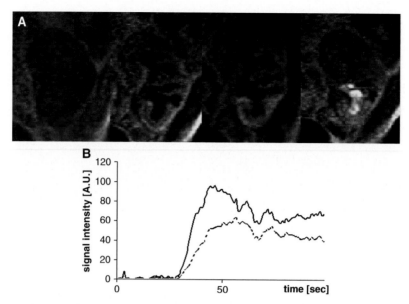

Fig. 3. (*A*) Images from a perfusion measurement of a 62-year-old patient who presented with rising serum creatinine levels 7 years after renal transplantation. The MR angiography (not shown) was unremarkable. MR perfusion measurements, however, show almost no perfusion and no excretion at the upper pole of the transplant kidney compared with the lower pole. (*B*) The SIVT curves of this patient show significantly lower perfusion at the upper pole (*dashed line*). Biopsy revealed chronic ischemic changes.

perimedial firboplasia, a rare subtype of FMD typically found in women aged 15 to 30 years, the beads are less numerous and are smaller than the vessel caliber. Adventitial hyperplasia and intimal fibroplasia are even less common. These two subtypes of FMD are mainly found in children and lead to smooth narrowing with concentric stenoses or sharply localized stenoses, respectively. Perimedial firboplasia, adventitial hyperplasia, and intimal fibroplasias can progress to vessel occlusion. FMD can be focal or can include the entire renal artery. Because of the vessel wall weakness in FMD, FMD accounts for 38% of all renal artery aneurysms (Fig. 5) and is responsible for a major part of renal artery dissections. Bilateral disease is present in 35% of cases; and involvement of an accessory artery is not uncommon.

Unlike atherosclerotic RAS, FMD affects mainly the middle and distal third of renal arteries. The proximal part is involved only in 30% of cases [18]. Visualizing FMD is still a challenge for 3-D CE MR angiography, because the distal part of the renal artery shows considerable motion from diaphragmatic random motion independent from the cardiac cycle [110]. The dysplastic vessel sections also can be very subtle and focal. Conventional angiography, the current reference standard, has a resolution of up to 300 μm, whereas even high-resolution 3-D CE MR angiography hardly surpasses 800 μm. In Fig. 6 the MR angiography reveals FMD, but the changes are obvious in the conventional angiography. Higher acceleration factors in parallel imaging together with higher field strengths will improve the performance of 3-D CE MR angiography. Shorter imaging times with parallel imaging can lead to improved image quality by diminishing the effect of inevitable renal artery motion [110]. FMD is a good example of the usefulness of MR-based flow and perfusion measurements. The latter may detect segmental reduced perfusion in case of segmental FMD, which, because of motion, is hard to appreciate in MR flow measurements and in the 3-D CE MR angiography. If the clinical differential diagnosis in a patient with FMD includes inflammatory diseases such as Takyasu arteriitis, a fat-suppressed T1W spin echo sequence should be performed after application of contrast agent to demonstrate the inflammatory enhancement (Fig. 7). Also, T2W images may be helpful, because they may show vessel wall edema in inflammatory diseases. Because FMD is a dysplastic disease without inflammatory components, contrast uptake in the vessel wall rules out a diagnosis of FMD.

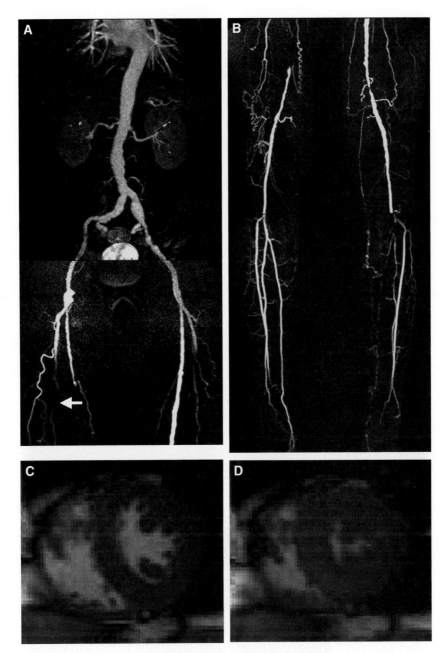

Fig. 4. Value of MR for identification of associated disease in a 68-year-old patient with severe atherosclerotic RAS. (*A*) The MR angiography of the abdomen and upper leg shows severe atherosclerotic disease with occlusion of the right superficial femoral artery (*arrow*) with multiple collateral vessels. (*B*) In the MR angiography of the lower leg, severe atherosclerotic changes are obvious with occlusion of the arteria tibialis posterior. The functional cardiac study shows a hypertrophy of the left wall in the diastole (*C*) and systole (*D*).

Renal artery dissection

Renal artery dissection (RAD) is a rare condition, with approximately 200 cases reported in the literature [111]. Clinical signs of RAD are progressive renovascular hypertension, decrease of the kidney function, and kidney infarction. If the false lumen re-enters the true lumen, the symptoms suddenly disappear. RAD typically affects patients in their fourth to sixth decade,

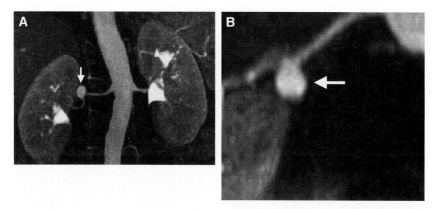

Fig. 5. (*A*) Coronal MIP view of a 45-year-old man suffering from severe hypertension. The MR angiography revealed normal proximal renal arteries bilateral, but a 1.2-cm aneurysm (*arrow*) of right renal artery was found. (*B*) The axial MIP view confirms the renal artery aneurysm (*arrow*).

and men are affected four times more often than women [111]. Bilateral RAD occurs in 10% to 15% of all patients [112]. The most frequent cause of RAD is FMD. Focal RADs can be detected in 9% of all patients with FMD [111]. Other reasons for RAD include atherosclerotic vessel disease, trauma [113], medial degeneration, Marfan's syndrome, Ehlers-Danlos syndrome, subadventitial angioma, and iatrogenic manipulation [114]. The typical imaging finding in RAD is the presence of

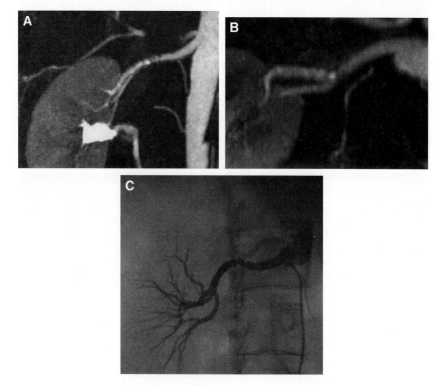

Fig. 6. (*A*) MIP view of a 35-year-old woman who presented with severe hypertension. The coronal view reveals wall irregularities in the distal part of the renal artery most consistent with medial fibroplasia. (*B*) The axial thin MIP view of the same patient reveals changes characteristic of FMD in the distal part of the renal artery. (*C*) This patient underwent subsequent conventional X-ray angiography to confirm the MR angiographic findings and to dilate the affected parts of the renal arteries. After the intervention, the blood pressure dropped markedly.

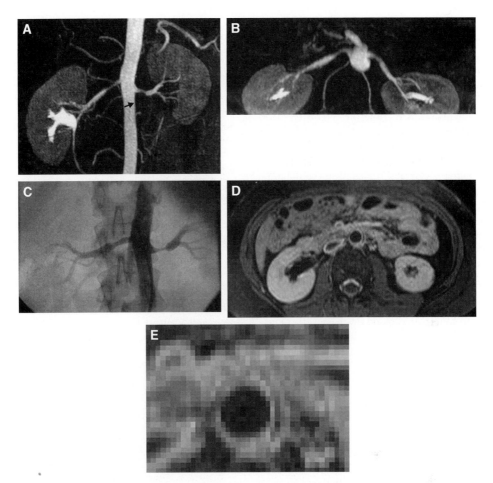

Fig. 7. (*A*) A coronal MIP view of a 25-year-old woman suffering from Takayasu arteriitis shows extensive bilateral RAS. (*B*) The axial MIP view confirms this finding. (*C*) The MR angiographoc findings were confirmed by conventional angiography performed for dilatation of the renal arteries. (*D*) A fat-suppressed, T1W black-blood contrast-enhanced image shows an enhancing and thickened aortic wall, indicating inflammation (ie, aortitis). (*E*) The close-up of the abdominal aorta better demonstrates the circumferential contrast enhancement of the aortic wall.

two lumens [112]; however, spatial resolution must be sufficient to prevent partial-volume effects, which may obscure the intimal flap. Because of the rarity of RAD, no studies have been published analyzing the value of MR angiography for the detection of RAD.

RAD can be isolated to the renal arteries but can also be secondarily involved as an extension of an abdominal aortic dissection. 3-D CE MR angiography is a valuable tool in the assessment of aortic aneurysm [115]. Because of the different blood flow velocities in the false and the true lumens, however, standard contrast-timing techniques may fail or produce artifacts, further limiting image interpretation. Renal involvement

by aortic dissection depends on the involvement of the renal artery by the disease process. MR flow and MR perfusion measurements may show delayed blood flow and delayed arrival of contrast agent in the renal parenchyma. MR flow measurements alone may fail to show renal involvement if the dissection leads to a small residual lumen. MR perfusion measurements, on the other hand, are more robust, because the information is acquired along the entire renal cortex. Another helpful approach in a dissecting aneurysm is the use of time-resolved multiphase MR angiography [59], which can show the arrival of the contrast agent bolus in the different lumens and thus identify the origins of the renal blood supply to be assessed.

Renal vein thrombosis

RVT is most common in patients with membranous glomerulonephritis, but it also occurs in patients with renal cell carcinomas, with a prior history of trauma, in sepsis, in states of dehydration [116], or with pancreatitis [117]. The thrombus may extend into the inferior vena cava. The classic diagnostic triad of a flank mass, gross hematuria, and thrombocytopenia is present in only 13% of all patients with RVT [118]. Therefore, imaging is essential to establish the diagnosis. Typical radiographic findings of RVT include swelling of the affected kidney, low signal intensity in both T1W and T2W pulse sequences, and compression of the collecting system [119]. The loss of signal intensity in the renal cortex in T2W pulse sequences is present from the first day [120]. Especially in acute RVT, a band of low signal intensity can be seen at the outer part of the medulla; this band is thought to represent hemorrhage from impaired blood drainage [119]. This imaging finding resembles the intrarenal changes seen in patients suffering from hemorrhagic fever with renal syndrome. Venous collateral vessels and dilatation of the left gonadal vein may be seen in chronic RVT [121]. The corticomedullary differentiation vanishes after the fifteenth day on T1W images, and the kidney becomes atrophic by 1 month [120]. The reference standard for diagnosis of RVT, conventional renal venography, is not popular and is rarely used in clinical practice [122]. MR angiography has been shown to be a useful and accurate test for the detection of RVT [121]. To detect RVT using 3-D CE MR angiography, MP perfusion views of the venous phase are most appropriate, as shown in Fig. 8. No studies comparing conventional X-ray venography with MR angiography exist, however.

Renal transplants

Because of its lack of nephrotoxicity, 3-D CE MR angiography has become a standard tool for the evaluation of renal transplants [31,123]. The ability to reformat 3-D MR data sets in any

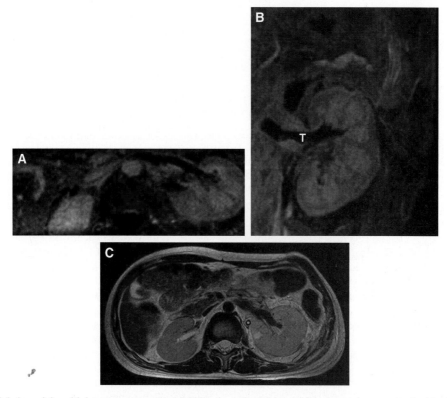

Fig. 8. (*A*) An axial multiplaner reconstruction (MPR) view of a 28-year-old woman who presented with abdominal swelling and pain reveals renal vein thrombosis up to the inferior vena cava. (*B*) In the coronal MPR view, the full extent of the thrombus (T) becomes visible. (*C*) The native T2W image reveals swelling of the affected left kidney with low signal from the affected kidney.

desired way is another advantage in the assessment of the often tortuous transplant arteries, as shown in Fig. 9. A standard 3-D CE MR angiography sequence can be used for the evaluation of the renal transplant arteries. Because of the pelvic position of the transplant organ and its decreased susceptibility to respiratory motion, longer scan times can used, enabling higher spatial resolution with 3-D CE MR angiography. Higher spatial resolution makes easier the detection of focal disease, which can occur with transplant rejection. Focal pathologies to be considered in patients with a renal transplant include renal infarction, cortical necrosis, acute tubular necrosis [31], and posttransplantation lymphoproliferative disease (PTLD). PTLD, which occurs in 1% of all renal transplants, arises in the setting of Epstein-Barr virus infection and high doses of immunosuppressive drugs [124]. In 75% of cases, PTLD is found near the allograft and presents as a hypointense lesion in T1W images with weak enhancement. T2W images show hypo- and hyperintense signal behavior of the mass [125]. The renal vessels themselves are rarely involved, but they can become encased [124,125].

In renal transplants, it is especially important to start the venous-phase scan immediately after the arterial-phase scan to enable evaluation of the renal vein for pathologic conditions. RVT in renal transplant patients may arise from kinking of the renal vein but also can arise from acute or chronic rejection. Another complication, RAS, is found commonly at the site of vascular anastomosis. The prevalence for RAS has been reported to be between 1% and 25%, occurring typically from

1 month to 2 years after transplantation [126]. RAS should be differentiated from suture-related narrowing or kinking. Like RAS, kinking of the transplant renal artery may lead to impaired renal blood supply, particularly in the early postoperative days [127].

MR angiography has been found to be a highly accurate modality for detecting and grading transplant RAS. Compared with digital subtraction angiography, sensitivities of 100% and specificities between 93% and 97% have been found [128]. Because the hemodynamic relevance can be hard to appreciate on the MR angiography images, MR flow measurements can be helpful. Because of the short and winding arterial segment, however, it often is difficult to position MR flow measurements perpendicular to the vessel axis. MR perfusion measurements can be positioned over the kidney itself and are not restricted by a short transplant renal artery. They have the further advantage of identifying parenchymal perfusion defects unrelated to vascular disease. Renal perfusion defects in a renal transplant can result from a variety of causes; in addition to vascular causes, these include transplant rejection, PTLD, and infections such as melanoplakia. With time-resolved perfusion techniques, decreased contrast ratios of the renal cortex and the medulla have been found in a variety of conditions, including acute tubular necrosis in which the contrast agent is contained in the medulla and is not excreted, cyclosporine tubulopathy, and acute rejection [129]. Affected kidneys usually show inhomogeneous, patchy parenchymal enhancement with focal areas of lower uptake of contrast agent. If the acquisition

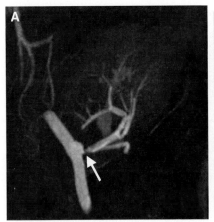
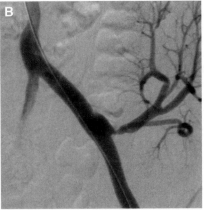

Fig. 9. (*A*) In the oblique MIP view of a 32-year-old patient with renal transplant, a 75% RAS (*arrow*) of the transplant artery is visible. (*B*) Conventional angiography confirmed the MR angiographic findings.

time of the perfusion measurement (using standard gadolinium chelate contrast agents) is long enough, excretion of the contrast agent into the calyceal system can be seen. Areas of delayed or no excretion are suspicious for parenchymal disease.

Imaging of hemodialysis shunts

Hemodialysis shunts are a prerequisite for vascular hemodialysis. In the United States, poly-etrafluoroethylene (PTFE) grafts account for 80% of hemodialysis shunts, whereas arteriovenous shunts make up the remaining 20% [130]. The direct arteriovenous bypass leads to an increased flow that reaches 350 to 400 mL/min in arteriovenous shunts and 800 to 1000 mL/min in PTFE grafts [130]. Hemodialysis shunts are prone to thrombosis, particularly at the anastomosis site, where a turbulent flow is present. The incidence of thrombosis is 0.5% to 2.5% of all hemodialysis shunts. The inflow volume and the inflow velocity have been found to be a good predictor of impending hemodialysis shunt failure [131]. Ultrasound and the conventional angiography are still considered the reference standards for imaging of hemodialysis shunts. 3-D CE MR angiography has been used in some studies to image hemodialysis shunts at the forearm, with interobserver agreement equal to that of conventional angiography [27–30]. Because of its 3-D volumetric nature, 3-D MR angiography can be beneficial in the work-up of suspected hemodialysis shunt pathology. The lack of inherent motion at the forearm allows prolongation of the acquisition times. The high flow in hemodialysis shunts, however, may lead to flow-related artifacts and false-positive results. To avoid flow-related artifacts, a blood pressure cuff can be inflated to decrease inflow into the hemodialysis shunts [28]. Han et al [28], who used a combined approach of flow measurements and MR angiography, report a sensitivity of 100% and a specificity of 94% [28]. An additional advantage of MR angiography in imaging hemodialysis shunts is the ability to depict a proximal stenosis or thrombus in the subclavian and brachial vessels. Despite these positive results, one must remember that all these studies included only a few patients. Further studies are needed to establish this application of MR angiography.

Summary

MR angiography, particularly 3-D CE MR angiography, has become a standard clinical tool in the evaluation of renovascular diseases. Virtually all scanners are able to perform a 3-D CE MR angiography that is the workhorse for most indications. Evaluations for renovascular diseases and renal transplant imaging have become routine examinations. Newer technical developments, such as parallel imaging and time-resolved imaging, will improve the quality and extend the spectrum of applications of CE MR angiography, improving both the spatial and the temporal resolution of CE MR angiography. Because of its advantages, CE MR angiography compares favorably with invasive conventional catheter X-ray angiography, which currently achieves a higher spatial resolution. Adding MR flow measurements and MR perfusion measurements complements 3-D CE MR angiography to yield a comprehensive renal examination that allows exact grading of RAS and differentiation between renovascular and renoparenchymal disease.

References

[1] Prince MR, Yucel EK, Kaufman JA, et al. Dynamic gadolinium-enhanced three-dimensional abdominal MR arteriography. J Magn Reson Imaging 1993;3(6):877–81.

[2] Prince MR. Gadolinium-enhanced MR aortography. Radiology 1994;191(1):155–64.

[3] Prince MR, Narasimham DL, Stanley JC, et al. Breath-hold gadolinium-enhanced MR angiography of the abdominal aorta and its major branches. Radiology 1995;197(3):785–92.

[4] Kent KC, Edelman RR, Kim D, et al. Magnetic resonance imaging: a reliable test for the evaluation of proximal atherosclerotic renal arterial stenosis. J Vasc Surg 1991;13(2):311–8.

[5] Dumoulin CL, Yucel EK, Vock P, et al. Two- and three-dimensional phase contrast MR angiography of the abdomen. J Comput Assist Tomogr 1990; 14(5):779–84.

[6] Textor SC, Canzanello VJ. Radiographic evaluation of the renal vasculature. Curr Opin Nephrol Hypertens 1996;5(6):541–51.

[7] Krestin GP. Magnetic resonance imaging of the kidneys: current status. Magn Reson Q 1994;10(1): 2–21.

[8] Thornton J, O'Callaghan J, Walshe J, et al. Comparison of digital subtraction angiography with gadolinium-enhanced magnetic resonance angiography in the diagnosis of renal artery stenosis. Eur Radiol 1999;9(5):930–4.

[9] Schoenberg SO, Rieger J, Nittka M, et al. Renal MR angiography: current debates and developments in imaging of renal artery stenosis. Semin Ultrasound CT MR 2003;24(4):255–67.

[10] Berg KJ. Nephrotoxicity related to contrast media. Scand J Urol Nephrol 2000;34(5):317–22.

[11] Rudnick MR, Goldfarb S, Wexler L, et al. Nephrotoxicity of ionic and nonionic contrast media in 1196 patients: a randomized trial. The Iohexol Cooperative Study. Kidney Int 1995;47(1):254–61.

[12] Rudnick MR, Berns JS, Cohen RM, et al. Contrast media-associated nephrotoxicity. Curr Opin Nephrol Hypertens 1996;5(2):127–33.

[13] Aspelin P, Aubry P, Fransson SG, et al. Nephrotoxic effects in high-risk patients undergoing angiography. N Engl J Med 2003;348(6):491–9.

[14] Prince MR, Arnoldus C, Frisoli JK. Nephrotoxicity of high-dose gadolinium compared with iodinated contrast. J Magn Reson Imaging 1996;6(1): 162–6.

[15] Textor SC. Epidemiology and clinical presentation. Semin Nephrol 2000;20(5):426–31.

[16] Safian RD, Textor SC. Renal-artery stenosis. N Engl J Med 2001;344(6):431–42.

[17] Olin JW. Renal artery disease: diagnosis and management. Mt Sinai J Med 2004;71(2):73–85.

[18] Slovut DP, Olin JW. Fibromuscular dysplasia. N Engl J Med 2004;350(18):1862–71.

[19] Romero JC, Feldstein AE, Rodriguez-Porcel MG, et al. New insights into the pathophysiology of renovascular hypertension. Mayo Clin Proc 1997; 72(3):251–60.

[20] Derkx FH, Schalekamp MA. Renal artery stenosis and hypertension. Lancet 1994;344(8917): 237–9.

[21] Sawicki PT, Kaiser S, Heinemann L, et al. Prevalence of renal artery stenosis in diabetes mellitus–an autopsy study. J Intern Med 1991;229(6): 489–92.

[22] Rihal CS, Textor SC, Breen JF, et al. Incidental renal artery stenosis among a prospective cohort of hypertensive patients undergoing coronary angiography. Mayo Clin Proc 2002;77(4):309–16.

[23] Harding MB, Smith LR, Himmelstein SI, et al. Renal artery stenosis: prevalence and associated risk factors in patients undergoing routine cardiac catheterization. J Am Soc Nephrol 1992;2(11): 1608–16.

[24] Olin JW, Melia M, Young JR, et al. Prevalence of atherosclerotic renal artery stenosis in patients with atherosclerosis elsewhere. Am J Med 1990; 88(1N):46N–51N.

[25] Wachtell K, Ibsen H, Olsen MH, et al. Prevalence of renal artery stenosis in patients with peripheral vascular disease and hypertension. J Hum Hypertens 1996;10(2):83–5.

[26] Scoble JE, Hamilton G. Atherosclerotic renovascular disease. BMJ 1990;300(6741):1670–1.

[27] Cavagna E, D'Andrea P, Schiavon F, et al. Failing hemodialysis arteriovenous fistula and percutaneous treatment: imaging with CT, MRI and digital subtraction angiography. Cardiovasc Intervent Radiol 2000;23(4):262–5.

[28] Han KM, Duijm LE, Thelissen GR, et al. Failing hemodialysis access grafts: evaluation of complete vascular tree with 3-D contrast-enhanced MR angiography with high spatial resolution: initial results in 10 patients. Radiology 2003;227(2):601–5.

[29] Planken RN, Tordoir JH, Dammers R, et al. Stenosis detection in forearm hemodialysis arteriovenous fistulae by multiphase contrast-enhanced magnetic resonance angiography: preliminary experience. J Magn Reson Imaging 2003;17(1):54–64.

[30] Waldman GJ, Pattynama PM, Chang PC, et al. Magnetic resonance angiography of dialysis access shunts: initial results. Magn Reson Imaging 1996; 14(2):197–200.

[31] Wiesner W, Pfammatter T, Krestin GP, et al. The MRT and MRA of kidney transplants—vascular and perfusion assessment. Rofo 1998;169(3):290–6.

[32] Huang AJ, Lee VS, Rusinek H. MR imaging of renal function. Radiol Clin North Am 2003;41(5): 1001–17.

[33] Helenon O, Correas JM, Thervet E, et al. [Imaging of vascular complications of renal transplantation]. J Radiol 1994;75(1):61–8.

[34] Hanna S, Helenon O, Legendre C, et al. MR imaging of renal transplant rejection. Acta Radiol 1991; 32(1):42–6.

[35] Martirosian P, Klose U, Mader I, et al. FAIR true FISP perfusion imaging of the kidneys. Magn Reson Med 2004;51(2):353–61.

[36] Wang JJ, Hendrich KS, Jackson EK, et al. Perfusion quantitation in transplanted rat kidney by MRI with arterial spin labeling. Kidney Int 1998; 53(6):1783–91.

[37] Prasad PV, Kim D, Kaiser AM, et al. Noninvasive comprehensive characterization of renal artery stenosis by combination of STAR angiography and EPISTAR perfusion imaging. Magn Reson Med 1997;38(5):776–87.

[38] Carvlin MJ, Arger PH, Kundel HL, et al. Use of Gd-DTPA and fast gradient-echo and spin-echo MR imaging to demonstrate renal function in the rabbit. Radiology 1989;170(3 Pt 1):705–11.

[39] Daly PF, Zimmerman JB, Gillen JS, et al. Rapid MR imaging of renal perfusion: a comparative study of GdDTPA, albumin-(GdDTPA), and magnetite. Am J Physiol Imaging 1989;4(4):165–74.

[40] Trillaud H, Grenier N, Degreze P, et al. First-pass evaluation of renal perfusion with TurboFLASH MR imaging and superparamagnetic iron oxide particles. J Magn Reson Imaging 1993;3(1): 83–91.

[41] Laissy JP, Faraggi M, Lebtahi R, et al. Functional evaluation of normal and ischemic kidney by means of gadolinium-DOTA enhanced TurboFLASH MR imaging: a preliminary comparison with 99Tc-MAG3 dynamic scintigraphy. Magn Reson Imaging 1994;12(3):413–9.

[42] Vosshenrich R, Kallerhoff M, Grone HJ, et al. Detection of renal ischemic lesions using Gd-DTPA

enhanced turbo FLASH MRI: experimental and clinical results. J Comput Assist Tomogr 1996; 20(2):236–43.

[43] Prasad PV, Cannillo J, Chavez DR, et al. Contrast-enhanced MR angiography and first-pass renal perfusion imaging using MS-325, an intravascular contrast agent. Acad Radiol 1998;5(Suppl 1): S219–22 [discussion: S26–7].

[44] Gandy SJ, Sudarshan TA, Sheppard DG, et al. Dynamic MRI contrast enhancement of renal cortex: a functional assessment of renovascular disease in patients with renal artery stenosis. J Magn Reson Imaging 2003;18(4):461–6.

[45] Schoenberg SO, Knopp MV, Bock M, et al. Renal artery stenosis: grading of hemodynamic changes with cine phase-contrast MR blood flow measurements. Radiology 1997;203(1):45–53.

[46] Bogren HG, Buonocore MH. Blood flow measurements in the aorta and major arteries with MR velocity mapping. J Magn Reson Imaging 1994;4(2): 119–30.

[47] Schoenberg SO, Bock M, Kallinowski F, et al. Correlation of hemodynamic impact and morphologic degree of renal artery stenosis in a canine model. J Am Soc Nephrol 2000;11(12):2190–8.

[48] Vexler VS, de Crespigny AJ, Wendland MF, et al. MR imaging of blood oxygenation-dependent changes in focal renal ischemia and transplanted liver tumor in rat. J Magn Reson Imaging 1993; 3(3):483–90.

[49] Prasad PV, Priatna A. Functional imaging of the kidneys with fast MRI techniques. Eur J Radiol 1999;29(2):133–48.

[50] Epstein FH, Veves A, Prasad PV. Effect of diabetes on renal medullary oxygenation during water diuresis. Diabetes Care 2002;25(3):575–8.

[51] Li L, Storey P, Kim D, et al. Kidneys in hypertensive rats show reduced response to nitric oxide synthase inhibition as evaluated by BOLD MRI. J Magn Reson Imaging 2003;17(6): 671–5.

[52] Vexler VS, Berthezene Y, Clement O, et al. Detection of zonal renal ischemia with contrast-enhanced MR imaging with a macromolecular blood pool contrast agent. J Magn Reson Imaging 1992;2(3): 311–9.

[53] Vexler VS, Roberts TP, Rosenau W. Early detection of acute tubular injury with diffusion-weighted magnetic resonance imaging in a rat model of myohemoglobinuric acute renal failure. Ren Fail 1996; 18(1):41–57.

[54] Sodickson DK, McKenzie CA, Li W, et al. Contrast-enhanced 3D MR angiography with simultaneous acquisition of spatial harmonics: a pilot study. Radiology 2000;217(1):284–9.

[55] Griswold MA, Jakob PM, Heidemann RM, et al. Generalized autocalibrating partially parallel acquisitions (GRAPPA). Magn Reson Med 2002; 47(6):1202–10.

[56] Weiger M, Pruessmann KP, Kassner A, et al. Contrast-enhanced 3D MRA using SENSE. J Magn Reson Imaging 2000;12(5):671–7.

[57] Pruessmann KP, Weiger M, Scheidegger MB, et al. SENSE: sensitivity encoding for fast MRI. Magn Reson Med 1999;42(5):952–62.

[58] Shetty AN, Bis KG, Vrachliotis TG, et al. Contrast-enhanced 3D MRA with centric ordering in k space: a preliminary clinical experience in imaging the abdominal aorta and renal and peripheral arterial vasculature. J Magn Reson Imaging 1998; 8(3):603–15.

[59] Schoenberg SO, Londy FJ, Licato P, et al. Multiphase-multistep gadolinium-enhanced MR angiography of the abdominal aorta and runoff vessels. Invest Radiol 2001;36(5):283–91.

[60] Korosec FR, Frayne R, Grist TM, et al. Time-resolved contrast-enhanced 3D MR angiography. Magn Reson Med 1996;36(3):345–51.

[61] Spuentrup E, Buecker A, Meyer J, et al. Navigator-gated free-breathing 3D balanced FFE projection renal MRA: comparison with contrast-enhanced breath-hold 3D MRA in a swine model. Magn Reson Med 2002;48(4):739–43.

[62] Coenegrachts KL, Hoogeveen RM, Vaninbroukx JA, et al. High-spatial-resolution 3D balanced turbo field-echo technique for MR angiography of the renal arteries: initial experience. Radiology 2004;231(1):237–42.

[63] Lundin B, Cooper TG, Meyer RA, et al. Measurement of total and unilateral renal blood flow by oblique-angle velocity-encoded 2D-cine magnetic resonance angiography. Magn Reson Imaging 1993;11(1):51–9.

[64] Debatin JF. MR quantification of flow in abdominal vessels. Abdom Imaging 1998;23(5): 485–95.

[65] Debatin JF, Ting RH, Wegmuller H, et al. Renal artery blood flow: quantitation with phase-contrast MR imaging with and without breath holding. Radiology 1994;190(2):371–8.

[66] Schoenberg SO, Just A, Bock M, et al. Noninvasive analysis of renal artery blood flow dynamics with MR cine phase-contrast flow measurements. Am J Physiol 1997;272(5 Pt 2):H2477–84.

[67] Westenberg JJ, Wasser MN, van der Geest RJ, et al. Variations in blood flow waveforms in stenotic renal arteries by 2D phase-contrast cine MRI. J Magn Reson Imaging 1998;8(3): 590–7.

[68] Binkert CA, Hoffman U, Leung DA, et al. Characterization of renal artery stenoses based on magnetic resonance renal flow and volume measurements. Kidney Int 1999;56(5):1846–54.

[69] Prince MR. Renal MR angiography. A comprehensive approach. J Magn Reson Imaging 1998; 8(3):511–6.

[70] Debatin JF, Leung DA, Wildermuth S, et al. Flow quantitation with echo-planar phase-contrast

velocity mapping: in vitro and in vivo evaluation. J Magn Reson Imaging 1995;5(6):656–62.

[71] Bock M, Schoenberg SO, Schad LR, et al. Interleaved gradient echo planar (IGEPI) and phase contrast CINE-PC flow measurements in the renal artery. J Magn Reson Imaging 1998;8(4): 889–95.

[72] Tsao J, Boesiger P, Pruessmann KP. k-t BLAST and k-t SENSE: dynamic MRI with high frame rate exploiting spatiotemporal correlations. Magn Reson Med 2003;50(5):1031–42.

[73] Baltes C, Tsao J, Kozerke S, et al. Accelerating PC-SSFP velocity mapping using k-t-BLAST. J Cardiov Mag Res 2004;6(1):48–9.

[74] Michaely HJ, Schoenberg SO, Ittrich C, et al. Renal disease: value of functional magnetic resonance imaging with flow and perfusion measurements. Invest Radiol 2004;39:698.

[75] Williams DS, Zhang W, Koretsky AP, et al. Perfusion imaging of the rat kidney with MR. Radiology 1994;190(3):813–8.

[76] Roberts DA, Detre JA, Bolinger L, et al. Renal perfusion in humans: MR imaging with spin tagging of arterial water. Radiology 1995;196(1):281–6.

[77] Karger N, Biederer J, Lusse S, et al. Quantitation of renal perfusion using arterial spin labeling with FAIR-UFLARE. Magn Reson Imaging 2000; 18(6):641–7.

[78] Gunther M, Bock M, Schad LR. Arterial spin labeling in combination with a look-locker sampling strategy: inflow turbo-sampling EPI-FAIR (ITS-FAIR). Magn Reson Med 2001;46(5):974–84.

[79] Michaely HJ, Schoenberg SO, Oesingmann N, et al. Renal artery stenosis: semiquantitative assessment of perfusion parameters with Gd-enhanced TurboFLASH sequences. Proceedings of the International Society for Magnetic Resonance in Medicine 2004. p. 599.

[80] Prasad PV, Cannillo J, Chavez DR, et al. First-pass renal perfusion imaging using MS-325, an albumin-targeted MRI contrast agent. Invest Radiol 1999; 34(9):566–71.

[81] Schoenberg SO, Aumann S, Just A, et al. Quantification of renal perfusion abnormalities using an intravascular contrast agent. Part 2: results in animals and humans with renal artery stenosis. Magn Reson Med 2003;49(2):288–98.

[82] Aumann S, Schoenberg SO, Just A, et al. Quantification of renal perfusion using an intravascular contrast agent. Part 1: results in a canine model. Magn Reson Med 2003;49(2):276–87.

[83] Choyke PL, Austin HA, Frank JA, et al. Hydrated clearance of gadolinium-DTPA as a measurement of glomerular filtration rate. Kidney Int 1992; 41(6):1595–8.

[84] Niendorf ER, Grist TM, Frayne R, et al. Rapid measurement of Gd-DTPA extraction fraction in a dialysis system using echo-planar imaging. Med Phys 1997;24(12):1907–13.

[85] Niendorf ER, Grist TM, Lee FT Jr. Rapid in vivo measurement of single-kidney extraction fraction and glomerular filtration rate with MR imaging. Radiology 1998;206(3):791–8.

[86] Ros PR, Gauger J, Stoupis C, et al. Diagnosis of renal artery stenosis: feasibility of combining MR angiography, MR renography, and gadopentetate-based measurements of glomerular filtration rate. AJR Am J Roentgenol 1995;165(6):1447–51.

[87] Prasad PV, Goldfarb J, Sundaram C, et al. MR renography in a swine model: toward a comprehensive evaluation of renal arterial stenosis. Radiology 2000;217(3):813–8.

[88] Lee VS, Rusinek H, Johnson G, et al. MR renography with low-dose gadopentetate dimeglumine: feasibility. Radiology 2001;221(2):371–9.

[89] Gates GF. Split renal function testing using Tc-99m DTPA. A rapid technique for determining differential glomerular filtration. Clin Nucl Med 1983; 8(9):400–7.

[90] Lee VS, Rusinek H, Noz ME, et al. Dynamic three-dimensional MR renography for the measurement of single kidney function: initial experience. Radiology 2003;227(1):289–94.

[91] Semelka RC, Corrigan K, Ascher SM, et al. Renal corticomedullary differentiation: observation in patients with differing serum creatinine levels. Radiology 1994;190(1):149–52.

[92] Gupta A, Tello R. Accessory renal arteries are not related to hypertension risk: a review of MR angiography data. AJR Am J Roentgenol 2004;182(6): 1521–4.

[93] Bude RO, Forauer AR, Caoili EM, et al. Is it necessary to study accessory arteries when screening the renal arteries for renovascular hypertension? Radiology 2003;226(2):411–6.

[94] Shetty AN, Bis KG, Kirsch M, et al. Contrast-enhanced breath-hold three-dimensional magnetic resonance angiography in the evaluation of renal arteries: optimization of technique and pitfalls. J Magn Reson Imaging 2000;12:912–23.

[95] Bakker J, Beek FJ, Beutler JJ, et al. Renal artery stenosis and accessory renal arteries: accuracy of detection and visualization with gadolinium-enhanced breath-hold MR angiography. Radiology 1998;207:497–504.

[96] Vasbinder GB, Nelemans PJ, Kessels AG, et al. Diagnostic tests for renal artery stenosis in patients suspected of having renovascular hypertension: a meta-analysis. Ann Intern Med 2001;135(6):401–11.

[97] Winterer JT, Strey C, Wolffram C, et al. Preoperative examination of potential kidney transplantation donors: value of gadolinium-enhanced 3D MR angiography in comparison with DSA and urography. Rofo 2000;172(5):449–57.

[98] Gupta SN, Solaiyappan M, Beache GM, et al. Fast method for correcting image misregistration due to organ motion in time-series MRI data. Magn Reson Med 2003;49(3):506–14.

[99] Textor SC, McKusick MA. Renal artery stenosis. Curr Treat Options Cardiovasc Med 2001;3(3): 187–94.

[100] Breyer JA, Jacobson HR. Ischemic nephropathy. Curr Opin Nephrol Hypertens 1993;2(2):216–24.

[101] Schreiber MJ, Pohl MA, Novick AC. The natural history of atherosclerotic and fibrous renal artery disease. Urol Clin North Am 1984;11(3): 383–92.

[102] Watson PS, Hadjipetrou P, Cox SV, et al. Effect of renal artery stenting on renal function and size in patients with atherosclerotic renovascular disease. Circulation 2000;102(14):1671–7.

[103] Klatte EC, Worrell JA, Forster JH, et al. Diagnostic criteria of bilateral renovascular hypertension. Radiology 1971;101(2):301–4.

[104] Prince MR, Schoenberg SO, Ward JS, et al. Hemodynamically significant atherosclerotic renal artery stenosis: MR angiographic features. Radiology 1997;205(1):128–36.

[105] Schoenberg SO, Rieger J, Weber C, et al. High-resolution MRA of the renal arteries using parallel acquisition techniques: value of isotropic cross-sectional reformats compared to digital subtraction angiography and intravascular ultrasound. Proceeedings of the International Society for Magnetic Resonance in Medicine. 2004. p. 235.

[106] Schoenberg SO, Knopp MV, Londy F, et al. Morphologic and functional magnetic resonance imaging of renal artery stenosis: a multireader tricenter study. J Am Soc Nephrol 2002;13(1): 158–69.

[107] Buller CE, Nogareda JG, Ramanathan K, et al. The profile of cardiac patients with renal artery stenosis. J Am Coll Cardiol 2004;43(9):1606–13.

[108] Edwards MS, Hansen KJ, Craven TE, et al. Associations between renovascular disease and prevalent cardiovascular disease in the elderly: a population-based study. Vasc Endovascular Surg 2004;38(1):25–35.

[109] Kennedy DJ, Colyer WR, Brewster PS, et al. Renal insufficiency as a predictor of adverse events and mortality after renal artery stent placement. Am J Kidney Dis 2003;42(5):926–35.

[110] Vasbinder GBC, Maki JH, Nijenhuis RJ, et al. Motion of the distal renal artery during three-dimensional contrast-enhanced breath-hold MRA. J Magn Reson Imaging 2002;16(6):685–96.

[111] Mudrick D, Arepally A, Geschwind JF, et al. Spontaneous renal artery dissection: treatment with coil embolization. J Vasc Interv Radiol 2003;14(4): 497–500.

[112] Lacombe M. Isolated spontaneous dissection of the renal artery. J Vasc Surg 2001;33(2):385–91.

[113] Bilge AK, Nisanci Y, Yilmaz E, et al. Renovascular hypertension secondary to spontaneous renal artery dissection and treatment with stenting. Int J Clin Pract 2003;57(5):435–6.

[114] Goldfarb R, Pool JL, Wheeler T. Isolated renal artery dissection secondary to medial degeneration. J Urol 1988;139(2):346–7.

[115] Schoenberg SO, Essig M, Hallscheidt P, et al. Multiphase magnetic resonance angiography of the abdominal and pelvic arteries: results of a bicenter multireader analysis. Invest Radiol 2002;37(1): 20–8.

[116] Jeong JY, Kim SH, Lee HJ, et al. Atypical low-signal-intensity renal parenchyma: causes and patterns. Radiographics 2002;22(4):833–46.

[117] Ma SK, Kim SW, Kim NH, et al. Renal vein and inferior vena cava thrombosis associated with acute pancreatitis. Nephron 2002;92(2):475–7.

[118] Zigman A, Yazbeck S, Emil S, et al. Renal vein thrombosis: a 10-year review. J Pediatr Surg 2000; 35(11):1540–2.

[119] Kim SH, Byun HS, Park JH, et al. Renal parenchymal abnormalities associated with renal vein thrombosis: correlation between MR imaging and pathologic findings in rabbits. AJR Am J Roentgenol 1994;162(6):1361–5.

[120] Sari A, Ozyavuz R, Demirci A, et al. MR imaging of renal vein occlusion in dogs. Invest Radiol 1999;34(8):523–9.

[121] Tempany CM, Morton RA, Marshall FF. MRI of the renal veins: assessment of nonneoplastic venous thrombosis. J Comput Assist Tomogr 1992;16(6): 929–34.

[122] Kanagasundaram NS, Bandyopadhyay D, Brownjohn AM, et al. The diagnosis of renal vein thrombosis by magnetic resonance angiography. Nephrol Dial Transplant 1998;13(1):200–2.

[123] Chan YL, Leung CB, Yu SC, et al. Comparison of non-breath-hold high resolution gadolinium-enhanced MRA with digital subtraction angiography in the evaluation of allograft renal artery stenosis. Clin Radiol 2001;56(2):127–32.

[124] Claudon M, Kessler M, Champigneulle J, et al. Lymphoproliferative disorders after renal transplantation: role of medical imaging. Eur Radiol 1998;8(9):1686–93.

[125] Ali MG, Coakley FV, Hricak H, et al. Complex posttransplantation abnormalities of renal allografts: evaluation with MR imaging. Radiology 1999;211(1):95–100.

[126] Bruno S, Remuzzi G, Ruggenenti P. Transplant renal artery stenosis. J Am Soc Nephrol 2004;15(1): 134–41.

[127] Frauchiger B, Bock A, Spoendlin M, et al. Early renal transplant dysfunction due to arterial kinking stenosis. Nephrol Dial Transplant 1994;9(1): 76–9.

[128] Huber A, Heuck A, Scheidler J, et al. Contrast-enhanced MR angiography in patients after kidney transplantation. Eur Radiol 2001;11(12):2488–95.

[129] Nakashima R, Yamashita Y, Tomiguchi S, et al. Functional evaluation of transplanted kidneys by

Gd-DTPA enhanced turbo FLASH MR imaging. Radiat Med 1996;14(5):251–6.

[130] Konner K, Nonnast-Daniel B, Ritz E. The arterio-venous fistula. J Am Soc Nephrol 2003;14(6): 1669–80.

[131] Smits JH, Bos C, Elgersma OE, et al. Hemodialysis access imaging: comparison of flow-interrupted contrast-enhanced MR angiography and digital subtraction angiography. Radiology 2002;225(3): 829–834.

[132] Holland GA, Dougherty L, Carpenter JP, et al. Breath-hold ultrafast three-dimensional gadolinium-enhanced MR angiography of the aorta and the renal and other visceral abdominal arteries. AJR Am J Roentgenol 1996;166(4):971–81.

[133] De Cobelli F, Vanzulli A, Sironi S, et al. Renal artery stenosis: evaluation with breath-hold, three-dimensional, dynamic, gadolinium-enhanced versus three-dimensional, phase-contrast MR angiography. Radiology 1997;205(3):689–95.

[134] Hany TF, Debatin JF, Leung DA, et al. Evaluation of the aortoiliac and renal arteries: comparison of breath-hold, contrast-enhanced, three-dimensional MR angiography with conventional catheter angiography. Radiology 1997;204(2):357–62.

[135] Leung DA, Hoffmann U, Pfammatter T, et al. Magnetic resonance angiography versus duplex sonography for diagnosing renovascular disease. Hypertension 1999;33(2):726–31.

[136] Shetty AN, Bis KG, Kirsch M, et al. Contrast-enhanced breath-hold three-dimensional magnetic resonance angiography in the evaluation of renal arteries: optimization of technique and pitfalls. J Magn Reson Imaging 2000;12(6):912–23.

ELSEVIER
SAUNDERS

Magn Reson Imaging Clin N Am
13 (2005) 153–160

MAGNETIC
RESONANCE
IMAGING CLINICS
of North America

Role of MR Angiography in Vascular Interventional Planning

Scott A. Koss, MD, E. Kent Yucel, MD*

Division of Cardiovascular Imaging, Department of Radiology, Brigham and Women's Hospital, Harvard Medical School, 75 Francis Street, Boston, MA 02115, USA

Peripheral vascular disease is a prevalent condition with marked variability in clinical presentation and treatment options. Clinical examination and noninvasive vascular laboratory studies can determine the presence of and, in many cases, the level of disease. The role of imaging is to provide a vascular roadmap to guide the vascular surgeon or interventional radiologist. Conventional angiography was considered the gold standard for evaluating the lower extremity arterial tree until the 1990s. Catheter-based techniques provide high-quality images; however, they are associated with the risks of percutaneous intervention. The first practical applications of MR angiography to peripheral vascular disease began with two-dimensional (2D) time-of-flight (TOF) imaging. This technique offered a noninvasive alternative to traditional angiography and removed the nephrotoxic effects of iodinated contrast and radiation exposure. 2D TOF MR angiography was found to be accurate in the diagnosis of hemodynamically significant stenosis and occlusions [1]; however, this technique presented serious limitations for MR angiography of peripheral vascular disease. One of the most significant limitations was the requirement for imaging in the axial plane, requiring hundreds of slices to cover the relevant territories from the infrarenal aorta to the foot. Artifacts were caused by arterial pulsation, slow flow, tortuous vessels, nonvisualization of retrograde flow from collaterals, and turbulent flow at stenoses.

Contrast-enhanced MR angiography has overcome many of these problems. As MR angiography has evolved into the contrast-enhanced era, there has been an improvement in examination speed, the signal-to-noise ratio (SNR), overall image quality, and diagnostic efficacy. Current advances in time-resolved imaging and venous compression strategies continue to improve this diagnostic tool for vascular intervention planning.

Clinical setting

Atherosclerotic disease of the lower extremity presents with a spectrum of clinical presentations ranging from claudication to rest pain and tissue loss. The advancement in percutaneous interventional therapies has resulted in more treatment options, especially for patients with claudication. MR angiography is a useful noninvasive diagnostic tool to plan for percutaneous interventional therapies or surgical bypass. Furthermore, MR angiography is an effective means of evaluating surgical bypass grafts.

Claudication is derived from the Latin word *claudus*, meaning lame. This term has been applied to patients with peripheral vascular disease who have symptoms of reproducible regional exertional pain that resolves at rest. Typically, the level of pain correlates with the level of vascular disease. For example, buttock and thigh claudication is typically referable to aortoiliac disease and calf claudication to superficial femoral occlusion. The duration that a patient needs to exercise to reproduce the pain sheds light on the severity of the disease. After taking a history and examining a patient's pulses, the experienced clinician will have a precise idea about the

---

* Corresponding author. 78 Howitt Road, West Roxbury, MA 02132.
E-mail address: ekyucel@partners.org (E.K. Yucel).

1064-9689/05/$ - see front matter © 2005 Elsevier Inc. All rights reserved.
doi:10.1016/j.mric.2004.12.008

mri.theclinics.com

location and severity of atherosclerotic disease. This precision is substantially increased by performing readily available noninvasive vascular laboratory tests, such as segmental Doppler pressures and pulse volume recordings. These diagnostic maneuvers indicate the hemodynamic significance and general level of disease. At this point, decisions about the need for treating peripheral vascular disease and the general treatment strategy (inflow versus outflow revascularization) can be made. The next step in the work-up of these patients includes an angiographic image to serve as a roadmap for treatment planning. Advances in endovascular treatment have changed the risk-benefit ratio and thresholds for revascularization therapy. Although the indications for revascularization in patients with claudication remain controversial, many more patients are eligible for percutaneous interventional therapies when the claudication may not be severe enough to merit bypass surgery. In these patients, the goal of angiography is to determine whether the patient has a lesion amenable to percutaneous interventional treatment. Minimally invasive MR angiography is more suitable for this purpose than conventional x-ray catheter angiography.

Limb-threatening ischemia is the other end of the peripheral vascular disease spectrum. These patients can present with rest pain, which is worse while lying supine and relieved by being upright. The severity of their disease is such that gravity improves perfusion to the foot. Further stages of disease include tissue loss, ulceration, and gangrene. Limb-threatening ischemia is an indication for relatively urgent revascularization. The goal of therapy is to restore a pulse in the foot to avoid limb loss.

Diagnostic tools

Conventional x-ray catheter angiography was the study of choice for arteriography until recently. This technique was improved with digital subtraction techniques to improve visualization of small runoff vessels. Potential complications were common, occurring at a rate of 5% to 10% for problems such as a groin hematoma, pseudoaneurysm, or arteriovenous fistula. Many patients with peripheral vascular disease also have chronic renal insufficiency or diabetes mellitus, which substantially increases the risk of the nephrotoxic effects of iodinated contrast. Radiation exposure is related to the overall length of the procedure

and, when combined with a prolonged endovascular intervention, can be substantial. There has been a need for an accurate noninvasive imaging study of the lower extremity arteries without catheterization, iodinated contrast, or radiation.

Magnetic resonance angiography began to offer a noninvasive alternative to conventional angiography with the 2D TOF technique. This method proved accurate enough to guide revascularization therapy as well as being cost effective [2,3]. MR angiography supplanted conventional x-ray catheter angiography as being sufficient alone for planning infrapopliteal surgical bypass grafts and percutaneous intervention [4–6]. A benefit of MR angiography is particularly evident in the identification of small runoff vessels in patients with limb-threatening ischemia. MR angiography has proved to be superior to conventional angiography in detecting small runoff vessels [4,7]. This difference is of critical importance in patients at risk for limb loss, because the identification of a suitable distal vessel for bypass may provide the only possibility of pulse restoration in the foot and, consequently, limb salvage. MR angiography has been found to improve surgical planning and limb salvage because of the ability to see potential bypass sites [8,9]. A multicenter trial involving six hospitals reported that MR angiography was as accurate as conventional angiography but improved the treatment plan in 13% of patients because of improved runoff vessel visualization [1].

Although 2D TOF techniques are accurate and in some instances better than conventional angiography, they are time consuming, with imaging times close to 2 hours for a complete examination [10]. The iliac arteries are especially subject to flow artifacts, which reduces the accuracy of diagnosis, owing to the fact that they are more often tortuous or aneurysmal and exhibit a higher degree of pulsatility in patients with peripheral vascular disease. The advent of three-dimensional (3D) contrast-enhanced (CE) MR angiography significantly reduced the imaging time necessary for a quality examination as well as minimizing artifact problems. 3D CE MR angiography, like 2D TOF MR angiography, has excellent accuracy when compared with conventional angiography [11–13]. In addition, 3D CE MR angiography demonstrates more target vessels than TOF imaging, and metallic susceptibility artifacts are less problematic [10]. Furthermore, TOF imaging tends to overestimate the degree of stenosis when compared with 3D CE MR angiography

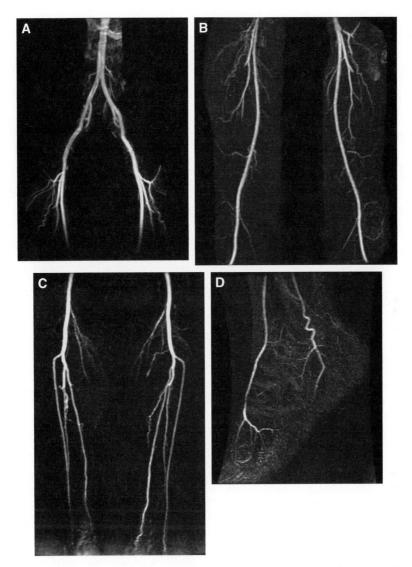

Fig. 1. (*A–D*) Normal hybrid contrast-enhanced MR angiography examination showing two-station runoff of the abdominal-pelvic station (*A*) and thighs (*B*) and stationary time-resolved MR angiography of the calf (*C*) and foot (*D*).

and conventional angiography [14]. 3D CE MR angiography techniques have become the non-invasive study of choice. Nevertheless, some shortcomings to this technique remain. Improvements are continually being made, and the imaging approach is not yet fully standardized across sites or equipment vendors.

Multistation bolus-chase techniques have been developed to improve speed and reduce the complexity of MR angiography [15]. There are inherent benefits to a technique that is limited to one contrast injection and one patient positioning with one coil. Bolus tracking techniques maintain

high sensitivity and specificity when compared with conventional angiography [16]. Nevertheless, there are challenges associated with timing the imaging during arterial windows to maximize arterial signal and avoid venous contamination. When compared with single-station 3D CE MR angiography, bolus-chase techniques have limited arterial visualization of the calves, with frequent venous contamination and reduced accuracy [17,18]. Using parallel imaging with sensitivity encoding (eg, sensitivity encoding [SENSE], array spatial sensitivity encoding technique, integrated parallel acquisition techniques) to shorten scan

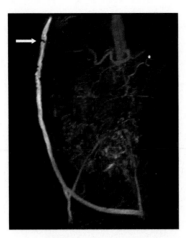

Fig. 2. This axillary bifemoral bypass graft (*arrow*) in a patient presenting for inflow treatment for aortic occlusion has a proximal weblike stenosis. Identification of this lesion facilitates proper catheter insertion for percutaneous interventional therapies.

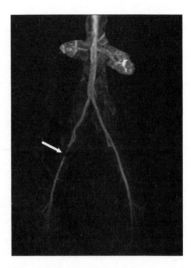

Fig. 3. MR angiography of the abdomen-pelvis station displays a focal, short segment, high-grade stenosis (*arrow*) of the distal right external iliac artery. This patient is an ideal candidate for percutaneous intervention to improve inflow. MR angiography road mapping permits ipsilateral or contralateral access, whereas clinical examination would only permit contralateral access.

times at the abdominal station, Maki et al [19] found themselves able to image the lower station more quickly, resulting in better resolution and decreased venous contamination. Early bolus tracking techniques were limited to fixed imaging parameters for all stations. Having flexible imaging parameters at each imaging level improves image quality by allowing the operator to optimize acquisition planes, spatial resolution, k-space trajectory, and scan times at each station [20]. Furthermore, the use of phased array coils versus a body coil provides better image quality for the lower legs and feet [15].

A meta-analysis of more than 1000 patients by Koelemay et al [21] determined that MR angiography was a highly accurate diagnostic tool for evaluating peripheral vascular disease, which has been further improved by 3D CE MR angiography. Technologic improvements continue to be made to reduce venous contamination and increase resolution. Venous signal is a particular problem in the lower legs in patients with limb-threatening ischemia whose hope for limb salvage rests on the identification of a patent runoff vessel in the lower calf and foot. In addition to advanced MR acquisition techniques, simple venous compression with a blood pressure cuff has been shown to produce a significant improvement in arterial visualization while reducing venous contamination [22,23]. A hybrid technique starting with a stationary examination of the calf with

a two-station runoff in the abdomen and thigh can minimize the problem of venous return.

Because of the dose of gadolinium (Gd)-chelate contrast agent required for the standard three-station examination, full examination of the ankle and foot generally requires time-consuming 2D TOF MR angiography. Time-resolved imaging, described by Grist et al [24], offers a technique that provides the appearance of an x-ray digital subtraction angiographic examination at a somewhat reduced temporal resolution but with good spatial resolution, no venous contamination, and reduced contrast dose. This technique has permitted the authors to obviate 2D TOF imaging by performing stationary time-resolved MR angiography at the pedal and calf levels, followed by an abdomen and thigh two-station examination with less than 80 mL of a Gd-chelate contrast agent (Fig. 1).

Postsurgical evaluation of bypass grafts is typically performed by duplex ultrasound; however, when the need arises, MR angiography can be a useful diagnostic tool for evaluating and localizing disease in bypass grafts [25]. Loewe et al [26] determined that MR angiography was equally accurate in detecting disease in bypass grafts and in native arteries. MR angiography provides remarkable sensitivity and specificity for disease

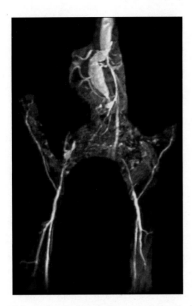

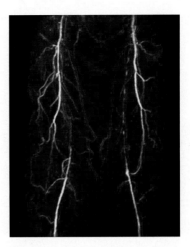

Fig. 4. This patient has an infrarenal abdominal aortic and bilateral common iliac arterial occlusion. Collateral flow fills the external iliac arteries in a retrograde fashion, precluding the patient from having endovascular therapy to improve inflow. The patient will most likely need a surgical bypass. Conventional angiography would require higher-risk transbrachial access.

Fig. 5. The thigh station on this 3D contrast-enhanced MR angiography demonstrates the importance of the profunda femoral artery in severe disease of the femoral popliteal arterial tree. There is bilateral superficial femoral artery occlusion with reconstitution of the above knee popliteal artery from profunda femoral collaterals. Given the length of occlusive segments, this patient will most likely require a surgical bypass as opposed to percutaneous intervention. The status of the profunda femoral artery and large collateral vessels is important to document.

detection in bypass grafts but is somewhat limited by susceptibility artifact owing to metallic clips (Fig. 2) [25].

What to report

The report should be divided into inflow and outflow sections divided at the inguinal ligament, because treatment decisions for these regions are relatively independent of each other, with inflow revascularization taking precedence over outflow. Important findings to report for all areas are patency (normal, stenotic, occlusion); the presence of occlusion; whether stenosis is focal or diffuse; and, in the presence of occlusion or diffuse stenosis, the level above which the artery is normal and the level of normal vessel reconstitution below to provide take-off and landing segments for a bypass graft.

The report on the lower extremity arterial examination should begin with an evaluation of the abdominal aorta and iliac arteries. Treatment algorithms for the iliac arteries depend on an accurate depiction and description of the number, severity, and length of stenoses [26]. Short segment stenosis of the iliac artery is an ideal candidate for angioplasty or stent deployment (Fig. 3); however, in lesions measuring up to 10 cm and even in unilateral common iliac artery occlusion, treatment with endovascular techniques will often be attempted. It is important to assure the interventionalist that disease does not extend into the common femoral artery, which would preclude endovascular treatment. Lesions that are not typically amenable to percutaneous intervention include diffuse disease of the common iliac arteries, external iliac arteries, and common femoral arteries, long segment occlusion of the common and external iliac arteries, diffuse disease involving the aorta and bilateral iliac arteries, and iliac stenosis with an abdominal aortic aneurysm (Fig. 4) [27].

The outflow report begins with the femoral-popliteal system. The common femoral artery has an important role as a common proximal anastomosis for bypass graft surgery, as well as serving as the puncture site for percutaneous intervention. Percutaneous interventional therapies are contraindicated in the common femoral artery; endarterectomy is the preferred technique for managing atherosclerotic disease at this level, often performed in conjunction with a bypass graft. In patients with superficial femoral artery disease,

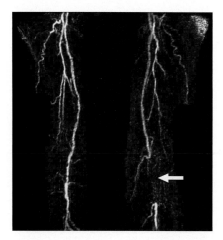

Fig. 6. This patient has an occlusion of the above knee left popliteal artery (*arrow*). The below knee popliteal artery will likely be the target vessel for bypass grafting with a venous conduit.

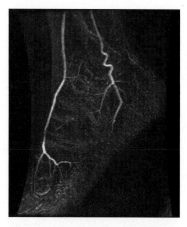

Fig. 8. Time-resolved, contrast-enhanced MR angiography of the foot clearly delineates the medial and lateral plantar branches and the plantar arch. This information has an important role in limb salvage planning; a single patent runoff vessel to the foot could restore a pulse and avoid amputation.

collateral flow is predominantly supplied by the profunda femoral artery, making its evaluation crucial in determining treatment planning for patients with progressive ischemia (Fig. 5). A stenosis at the origin of the profunda femoral artery with superficial femoral artery occlusion may be treated with a percutaneous or surgical

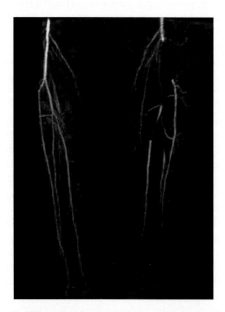

Fig. 7. This patient has an occlusion of the below knee left popliteal artery and proximal tibial vessels. The posterior tibial artery appears to be the dominant runoff to the left ankle, making it a suitable target for bypass graft planning.

profundoplasty to improve collateral flow. The superficial femoral artery is a common site for atherosclerotic disease, particularly at the adductor canal. It is of paramount importance when describing popliteal disease to note the relationship of the disease or reconstitution to the level of the knee (above the knee, at the knee, below the knee). This relationship can alter the treatment plan substantially; above the knee bypass can be performed with synthetic materials, whereas below the knee bypass requires harvesting of vein (Fig. 6).

Runoff vessels to the feet are important to document, particularly in patients who have limb-threatening ischemia. Vascular surgeons are interested in the level at which there is no longer disease in the runoff vessel and where, if a bypass is performed, a pedal pulse will be restored (Fig. 7). Imaging of the foot with contrast-enhanced MR angiography provides visualization of the plantar branches and arch (Fig. 8). Determining which runoff vessel is contiguous with the plantar branches and arch is helpful information for the surgeon who is searching for a way to avoid an amputation in a patient with limb-threatening ischemia.

Future advances

The continuing advances in multichannel systems with whole-body multidetector arrays in combination with SENSE-like acquisition will substantially reduce acquisition times with maintenance of spatial resolution and the SNR. The development of time-resolved acquisitions may eventually permit multiple sequential station acquisitions comparable with x-ray digital subtraction angiography, eliminating issues of bolus timing and venous contamination. Several blood-pool contrast agents are also in various stages of clinical development. In conjunction with arteriovenous segmentation or suppression techniques implemented on imaging workstations, these advances have the potential to eliminate the current need for imaging during the brief arterial transit phase of the contrast agent, raising the achievable level of spatial resolution.

Summary

Peripheral vascular disease is a common problem in the United States. MR angiography is a high-quality noninvasive imaging tool for planning vascular intervention. This technique has supplanted conventional angiography as the tool of choice for planning surgery and percutaneous intervention. The evolution from 2D TOF MR angiography to 3D CE MR angiography has provided improved imaging quality and reduced examination times. Further advancements in the field will continue to improve this technique.

References

[1] Baum R, Rutter C, Sunshine J, et al. Multicenter trial to evaluate vascular magnetic resonance angiography of the lower extremity. JAMA 1995; 274(11):875–80.

[2] Hoch J, Tullis M, Kennell T, et al. Use of magnetic resonance angiography for the preoperative evaluation of patients with infrainguinal arterial occlusive disease. J Vasc Surg 1996;23(5):792–800.

[3] Carpenter J, Baum R, Holland G, et al. Peripheral vascular surgery with magnetic resonance angiography as the sole preoperative imaging modality. J Vasc Surg 1994;20(6):861–70.

[4] Carpenter J, Owen R, Baum R, et al. Magnetic resonance angiography of the peripheral runoff vessels. J Vasc Surg 1992;16(6):807–14.

[5] Cambria R, Yucel E, Brewster D, et al. The potential for lower extremity revascularization without contrast angiography: experience with magnetic resonance angiography. J Vasc Surg 1993;17(6):1050–6.

[6] Levy M, Baum R, Carpenter J. Endovascular surgery based solely on noninvasive preprocedural imaging. J Vasc Surg 1998;28(6):995–1003.

[7] Unger E, Schilling J, Awad A, et al. MR angiography of the foot and ankle. J Magn Reson Imaging 1995;5(1):1–5.

[8] Carpenter J, Golden M, Barker C, et al. The fate of bypass grafts to angiographically occult runoff vessels detected by magnetic resonance angiography. J Vasc Surg 1996;23(3):483–9.

[9] Owen R, Carpenter J, Baum R, et al. Magnetic resonance imaging of angiographically occult runoff vessels in peripheral arterial occlusive disease. N Engl J Med 1992;326(24):1577–81.

[10] Sharafuddin M, Stolpen A, Sun S, et al. High resolution multiphase contrast-enhanced three-dimensional MR angiography compared with two-dimensional time-of flight MR angiography for the identification of the pedal vessels. J Vasc Interv Radiol 2002;13(7):695–702.

[11] Huber A, Hueck A, Baur A, et al. Dynamic contrast-enhanced MR angiography from the distal aorta to the ankle joint with a step-by-step technique. Am J Radiol 2000;175:1291–8.

[12] Ruehm S, Hany T, Pfammatter T, et al. Pelvic and lower extremity arterial imaging: diagnostic performance of three-dimensional contrast-enhanced MR angiography. Am J Radiol 2000; 174:1127–35.

[13] Reid S, Pagan-Marin H, Menzoian J, et al. Contrast-enhanced moving-table MR angiography: prospective comparison to catheter angiography for treatment planning in peripheral arterial occlusive disease. J Vasc Interv Radiol 2001; 12(1):45–53.

[14] Poon E, Yucel E, Pagan-Marin H, et al. Iliac artery stenosis measurements: comparison of two-dimensional time-of-flight and three-dimensional dynamic gadolinium-enhanced MR angiography. Am J Radiol 1997;169:1139–44.

[15] Ho K, Leiner T, de Haan M, et al. Peripheral vascular tree stenoses: evaluation with moving-bed infusion-tracking MR angiography. Radiology 1998;206(3):683–92.

[16] Loewe C, Schoder M, Rand T, et al. Peripheral vascular occlusive disease: evaluation with contrast-enhanced moving-bed MR angiography versus digital subtraction angiography in 106 patients. Am J Radiol 2002;179:1013–21.

[17] Hood M, Ho V, Foo T, et al. High-resolution gadolinium-enhanced 3D MRA of the infrapopliteal arteries: lessons for improving bolus-chase peripheral MRA. Magn Reson Imaging 2002;20: 543–9.

[18] Binkert C, Baker P, Petersen B, et al. Peripheral vascular disease: blinded study of dedicated calf MR angiography versus standard bolus-chase MR angiography and film hard-copy angiography. Radiology 2004;232(3):860–6.

[19] Maki J, Wilson G, Eubank W, et al. Utilizing SENSE to achieve lower station sub-millimeter isotropic resolution and minimal venous enhancement

in peripheral MR angiography. J Magn Reson Imaging 2002;15:484–91.

[20] Leiner T, Ho K, Nelemans P, et al. Three-dimensional contrast-enhanced moving-bed infusion-tracking (MoBI-Track) peripheral MR angiography with flexible choice of imaging parameters for each field of view. J Magn Reson Imaging 2000;11:368–77.

[21] Koelemay M, Lijmer J, Stoker J, et al. Magnetic resonance angiography for the evaluation of lower extremity arterial disease: a meta-analysis. JAMA 2001;285(10):1338–45.

[22] Bilecen D, Schulte A, Bongartz G, et al. Infragenual cuff-compression reduces venous contamination in contrast-enhanced MR angiography of the calf. J Magn Reson Imaging 2004;20:347–51.

[23] Herborn C, Ajaj W, Goyen M, et al. Peripheral vasculature: whole-body MR angiography with midfemoral venous compression—initial experience. Radiology 2004;230(3):872–8.

[24] Grist T, Swan J, Kennell T, et al. Time-resolved three-dimensional contrast-enhanced MR angiography of the peripheral vessels. Radiology 2001;225(1):43–52.

[25] Bertschinger K, Cassina P, Debatin J, et al. Surveillance of peripheral arterial bypass grafts with three-dimensional MR angiography: comparison with digital subtraction angiography. Am J Radiol 2001; 176:215–20.

[26] Loewe C, Cejna M, Schoder M, et al. Contrast material-enhanced, moving-table MR angiography versus digital subtraction angiography for surveillance of peripheral arterial bypass grafts. J Vasc Interv Radiol 2003;14(9):1129–37.

[27] TransAtlantic Inter-Society Consensus (TASC). Management of peripheral arterial disease. J Vasc Surg Suppl 2000;31(1).

ELSEVIER
SAUNDERS

Magn Reson Imaging Clin N Am
13 (2005) 161–170

MAGNETIC
RESONANCE
IMAGING CLINICS
of North America

Contrast-Enhanced MR Angiography in Infants and Children

Taylor Chung, MD[a,b,c],*, Rajesh Krishnamurthy, MD[a,c]

[a]Department of Radiology, Baylor College of Medicine, 1200 Moursund, Houston, TX 77030, USA
[b]Department of Pediatrics, Baylor College of Medicine, 1200 Moursund, Houston, TX 77030, USA
[c]Edward B. Singleton Department of Diagnostic Imaging, Texas Children's Hospital,
6621 Fannin Street, Houston, TX 77030, USA

MR imaging of vascular structures began with techniques such as time-of-flight and phase contrast that do not require administration of intravenous contrast. At the time, these techniques were considered advantageous when compared with other imaging modalities such as CT that required use of an intravenous contrast agent. Since the introduction of contrast-enhanced MR angiography in the early 1990s [1], however, contrast-enhanced MR angiography has become the most widely used MR angiographic technique. The clinical application of contrast-enhanced MR angiography in the pediatric population has lagged behind that in the adult population, especially in infants and children. The earliest references did not appear in the literature until in 1998 [2]. This delay is probably related, in part, to technical issues such as relatively long scan time and need for breath-holding. With newer high-performance gradients, MR imaging can now be performed much more rapidly, and these faster MR systems have become more widely available. Using current techniques, contrast-enhanced MR angiography can be performed safely even in infants and children, yielding clinically relevant data.

Technical considerations

The truism in pediatric radiology that children are not small adults clearly applies to contrast-enhanced MR angiography. There are some technical challenges in performing contrast-enhanced MR angiography in children. Children may not be able to suspend respiration for a long time, if at all. Depending on their ages, children may require sedation and therefore be unable to hold their breath unless they are fully anesthetized and paralyzed. Children have faster heart rates and more rapid circulation times. Moreover, the volume of contrast agent is limited by their weight and can therefore be quite small (a double dose of contrast in a 5-kg infant is 2 mL). Thus, timing the arrival of the contrast agent can be problematic. For example, small doses of contrast agent do not allow for the use of a test bolus for timing. Moreover, in the practical setting, the intravenous access site can be variable, and often manual injection of contrast is necessary rather than the more controlled administration of contrast by automated injector. The vascular structures are proportionally smaller, putting a certain constraint on the needed spatial resolution.

The use of contrast-enhanced MR angiography in the pediatric population has been reported since the late 1990s [2–19]. Review of the literature shows various techniques are used: free breathing or breath-holding; test-bolus timing scan or best estimate for contrast arrival time, a single dose (ie, 0.1 mmol/kg) or higher doses of contrast agent. Most of the authors reported favorable results, but study methodologies differ, and there is no

* Corresponding author. Edward B. Singleton Department of Diagnostic Imaging, Texas Children's Hospital, 6621 Fannin Street MC2-2521, Houston, TX 77030.

E-mail address: txchung@texaschildrenshospital.org (T. Chung).

accepted reference standard. It seems logical that a contrast-enhanced MR angiography performed with breath-holding will be superior to one performed with free breathing. As Kondo et al [10] had quantified, more peripheral branch pulmonary arteries were visualized on MR angiography with breath-holding than on MR angiography with free breathing. On the other hand, if the goal of the examination is to determine the anatomy or the presence or absence of anomalies of the major vasculature in the body rather than to quantify varying degrees of stenosis of a particular vessel, free-breathing techniques are adequate. Successful visualization of all major thoracic vessels with contrast-enhanced MR angiography during free breathing has been systemically studied with an animal model using baboons with mean weight of 5.7 kg and also in pediatric patients [4,12].

What, then, is the optimal technique for contrast-enhanced MR angiography in infants and children? The answer depends on practical issues such as the MR hardware and software and the level of sedation/anesthesia support available and on the clinical question to be answered. These factors will dictate the trade-off between temporal resolution and spatial resolution. As an extreme example, if the clinical question is to assess differential pulmonary blood flow qualitatively, one can perform a MR angiography with subsecond temporal resolution by significantly compromising the spatial resolution (Fig. 1).

One approach: time-resolved MR angiography

The following discussion describes the authors' approach to performing contrast-enhanced MR angiography in the pediatric population. It is by no means the only approach. Given the particular MR scanner available (1.5-T NT-Intera, Philips Medical Systems, Best, Netherlands; 30-mT/m gradient strength, 150-mT/m/s slew rate) and the authors' desire to have a simple protocol for the technologists to use, they implemented a time-resolved

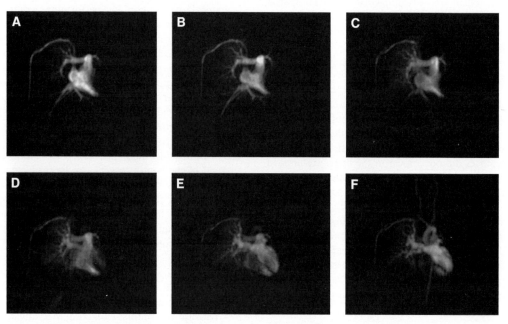

Fig. 1. Subsecond MR angiography. The patient is a sedated, free-breathing, 6-year-old girl with history of left pulmonary vein stenosis following surgical repair of total anomalous pulmonary venous return. (A–F) This multiphase contrast-enhanced MR angiography was performed with the intention to assess qualitatively the differential pulmonary flow between the right and the left lungs. Temporal resolution of 680 milliseconds was achieved by compromising on the spatial resolution (3.7 mm × 1.8 mm × 12 mm) and the use of SENSE factor of three. (Other parameters are TR = 3 milliseconds; TE = 1 millisecond; flip angle = 35°). 0.05 mmol/kg of gadolinium was administered through an automated injector. A through F are full-volume MIP images after subtraction of sequential dynamics illustrating the first pass of contrast through the pulmonary vasculature. There is essentially no gross perfusion to the left lung and no opacification of left pulmonary veins. Cine phase contrast evaluation of the right and left pulmonary arteries (not shown) indicated 99% flow through the right pulmonary artery.

approach [17,19]. This approach has proven to be clinically robust in the past 3 years and can be applied easily for pediatric body MR angiography. Strict bolus timing is not necessary with a time-resolved approach, and it can be applied with or without breath-holding. For a bolus-timing approach, the reader is referred to the excellent work of Holmqvist et al [9].

The basic premise for time-resolved contrast-enhanced MR angiography in the pediatric patient is based on the ability to collect data rapidly while maintaining adequate spatial resolution.

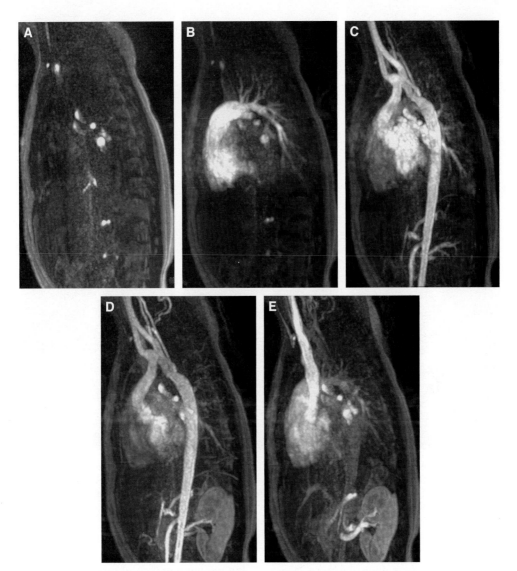

Fig. 2. Time-resolved contrast-enhanced MR angiography with SENSE. The patient is a sedated, freely breathing 4-year-old boy with a tortuous left-sided aortic arch with aberrant right subclavian artery and coarctation of the aorta. The scan time per dynamic scan or the temporal resolution was 4.7 seconds with an acquired spatial resolution of 1.1 mm × 1.9 mm × 2.6 mm reconstructed to 0.5 mm × 0.5 mm × 1.3 mm. Seven dynamic scans were obtained with a total scan time of 33 seconds. (Other parameters are TR = 4.8 milliseconds; TE = 1.4 milliseconds; flip angle = 35°; SENSE factor = 3). 0.2 mmol/kg of gadolinium was administered intravenously using an automated injector. (A–E) Full-volume MIP images of the second through sixth dynamic scans, respectively, without any other forms of postprocessing. Note that the pulmonary arterial phase (B), pulmonary venous phase (C), the systemic arterial phase (D), and the systemic venous phase (E) can be separated.

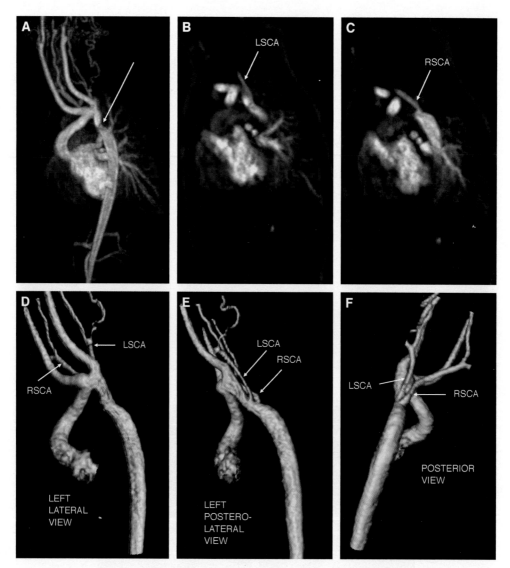

Fig. 3. (*A*) MIP image after subtraction indicating area of coarctation (*arrow*). (*B, C*) MPR images and (*D–G*) 3-D surface-rendered images reconstructed using the fourth dynamic of the contrast-enhanced MR angiogram shown in Fig. 2C. The origins of the left subclavian artery (LSCA) and the aberrant right subclavian artery (RSCA) can be seen immediately adjacent to each other and to the site of discrete coarctation and are best appreciated on the surface-rendered 3-D images.

Theoretically, faster acquisition ought to minimize respiratory and cardiovascular pulsation artifacts. Given the fixed parameters of strength and speed of the gradients in a MR scanner, parallel imaging is most helpful in this regard [20,21]. Parallel imaging can allow decreased scan time without compromise of spatial resolution, or vice versa [22]. The disadvantage of parallel imaging is a decreased signal-to-noise ratio (S/N).

Intravenous injections of gadolinium chelate contrast agent have been shown clinically to boost the vascular S/N efficiently, even with the variable injection rates and small volume used in infants and children [17]. There are methods other than parallel imaging reconstruction for shortening scan time; these methods include various clever schemes of k-space filling such as undersampled projection methods [23,24].

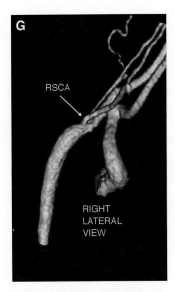

Fig. 3 (*continued*)

For contrast-enhanced MR angiography, the authors use a three-dimensional (3-D) T1-weighted fast gradient echo sequence with a flip angle of 30° to 40° and shortest repetition time (TR) and echo time (TE). By applying sensitivity encoding (SENSE), a parallel-imaging technique [21], with a SENSE factor of two to three in the in-plane phase-encoding direction or a SENSE factor of two in both the slice direction and the in-plane phase-encoding direction, one can achieve a two- to fourfold acceleration of scan speed in a 3-D acquisition without compromising spatial resolution. The authors typically adjust the in-plane resolution and slice-direction partition thickness for a particular required volume of coverage to achieve a scan time of 4 to 6 seconds for each dataset. Usually, the first 3-D image set is acquired before injection of contrast. This image set is used as the image mask for subtraction in postprocessing. They typically use double-dose contrast, 0.2 mmol/kg of a gadolinium chelate. (The use of gadolinium chelate contrast agents for contrast-enhanced MR angiography in pediatric patients is

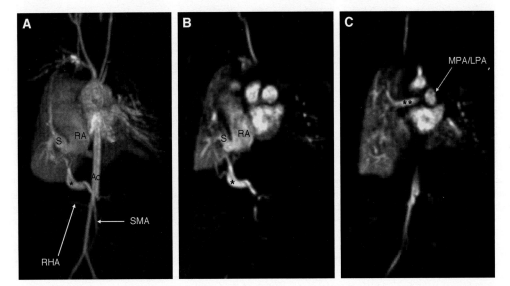

Fig. 4. A 2-month-old infant with scimitar syndrome. For medical reasons, the patient was under general anesthesia for this MR examination; therefore respirations were suspended during the contrast-enhanced MR angiogram. (*A*) A full-volume MIP image after subtraction. The 'scimitar' vein (S) can be seen entering into inferior-lateral aspect of the right atrium (RA). The systemic arterial feeder (*) is seen originating from the proximal celiac axis. Note the relatively large upper abdominal aorta (Ao) when compared with the infraceliac abdominal aorta. There is an incidental finding of a replaced right hepatic artery (RHA) from the superior mesenteric artery (SMA). (*B, C*) Selected thin subvolume MIP images. (*B*) The systemic arterial feeder (*) is shown in better detail. (*C*) The right pulmonary artery (**) is smaller than the left pulmonary artery. The junction of the main pulmonary artery and the left pulmonary artery (MPA/LPA) can be seen on this thin MIP image.

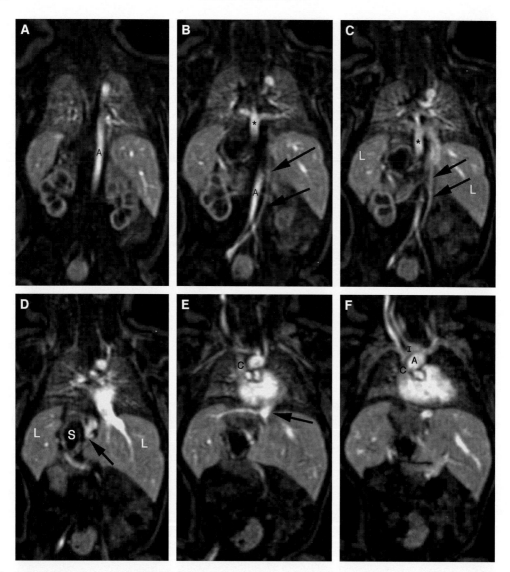

Fig. 5. Selected postprocessed images from a time-resolved contrast-enhanced MR angiogram performed on a newborn infant with heterotaxy. This infant was under general anesthesia for the MR examination because of his general medical condition, and the contrast-enhanced MR angiogram was performed with respiration suspended. By analyzing the source images, nearly all the extracardiac vascular anomalies in this infant with heterotaxy (asplenia) can be detected. (*A–G*) Selected coronal sections from a mixed arterial and venous dynamic scan from the contrast-enhanced MR angiogram arranged from posterior to anterior. Scan time for each dynamic image set was 6 seconds. (*A*) A left-sided descending aorta (A). (*B*, *C*) The total anomalous pulmonary venous return (TAPVR) below the diaphragm (*) and a left-sided inferior vena cava (*black arrows*) traversing a transverse liver (L). (*D*) A right-sided stomach (S) with the transverse liver (L) and the TAPVR entering into a branch of the portal venous system (*black arrow*). (*E* and *F*) The confluence of hepatic veins entering into the left side of the floor of the atrium (*black arrow*). A right-sided superior vena cava (C) with a patent left innominate vein (I) and a right-sided ascending aorta (A). (*G*) The main portal vein (PV) spanning the transverse liver. (*From* Chung T. Magnetic Resonance angiography of the body in pediatric patients: experience with contrast-enhanced time-resolved technique. Pediatr Radiol, in press; with permission.)

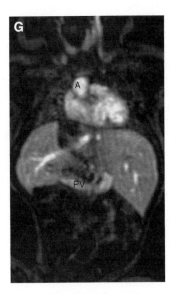

Fig. 5 (*continued*)

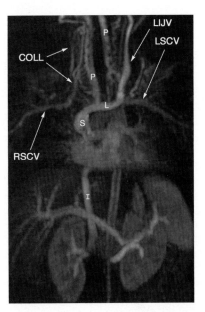

Fig. 6. A 2-year-old girl with history of multiple central venous catheter placements. The contrast-enhanced MR angiogram was performed for presurgical evaluation of the anatomy of the central venous system in the chest before placement of another central venous catheter. The full-volume MIP of the venous dynamic after subtraction shows large paraspinal venous collaterals (P) posteriorly and right-sided cervical venous collaterals (COLL) with nonopacification of the presumably thrombosed right internal jugular vein. The right sub-clavian vein (RSCV) is no longer in communication with the superior vena cava (S). The left internal jugular vein (LIJV), the left subclavian vein (LSCV), and the left innominate vein (L) are all patent to the superior vena cava. The suprarenal inferior vena cava (I) is also patent.

an off-label usage). Then contrast is injected simultaneously with the start of the acquisition of the remainder of the dynamic scans. There is no pause between the acquisitions of each of the subsequent dynamic scans. Arterial and venous phases tend to be resolved in most cases (Fig. 2).

The degree of spatial resolution versus temporal resolution one can achieve depends on the particular strength and speed of the gradients and the strength of the magnet. For example, Balci et al [16] reported on their evaluation of anomalous pulmonary circulation by dynamic contrast-enhanced MR angiography (using a single dose of gadolinium-based intravenous contrast agent) in 10 freely breathing patients (ages, 1–8 years; mean age, 2.8 years). They achieved acquisition times of 2 to 3 seconds with a TR of 1.85 to 2 milliseconds and a TE of 0.6 milliseconds on a 1.5-T MR scanner with gradient strength of 40 mT/m and slew rate of 200 mT/m/s. Adequate spatial resolution was achieved.

Depending on the clinical situation, various datasets of different vascular phases can be analyzed retrospectively by using two-dimensional techniques such as multiplanar reformat (MPR), maximum intensity projection (MIP), and 3-D volume rendering. (Fig. 3) With the advent of the latest 3-D workstations by various vendors, the time required for postprocessing has significantly decreased. It typically takes no longer than 5 to 10 minutes to generate a 3-D volume-rendered, animated movie file for display purposes for the referring physicians.

Clinical applications

In the authors' clinical practice, the most common referral for body MR angiography is MR angiography of the chest related to congenital heart disease (see Figs. 1–4). Although echocardiography is an excellent, noninvasive, mobile imaging modality for imaging the heart and the great vessels of the chest, there are many instances in which the transverse arch, the proximal descending thoracic aorta, or the pulmonary arteries and veins cannot be well seen, especially in older children and young adolescents and in postoperative patients after median sternotomy. Multidetector-row CT scanning also is an excellent imaging modality. In addition, the acquisition time is so fast that sedation is not needed in some children. The disadvantages of CT are the need for iodinated intravenous contrast agent and ionization radiation. The discussion here is limited to contrast-enhanced MR angiography, one of the many MR pulse sequences available. In general, MR offers a much more comprehensive examination, with the ability to obtain functional information such as ventricular function and flow quantification.

Although most referring physicians have come to expect 3-D displays of the MR angiography data, it is the raw data or source images that contain detailed morphologic information. With MPR and thin, subvolume MIP images, all MR angiography data can be scrutinized. This ability proves most helpful in complex cases, such as in patients with heterotaxy syndrome (Fig. 5).

Another clinical use of MR angiography is to evaluate the systemic venous anatomy. The systemic venous anatomy is easily demonstrated in the venous phases of a MR angiography of the chest (Fig. 6). This information can be most helpful in the preoperative evaluation of a patient with difficult venous access because of prior central lines. MR angiography provides the surgeon or interventional radiologist a global view of

the systemic venous anatomy in any desired orientation.

Other reported clinical applications of MR angiography in the pediatric population include oncologic imaging and evaluation before liver transplantation (Fig. 7) [3,6,8]. Contrast-enhanced MR angiography allows improved assessment of the anatomic relationship of the vascular anatomy with the solid tumor and other vital structures and was thought to be superior to other imaging modalities, although the study population was quite small. In the later phases of the MR angiography of the abdomen, the portal venous anatomy typically is well depicted in a global fashion for the transplant surgeon (Fig. 8).

Because of its relative noninvasive nature, contrast-enhanced MR angiography has been requested for various other clinical scenarios. These requests have included renal MR angiography for evaluation of renal artery stenosis for the work-up of hypertension and total-body MR angiography for evaluation of systemic vascular disease such as Kawasaki disease. There are limitations to the use of MR angiography in these

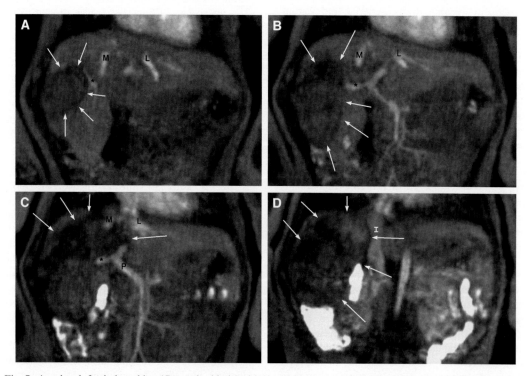

Fig. 7. A sedated, freely breathing 17-month-old girl with hepatoblastoma. (A–D) selected coronal MPR images from the venous dynamic scan of a contrast-enhanced MR angiogram showing the spatial relationship between the margin of the tumor (arrows) and the major hepatic vessels. *, right portal vein and branch; I, inferior vena cava; L, left hepatic vein; M, middle hepatic vein; P, main portal vein.

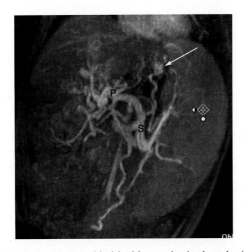

Fig. 8. An 11-year-old girl with portal vein thrombosis and cavernous transformation and massive splenomegaly. This subvolume MIP image in the portal venous phase demonstrates many irregular collateral vessels representing cavernous transformation at the porta hepatis. Other portal venous collaterals between the massive spleen and the stomach are also depicted (*arrow*). The splenic vein (S) and the proximal portal vein (P) are patent.

clinical settings. Given the achievable spatial resolution, only gross disease states can be determined. In renal artery stenosis, time-resolved MR angiography will be useful only for evaluating the narrowing of the main renal arteries. Stenosis in a branch renal artery that can be the cause of hypertension is best assessed by conventional angiography. In Kawasaki disease, serial examinations can demonstrate regression of gross aneurysms (Fig. 9), but fine irregularities of the vessel wall are not detected.

Summary

With the availability of faster and stronger gradients in MR scanner hardware and advances in MR scanner software, contrast-enhanced MR angiography can be successfully performed even in infants and children despite the technical challenges detailed earlier in this discussion. As the speed of rapid MR imaging approaches real time [25–27], the technique of vascular imaging of infants and children by MR will continue to improve. The current challenges of rapid physiologic motions and the inability of a child to hold breath may not be significant issues in the near future.

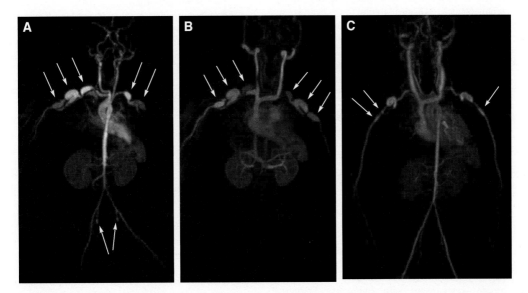

Fig. 9. An 11-month-old infant with Kawasaki disease and giant coronary aneurysms (not shown). (*A, B*) Full-volume MIP images from two consecutive dynamic scans of a time-resolved contrast-enhanced MR angiogram with 5-second temporal resolution. Multiple bilateral large subclavian/branchial artery aneurysms and bilateral small internal iliac artery aneurysms are present (*arrows*). (*C*) A full-volume MIP image from a follow-up contrast-enhanced MR angiogram on the same patient 5 months later showing significant improvement of the aneurysms. Arrows point to subtle focal dilations along the bilateral subclavian/branchial arteries, which are not visualized as well because of the limited spatial resolution of the sequence. Note that the internal iliac aneurysms are no longer detectable.

References

[1] Prince MR, Yucel E, Kaufman J, et al. Dynamic gadolinium-enhanced three-dimensional abdominal MR arteriography. J Magn Reson Imaging 1993;3: 877–81.

[2] Lam WWM, Chan JHM, Hui Y, et al. Technical innovation: non-breath-hold gadolinium-enhanced MR angiography of the thoracoabdominal aorta: experience in 18 children. AJR 1998;170: 478–80.

[3] Haliloglu M, Hoffer FA, Gronemeyer SA, et al. Applications of 3D contrast enhanced MR angiography in pediatric oncology. Pediatr Radiol 1999; 29:863–8.

[4] Pawlik HN, Chung T. Initial clinical experience with non-breath-hold gadolinium-enhanced 3D-MR angiography of thorax and abdomen in infants and children with pathology. Proceedings of the International Society for magnetic Resonance in Medicine 1999;7:1221.

[5] Teo EHJ, Strouse PJ, Prince MR. Applications of magnetic resonance imaging and magnetic resonance angiography to evaluate the hepatic vasculature in the pediatric patient. Pediatr Radiol 1999; 29:238–43.

[6] Haliloglu M, Hoffer FA, Gronemeyer SA, et al. 3D gadolinium-enhanced MRA: evaluation of hepatic-vasculature in children with hepatoblastoma. J Magn Reson Imaging 2000;11:65–8.

[7] Masui T, Katayama M, Kobayashi S, et al. Gadolinium-enhanced MR angiography in the evaluation of congenital cardiovascular disease pre- and post-operative states in infants and children. J Magn Reson Imaging 2000;12:1034–42.

[8] Ng KK, Cheng YF, Wong HF, et al. Gadolinium-enhanced magnetic resonance portography: application in paediatric liver transplant recipients. Transplant Proc 2000;21:2099–100.

[9] Holmqvist C, Larrsson E-M, Stahlberg F, et al. Contrast-enhanced thoracic 3D-MR angiography in infants and children. Acta Radiol 2001;42: 50–8.

[10] Kondo C, Takada K, Yokoyama U, et al. Comparison of three-dimensional contrast-enhanced magnetic resonance angiography and axial radiographic angiography for diagnosing congenital stenoses in small pulmonary arteries. Am J Cardiol 2001;87: 420–4.

[11] Kuroiwa M, Suzuki N, Hatakeyama S, et al. Magnetic resonance angiography of portal collateral pathways after hepatic portoenterostomy in biliary atresia: comparisons with endoscopic findings. J Ped Surg 2001;36:1012–6.

[12] Hernandez RJ, Strouse PJ, Londy FJ, et al. Gadolinium-enhanced MR angiography (Gd-MRA) of thoracic vasculature in an animal model using double-dose gadolinium and quiet breathing. Pediatr Radiol 2001;31:589–93.

[13] Hernandez RJ. Magnetic resonance imaging of mediastinal vessels. Magn Reson Imaging Clin N Am 2002;10(2):237–51.

[14] Geva T, Greil GF, Marshall AC, et al. Gadolinium-enhanced 3-dimensional magnetic resonance angiography of pulmonary blood supply in patients with complex pulmonary stenosis or atresia: comparison with X-ray angiography. Circulation 2002; 106(4):473–8.

[15] Valsangiasomo ER, Levasseur S, McCrindle BW, et al. Contrast-enhanced MR angiography of pulmonary venous abnormalities in children. Pediatr Radiol 2003;33:92–8.

[16] Balci NC, Yalsin Y, Tunaci A, et al. Assessment of the anomalous pulmonary circulation by dynamic contrast-enhanced MR angiography in under four seconds. Magn Reson Imaging 2003;21:1–7.

[17] Muthupillai R, Vick GW III, Flamm SD, et al. Free breathing time resolved contrast enhanced MRA in pediatric patients with sensitivity encoding. J Magn Reson Imaging 2003;17:559–64.

[18] Caseiro-Alves F, Gil-Agostinho P, Ramalheiro G, et al. Contrast-enhanced MR angiography of thoracic vascular malformations in a pediatric population. AJR Am J Roentgenol 2003;181:729–35.

[19] Chung T. Magnetic resonance angiography of the body in pediatric patients: experience with a contrast-enhanced time-resolved technique. Pediatr Radiol, in press.

[20] Sodickson DK, Manning WJ. Simultaneous acquisition of spatial harmonics (SMASH): fast imaging with radiofrequency coil arrays. Magn Reson Med 1997;38:591–603.

[21] Pruessmann KP, Weiger M, Schiedegger MB, et al. SENSE: sensitivity encoding for fast MRI. Magn Reson Med 1999;42:952–62.

[22] Weiger M, Pruessmann KP, Kassner A, et al. Contrast-enhanced 3D MRA using SENSE. J Magn Reson Imaging 2000;12:671–7.

[23] Vigen KK, Peters DC, Grist TM, et al. Under-sampled projection-reconstruction imaging for time-resolved contrast-enhanced imaging. Magn Reson Med 2000;43:170–6.

[24] Barger AV, Block WF, Toropov Y, et al. Time-resolved contrast-enhanced imaging with isotropic resolution and broad coverage using an under-sampled 3D projection trajectory. Magn Reson Med 2002;48:297–305.

[25] Tsao J, Behnia B, Webb AG. Unifying linear prior-information-driven method for accelerated image acquisition. Mag Reson Med 2001;46:652–60.

[26] Tsao J, Kozerke S, Boesiger P, et al. Eight-fold acceleration in real-time cardiac imaging using k-t BLAST and k-t SENSE with SSFP and segmented EPI. Proc Intl Soc Mag Reson Med 2003;11:209.

[27] Tsao J, Boesiger P. Pruessmann. MR angiography at high acceleration using feedback regularized SENSE and variable density k-space sampling. Proc Intl Soc Mag Reson Med 2003;11:484.

ELSEVIER
SAUNDERS

Magn Reson Imaging Clin N Am
13 (2005) 171–180

MAGNETIC
RESONANCE
IMAGING CLINICS
of North America

Atherosclerosis Imaging Using MR Imaging: Current and Emerging Applications

Milind Y. Desai, MD[a,b], David A. Bluemke, MD, PhD[b,*]

[a]National Institute of Biomedical Imaging and Bioengineering, National Institutes of Health,
6707 Democracy Boulevard, Bethesda, MD 20892-5477, USA
[b]Russell H. Morgan Department of Radiology and Radiologic Sciences, Johns Hopkins University,
600 North Wolfe Street, Baltimore, MD 21287, USA

Atherosclerosis remains the leading cause of death in industrialized societies, and its incidence is projected to increase worldwide in the next 2 decades [1]. It is recognized as a systemic disease affecting the vessel walls of all the major arteries, including the aorta, coronary, carotid, and peripheral arteries, and leads to a myriad of diseases, including stroke, myocardial infarction, peripheral vascular disease, aortic aneurysms, and sudden death [2]. Traditionally, clinicians have focused on atherosclerotic lesions that cause flow-limiting stenoses. During the last 2 decades, however, it has been shown that the process of atherosclerosis begins as an extraluminal phenomenon in the blood vessel wall, and the flow-limiting stenoses constitute a much later stage in the process of atherosclerosis [3]. Also, studies have demonstrated that the benefits of therapy-related decreased clinical events are not proportional to parallel reductions in vessel stenoses [4]. Therefore, the concept of flow-limiting stenoses has been challenged, and studies now focus more on the progressively atherosclerotic vessel wall. The American Heart Association created a detailed classification scheme designed to be used as a histologic template for images obtained by a variety of invasive and noninvasive techniques in the clinical setting [5,6]. It has been demonstrated that a vast majority of the thromboembolic events result from plaque rupture or erosion [7,8], which is characterized by thinning and rupture of the fibrous cap overlying the thrombogenic lipid core [9,10]. Accurate in vivo tracking of progressive lesions would be extremely useful clinically to determine the status of patients' atherosclerotic disease.

Because a major limitation of X-ray angiography is being a "luminogram," alternative imaging modalities to detect atherosclerotic plaque have been investigated. Intravascular ultrasound has been used to discern plaque components accurately [11], but it is an invasive procedure and is associated with procedure-related complications, and its ability to image the vessel wall downstream from a stenosis is limited. Furthermore, because of its high cost, intravascular ultrasound cannot be justified as a screening tool in an asymptomatic population. B-mode ultrasonography has been used to measure plaque volume in the carotid arteries, but its accuracy is limited by the plane of acquisition and the fact that atherosclerosis is a focal process [12,13]. CT has been used to detect and quantify coronary calcification, but its ability to detect soft, noncalcified plaques is not yet fully determined [14]. MR imaging, because of its high resolution, three-dimensional (3-D) capabilities, noninvasive nature, and capacity for soft tissue characterization, is emerging as a powerful modality to assess the atherosclerotic plaque burden in the arterial wall and has been used to monitor atherosclerosis in vivo [15,16]. This article reviews the technical principles and current status of in vivo MR imaging of atherosclerosis in various arterial beds and briefly discusses ongoing research in this field.

* Corresponding author.
E-mail address: dbluemke@jhmi.edu
(D.A. Bluemke).

Technical considerations for MR imaging of atherosclerosis

To visualize the atherosclerotic plaque by MR imaging accurately, many factors need to be taken into consideration. Accurate imaging must obtain adequate spatial resolution and adequate tissue contrast, avoid or minimize artifacts, be highly reproducible to facilitate longitudinal studies, and at the same time cause little or no discomfort to the subjects.

A normal artery wall is extremely thin (around 1 mm for the coronaries and thicker for the aorta and carotids), but with progressive arterial remodeling this thickness can vary from a few millimeters to more than a centimeter. An important imaging consideration is the ability to discern different plaque components, including the fibrous cap, lipid core, hemorrhage, and calcification. To do so, a spatial resolution in the submillimeter range is necessary. With the advent of sophisticated receiver coils and improvements in hardware, it is now possible to achieve an in-plane resolution in the order of 0.25×0.25 mm^2 in the carotids, 0.8×0.8 mm^2 in the aorta, and 0.46×0.46 mm^2 in the coronaries, with a 2- to 5-mm slice thickness [17–19] on a 1.5-T MR scanner. In 3-D coronary vessel wall imaging, an isotropic resolution of $1.0 \times 1.0 \times 1.0$ mm^3 has also been reported [20]. The use of phased-array surface coil techniques has proven to be effective in improving the signal-to-noise ratio (S/N) [21,22]. The widespread availability of 3-T MR scanners will probably help improve the S/N, which can be partially traded for an improved spatial resolution.

Histologic studies have shown that different plaque components co-exist, and these different components produce differences in the MR signal based upon their physical properties [23]. T1 and T2 relaxation times vary among tissue types, enabling the generation of tissue contrast. Thus, to achieve tissue contrast and hence plaque characterization, images obtained using different weightings are necessary [18,24]. Another technical aspect to consider is the suppression of the signal obtained from the blood flow; this suppression enhances the conspicuity of the vessel wall and its components against the backdrop of a hypointense lumen. Currently, the most effective flow-suppression (black-blood) method in plaque imaging is thought to be the double inversion recovery (IR) technique [25]. IR, in combination with fast spin echo (FSE) techniques, has been used to image the carotid, aortic, and coronary vessel wall [17–19,26]. To reduce the scan time related to this technique, multislice techniques have been developed that reduce the imaging time by two- to fourfold without significantly compromising the S/N [27,28].

The next technical issue to consider is that of artifacts, including those caused by cardiac contraction, breathing, blood flow, and random motion such as swallowing or tremors, all of which can significantly deteriorate image quality. To counter these artifacts, cardiac gating is used to improve the quality of the scan. For aortic and coronary imaging, along with cardiac gating, breathing also is an issue, which is countered by breath-holding or use of respiratory navigators [18–20]. Also, perivascular fat, which can obscure signal from the vessel wall, particularly in the coronaries, needs to be suppressed [29]. An interesting development is the use of contrast agents to enhance plaque components. Usually gadolinium-based agents are used in association with double IR imaging or spoilt gradient echo sequences [30,31]. With the use of novel contrast agents such as ultrasmall paramagnetic particles of iron oxide (USPIOs) or fibrin-specific agents, new data are being acquired rapidly [32–34].

The final technical aspect that needs to be considered is the processing of the MR images that are obtained. Plaque analysis is generally separated into two domains: assessment of morphology (plaque dimensions) and assessment of tissue characteristics. In general, these variables are considered in continuous rather than categorical form so that inferences can be drawn about the longitudinal regression or progression of plaque.

Assessment of plaque morphology using MR imaging

Accurate quantification of vessel wall dimensions depends upon the ability to discern the inner and outer boundaries of the vessel wall. Once these boundaries have been determined, the dimensions can be recorded as thickness or area (difference between outer contour and inner contour). Several semiautomatic image-processing tools have been proposed for vessel boundary detection [35,36]. Atherosclerosis, however, is generally not a uniform process, and there can be sudden variations in regional plaque surfaces. The measurements of thickness and area are less accurate and more vulnerable to anatomic mismatches because only a single slice is measured, and an entire anatomic rematch of the patient's prior scanning position is virtually impossible. Thus, to reduce the variation in plaque dimensions from study to study, plaque volume becomes the morphologic assessment of choice. Generally, multiple (five or six) slices are obtained with the center slice in the middle of the thickest part of the plaque. A modification of Simpson's formula is used to calculate plaque volume. In this process, the emphasis is on the middle slices rather than the outer slices, and minimal errors of registration do not significantly alter the volume measurements. In a carotid artery study, the variability in plaque volume assessment was found to be between 4% and 6% [37]. In a recent study of aortic atherosclerosis, the authors were able to demonstrate that the reproducibility of plaque volume assessment (intraclass correlation coefficient, 0.95; coefficient of variation, 5.7%) was significantly superior to that of plaque thickness (intraclass correlation coefficient, 0.82; coefficient of variation, 18.9%) or plaque area (intraclass correlation coefficient, 0.90; coefficient of variation, 21.3%). Based on these findings, the authors concluded that changes of less than 4.6% in aortic plaque volume could be considered as accurately measured by MR imaging [38].

Characterizing plaque using MR imaging

The difference in MR signal between hydrogen protons in different chemical environments make it ideally suited for noninvasive characterization of the different components of a given plaque. Techniques focused on lipid assessment using spectroscopy and chemical-shift imaging have been found less useful in the in vivo setting because of the relatively low lipid concentration in the tissue and hence poor S/N [39–41]. Most of the newer techniques use water protons to generate the MR signal. Different plaque components have been characterized by T1, T2, and proton-density weightings in animals [42,43], ex vivo specimens [41,44], in vivo carotids [44,45], in vivo aortas [18], and, more recently, the coronaries [19,22].

The characteristic appearance of different plaque components on MR imaging has been previously validated (Figs. 1 and 2) [17,23,44]. Generally, lipid components appear as isointense regions within the plaque on T1- and proton density–weighted images but hypointense on T2-weighted images. On the other hand, the fibrous cap appears bright, and calcium appears very

hypointense on all three weightings. Thrombus appears hyperintense (albeit less so than fibrous cap) on all three weightings. Perivascular fat, which predominantly consists of triglycerides, has a different MR appearance than the lipid core, which generally consists of unesterified cholesterol and cholesterol esters [23,41].

Recent studies have demonstrated that the use of paramagnetic contrast agents, such as gadolinium, enables subtle distinctions between different plaque components to be detected (Fig. 3). Increases in T1 relaxation by gadolinium leads to increased contrast enhancement on T1-weighted pulse sequences. There is evidence of neovascularization and inflammation in atherosclerotic plaque [46], and it has been proposed that contrast-enhanced MR imaging can aid in plaque characterization by helping to detect these changes [30,31]. These studies demonstrated that pre- and postcontrast MR imaging helped differentiate between the necrotic core and fibrous tissue. In the study by Wasserman et al [31] the S/N of fibrous cap was twice that of the lipid core. Another study demonstrated that postcontrast signal enhancement in carotid arteries and aorta is associated with elevated serum levels of interleukin-6, C-reactive protein, and cell adhesion molecules [47].

USPIOs alter the relaxation times of adjacent tissue and are avidly taken up by macrophages. It has been demonstrated that injection of USPIO into hyperlipidemic rabbits is associated with the appearance of signal voids on the luminal surface of the aorta [48]. Another active area of research is the detection of thrombus or fibrin, which has been demonstrated to play a role in plaque progression [7]. Contrast agents that can detect and characterize thrombi have been developed, and fibrin has been identified by lipid-encapsulated perfluorocarbon paramagnetic nanoparticles in vitro [33,49] as well as in vivo [33]. In a recent report, the feasibility of a gadolinium-based fibrin-binding contrast agent, EP-2104R (EPIX Medical, Inc., Cambridge, Massachusetts) was demonstrated in a swine model of coronary thrombus and in-stent thrombosis (Fig. 4) [34]. Potential applications include detection of coronary in-stent thrombosis or thrombus burden in patients with acute coronary syndromes.

MR imaging of carotid atherosclerosis

The carotid artery has become the most common target vessel for MR imaging of

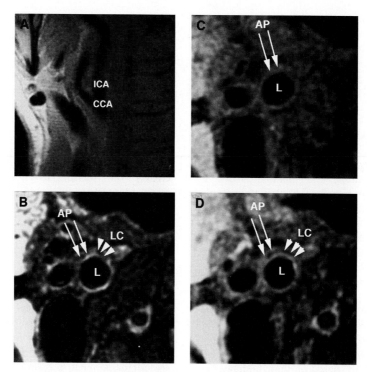

Fig. 1. High-resolution MR images of the right carotid artery of a 72-year-old man with advanced atherosclerosis. (*A*) Oblique proton-density image through the proximal internal and external carotid arteries. This image was used to prescribe subsequent images. CCA, common carotid artery ICA, internal carotid artery. (*B*) T2-weighted precontrast, (*C*) T1-weighted precontrast and (*D*) T1-weighted postcontrast FSE images of the right internal carotid artery demonstrating arterial wall remodeling caused by atherosclerotic plaque (AP). Note the lipid core (LC) within the atherosclerotic plaque on T2-weighted and postcontrast T1-weighted images. L, lumen.

atherosclerosis (see Figs. 1–3). This application has become widespread because of the use of phased-array coils, well-validated multicontrast imaging protocols [17,44], and the existence of a reference based on histologic examination of atherosclerotic lesions obtained surgically during carotid endarterectomy [50].

MR imaging accurately identifies the adventitial layer of the carotid artery and thus aids in measurement of vessel wall dimensions with high accuracy (4%–6% error of vessel volume measurement) [16,37,51]. MR imaging has also been used to demonstrate the state of carotid plaque substructure, including the fibrous cap. In one study, the in vivo state of the fibrous cap was characterized based on its appearance on MR images (intact and thin, intact and thick, or ruptured), and there was a high level of agreement between the MR images and the histologic state of the fibrous cap [45]. When multicontrast MR imaging has been compared with histology, a sensitivity of 81% and specificity of 90% has been

demonstrated for identification of an unstable fibrous cap [52]. A ruptured fibrous cap identified on MR imaging was highly associated with a stroke or a transient ischemic attack [53]. MR imaging also has a high sensitivity and specificity in detecting lipid core, hemorrhage, and calcification in ex vivo imaging of endarterectomy specimens (90%–100%) [54] and in vivo imaging (85%–92%) [24,55]. The role of contrast-enhanced MR imaging in characterizing carotid plaque has been described previously in this article.

MR imaging of aortic atherosclerosis

The feasibility of detecting atherosclerosis of the thoracic aorta using surface receiver coils has been demonstrated, using transesophageal echocardiography (TEE) as a reference [18]. MR assessment of the aorta correlated well with TEE for assessment of plaque thickness, extent, and composition. This technique has been found to be

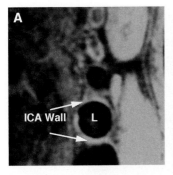 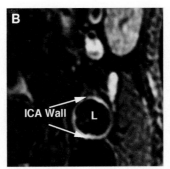 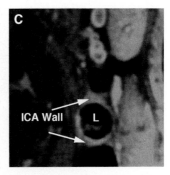

Fig. 2. High-resolution MR images of the right carotid artery of a 75-year-old man with advanced atherosclerosis. (*A*) T2-weighted precontrast, (*B*) T1-weighted precontrast, and (*C*) T1-weighted postcontrast FSE images of the right internal carotid artery (ICA) demonstrating only arterial wall remodeling caused by atherosclerotic plaque (*arrows*). Note the lipid core is absent. L, lumen.

highly reproducible [26]. In subjects from the Framingham heart study, aortic plaque burden increases with age [56]. After 1 year of lipid-lowering therapy, MR imaging of the aorta has demonstrated plaque regression by 8% without a change in the cross-sectional area of the arterial lumen [15,57].

Transesophageal MR imaging (TEMRI) using a loopless antenna coil has been developed for aortic MR imaging. The rationale behind TEMRI comes from a specific limitation for surface MR receiver coils: the trade-off between depth of penetration and S/N. To detect and visualize distant structures such the thoracic aorta adequately, a strong local signal could be of paramount importance; such a signal was achieved by using a TEMRI coil [58]. The feasibility and utility of this technique was demonstrated in patients with aortic atherosclerosis [59]. The authors have

recently demonstrated that the addition of the TEMRI coil increases the signal in the aortic arch and descending aorta by 157% to 225% above that attained by surface coils alone (Fig. 5) [38]. Furthermore, using the combined surface MR imaging and TEMRI, the authors also have demonstrated recently that aortic plaque regression of about 12% can be detected as early as 6 months (as compared with 1 year or longer) following lipid-lowering therapy [60]. The disadvantage of this approach is that the technique is invasive and requires a skilled operator to position the TEMRI probe.

MR imaging of coronary atherosclerosis

Until recently, the acceptance of MR imaging for coronary imaging has been hampered by many

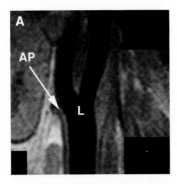 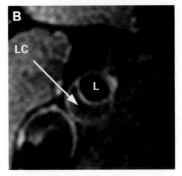

Fig. 3. High-resolution MR images of the right carotid artery of another patient with advanced atherosclerosis. (*A*) Oblique proton density image through the proximal internal and external carotid arteries. This image was used to prescribe subsequent images. AP, atherosclerotic plaque; L, lumen. (*B*) T1-weighted postcontrast FSE image of the right internal carotid artery demonstrating significant arterial wall remodeling caused by atherosclerotic plaque with an excellent postcontrast delineation of the lipid core (LC). L, lumen.

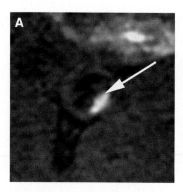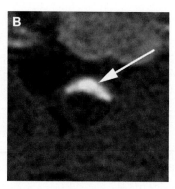

Fig. 4. (*A* and *B*) Two mural thrombi (*arrows*) observed at different levels of the aorta, with good contrast between thrombus (*arrow*), arterial lumen, and vessel wall, 20 hours after administration of EP-1873 contrast agent. (Courtesy of Dr. Phillip Graham, EPIX Medical Inc, Cambridge, MA.)

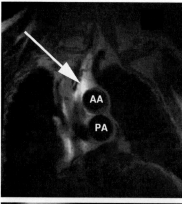
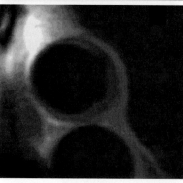

Fig. 5. Double IR FSE proton-density images of the aortic arch, in a patient with advanced atherosclerosis, obtained using a combination of surface and transesophageal MR imaging, demonstrating excellent delineation of the atherosclerotic plaque. The arrow points to the hyperintense signal related to the transesophageal receiver coil. AA, aortic arch; PA, pulmonary artery.

technical limitations, including constant cardiac motion caused by contraction/relaxation, diaphragmatic/chest wall motion caused by respiration, the small caliber of the coronary vessels, the tortuosity of the coronary arteries, and signal from surrounding epicardial fat and myocardium [61]. With the following refinements of MR techniques, however, coronary imaging has become technically feasible. To account for bulk cardiac motion, ECG gating (particularly the vector ECG approach) has been used with unprecedented results [62]. Because coronary artery motion is minimal at mid-diastole, it has become the preferred time for imaging [61]. Several different approaches have been used to minimize the effect of respiratory motion. These methods include sustained or multiple brief breath-holds, coached breathing, free breathing using multiple averages, and chest wall bellows. A more recent innovation is the positioning of MR navigators at any interface that accurately depicts respiratory motion (eg, the dome of the right hemidiaphragm) [61,63]. Advanced MR pulse sequences have been developed that can suppress the signal from surrounding epicardial fat and the myocardium, thus enabling visualization of the coronary arteries with contrast [29]. Finally, to improve in-plane spatial resolution to image the coronaries, newer cardiac-specific coils have been developed that support an improved S/N [61].

Fayad et al [19] have demonstrated the feasibility of in vivo imaging of the coronary vessel wall using a 2-D black-blood technique [19]. The reproducibility of this technique, which must be excellent for this imaging method to become a useful clinical tool, has only recently been studied at John Hopkins University. The authors have recently demonstrated that coronary vessel wall imaging (Fig. 6) using the double IR FSE (2-D black-blood pulse sequence) was reproducible (r = 0.87) with good inter- and intraobserver agreement [64]. This technique allows only limited spatial coverage, however. To overcome this problem, Botnar et al [65] have attempted to image the coronary vessel wall using 3-D black-blood coronary MR imaging, along with a local inversion prepulse to suppress unwanted signal (ventricular blood, myocardium, and chest wall tissue) outside a user-defined region of interest, and a spiral imaging technique. They were able to show the phenomenon of outward arterial remodeling noninvasively [20]. This technique enables the imaging of a long segment of the coronary artery wall and might be a useful screening technique for measuring plaque burden.

Role of intravascular MR imaging

The ability of MR imaging to generate high-resolution images of the vessel wall, delineate perivascular soft tissue structures, and generate multiplanar images in real time have generated interest in MR imaging as a replacement for X-ray angiography [66]. In a recent study on swine, an intravascular MR coil/guide wire (Surgi-Vision, Gaithersburg, Maryland), introduced through the external iliac vein into the inferior vena cava generated excellent images in vivo that correlated well with histologic findings (Fig. 7) [67]. Preliminary studies have also demonstrated the feasibility of MR-guided percutaneous angioplasty in rabbit aorta [68], stent deployment in pig femoral arteries [69] and pig coronary arteries

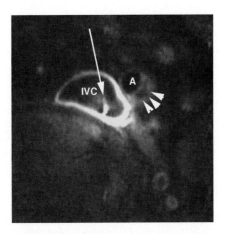

Fig. 7. Double IR FSE image of the abdominal aorta (A) in a patient with advanced atherosclerosis, obtained using an intravascular coil positioned in the inferior vena cava (IVC). Notice the bright signal emanating from the coil (*arrow*). The atherosclerotic changes in the aortic wall (*arrowheads*) are well delineated.

[70], and monitoring of catheter-based gene therapy in pig femoral arteries [71].

Future of MR-based atherosclerosis imaging

As described in this article, the past decade has seen significant developments in the MR imaging of atherosclerosis. Most of the studies, however, have involved a small number of subjects, and there is paucity of multicenter data. Because there is considerable institutional variation in acquisition and in analysis techniques, it is difficult to classify current findings as anything other than preliminary. Nonetheless, current results open an exciting window of opportunity that can be used to devise an optimal treatment strategy, monitor the effect of therapy, and understand better the pathophysiology of atherosclerosis.

Potential applications of MR atherosclerosis imaging might include its use in longitudinal studies looking at the effects of newer drug therapies on plaque composition and morphology. Advantages would include noninvasive or minimally invasive monitoring of plaque regression with MR imaging and the potential to reduce the sample size compared with intravascular ultrasound. MR imaging also can be used to monitor disease progression in high-risk patients. Further refinements of the technique and in image analysis will be necessary before the use of MR imaging for this purpose becomes widespread.

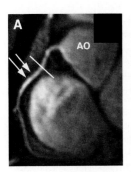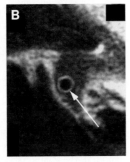

Fig. 6. (*A*) MR angiogram of the right coronary artery (*arrows*). AO, aorta. The bold line indicates where the image of the vessel wall was obtained. (*B*) Double IR FSE image of the right coronary artery (*arrow*) in a healthy volunteer.

Other potential applications include individually tailored therapy for patients based on their plaque characteristics and plaque burden. Because of advances in MR hardware and software, MR imaging could be used as a screening tool to stratify patients based on their cardiovascular risk. Finally, the high resolution of MR imaging and the development of sophisticated contrast agents offer tremendous promise of in vivo molecular imaging of the atherosclerotic plaque.

Summary

Because of its high resolution, 3-D capabilities, noninvasive nature, and capacity for soft tissue characterization, MR imaging has emerged as a powerful modality to assess the process of atherosclerosis comprehensively in different arterial beds, including the coronary arteries. It holds great promise in studies involving longitudinal follow-up of plaque progression and for detection of therapeutic intervention-related changes. With the development of newer, target-specific contrast agents and molecular imaging applications, an exponential growth in its current applications is anticipated.

Acknowledgments

The authors thank Dr. Phillip Graham of Epix Medical Inc, Cambridge, MA, for providing the images in Fig. 4.

References

[1] Michaud CM, Murray CJ, Bloom BR. Burden of disease–implications for future research. JAMA 2001;285(5):535–9.
[2] Ross R. Atherosclerosis–an inflammatory disease. N Engl J Med 1999;340(2):115–26.
[3] Glagov S, Weisenberg E, Zarins CK, et al. Compensatory enlargement of human atherosclerotic coronary arteries. N Engl J Med 1987;316(22):1371–5.
[4] Brown BG, Zhao XQ, Chait A, et al. Simvastatin and niacin, antioxidant vitamins, or the combination for the prevention of coronary disease. N Engl J Med 2001;345(22):1583–92.
[5] Stary HC, Chandler AB, Dinsmore RE, et al. A definition of advanced types of atherosclerotic lesions and a histological classification of atherosclerosis. A report from the Committee on Vascular Lesions of the Council on Arteriosclerosis, American Heart Association. Circulation 1995;92(5):1355–74.
[6] Stary HC, Chandler AB, Glagov S, et al. A definition of initial, fatty streak, and intermediate lesions of atherosclerosis. A report from the Committee on Vascular Lesions of the Council on Arteriosclerosis, American Heart Association. Arterioscler Thromb 1994;14(5):840–56.
[7] Virmani R, Kolodgie FD, Burke AP, et al. Lessons from sudden coronary death: a comprehensive morphological classification scheme for atherosclerotic lesions. Arterioscler Thromb Vasc Biol 2000;20(5):1262–75.
[8] Shah PK. Pathophysiology of coronary thrombosis: role of plaque rupture and plaque erosion. Prog Cardiovasc Dis 2002;44(5):357–68.
[9] Falk E. Why do plaques rupture? Circulation 1992;86(6 Suppl):III30–42.
[10] Davies MJ, Thomas AC. Plaque fissuring–the cause of acute myocardial infarction, sudden ischaemic death, and crescendo angina. Br Heart J 1985;53(4):363–73.
[11] Nissen SE, Yock P. Intravascular ultrasound: novel pathophysiological insights and current clinical applications. Circulation 2001;103(4):604–16.
[12] O'Leary DH, Polak JF. Intima-media thickness: a tool for atherosclerosis imaging and event prediction. Am J Cardiol 2002;90(10C):18L–21L.
[13] Spence JD. Ultrasound measurement of carotid plaque as a surrogate outcome for coronary artery disease. Am J Cardiol 2002;89(4A):10B–5B [discussion: 15B–16B].
[14] Fayad ZA, Fuster V, Nikolaou K, et al. Computed tomography and magnetic resonance imaging for noninvasive coronary angiography and plaque imaging: current and potential future concepts. Circulation 2002;106(15):2026–34.
[15] Corti R, Fuster V, Fayad ZA, et al. Lipid lowering by simvastatin induces regression of human atherosclerotic lesions: two years' follow-up by high-resolution noninvasive magnetic resonance imaging. Circulation 2002;106(23):2884–7.
[16] Yuan C, Beach KW, Smith LH Jr, et al. Measurement of atherosclerotic carotid plaque size in vivo using high resolution magnetic resonance imaging. Circulation 1998;98(24):2666–71.
[17] Yuan C, Mitsumori LM, Beach KW, et al. Carotid atherosclerotic plaque: noninvasive MR characterization and identification of vulnerable lesions. Radiology 2001;221(2):285–99.
[18] Fayad ZA, Nahar T, Fallon JT, et al. In vivo magnetic resonance evaluation of atherosclerotic plaques in the human thoracic aorta: a comparison with transesophageal echocardiography. Circulation 2000;101(21):2503–9.
[19] Fayad ZA, Fuster V, Fallon JT, et al. Noninvasive in vivo human coronary artery lumen and wall imaging using black-blood magnetic resonance imaging. Circulation 2000;102(5):506–10.
[20] Kim WY, Stuber M, Bornert P, et al. Three-dimensional black-blood cardiac magnetic resonance coronary vessel wall imaging detects positive arterial remodeling in patients with nonsignificant

coronary artery disease. Circulation 2002;106(3): 296–9.

[21] Hayes CE, Mathis CM, Yuan C. Surface coil phased arrays for high-resolution imaging of the carotid arteries. J Magn Reson Imaging 1996;6(1):109–12.

[22] Botnar RM, Stuber M, Kim WY, et al. Magnetic resonance coronary lumen and vessel wall imaging. Rays 2001;26(4):291–303.

[23] Yuan C, Petty C, O'Brien KD, et al. In vitro and in situ magnetic resonance imaging signal features of atherosclerotic plaque-associated lipids. Arterioscler Thromb Vasc Biol 1997;17(8):1496–503.

[24] Yuan C, Mitsumori LM, Ferguson MS, et al. In vivo accuracy of multispectral magnetic resonance imaging for identifying lipid-rich necrotic cores and intraplaque hemorrhage in advanced human carotid plaques. Circulation 2001;104(17):2051–6.

[25] Edelman RR, Chien D, Kim D. Fast selective black blood MR imaging. Radiology 1991;181(3): 655–60.

[26] Chan SK, Jaffer FA, Botnar RM, et al. Scan reproducibility of magnetic resonance imaging assessment of aortic atherosclerosis burden. J Cardiovasc Magn Reson 2001;3(4):331–8.

[27] Song HK, Wright AC, Wolf RL, et al. Multislice double inversion pulse sequence for efficient blackblood MRI. Magn Reson Med 2002;47(3):616–20.

[28] Yarnykh VL, Yuan C. Multislice double inversionrecovery black-blood imaging with simultaneous slice reinversion. J Magn Reson Imaging 2003; 17(4):478–83.

[29] Li D, Paschal CB, Haacke EM, et al. Coronary arteries: three-dimensional MR imaging with fat saturation and magnetization transfer contrast. Radiology 1993;187(2):401–6.

[30] Yuan C, Kerwin WS, Ferguson MS, et al. Contrastenhanced high resolution MRI for atherosclerotic carotid artery tissue characterization. J Magn Reson Imaging 2002;15(1):62–7.

[31] Wasserman BA, Smith WI, Trout HH III, et al. Carotid artery atherosclerosis: in vivo morphologic characterization with gadolinium-enhanced doubleoblique MR imaging initial results. Radiology 2002; 223(2):566–73.

[32] Kooi ME, Cappendijk VC, Cleutjens KB, et al. Accumulation of ultrasmall superparamagnetic particles of iron oxide in human atherosclerotic plaques can be detected by in vivo magnetic resonance imaging. Circulation 2003;107(19):2453–8.

[33] Flacke S, Fischer S, Scott MJ, et al. Novel MRI contrast agent for molecular imaging of fibrin: implications for detecting vulnerable plaques. Circulation 2001;104(11):1280–5.

[34] Botnar RM, Buecker A, Wiethoff AJ, et al. In vivo magnetic resonance imaging of coronary thrombosis using a fibrin-binding molecular magnetic resonance contrast agent. Circulation 2004;110:1463–6.

[35] Yuan C, Lin E, Millard J, et al. Closed contour edge detection of blood vessel lumen and outer wall boundaries in black-blood MR images. Magn Reson Imaging 1999;17(2):257–66.

[36] Ladak HM, Thomas JB, Mitchell JR, et al. A semiautomatic technique for measurement of arterial wall from black blood MRI. Med Phys 2001;28(6): 1098–107.

[37] Zhang S, Hatsukami TS, Polissar NL, et al. Comparison of carotid vessel wall area measurements using three different contrast-weighted black blood MR imaging techniques. Magn Reson Imaging 2001;19(6):795–802.

[38] Steen H, Warren W, Desai MY, et al. Combined transesophageal and surface MRI provides optimal imaging and high reproducibility of aortic atherosclerosis imaging. J Cardiovasc Magn Reson, in press.

[39] Mohiaddin RH, Firmin DN, Underwood SR, et al. Chemical shift magnetic resonance imaging of human atheroma. Br Heart J 1989;62(2):81–9.

[40] Vinitski S, Consigny PM, Shapiro MJ, et al. Magnetic resonance chemical shift imaging and spectroscopy of atherosclerotic plaque. Invest Radiol 1991; 26(8):703–14.

[41] Toussaint JF, Southern JF, Fuster V, et al. T2-weighted contrast for NMR characterization of human atherosclerosis. Arterioscler Thromb Vasc Biol 1995;15(10):1533–42.

[42] Skinner MP, Yuan C, Mitsumori L, et al. Serial magnetic resonance imaging of experimental atherosclerosis detects lesion fine structure, progression and complications in vivo. Nat Med 1995;1(1): 69–73.

[43] Helft G, Worthley SG, Fuster V, et al. Atherosclerotic aortic component quantification by noninvasive magnetic resonance imaging: an in vivo study in rabbits. J Am Coll Cardiol 2001;37(4):1149–54.

[44] Toussaint JF, LaMuraglia GM, Southern JF, et al. Magnetic resonance images lipid, fibrous, calcified, hemorrhagic, and thrombotic components of human atherosclerosis in vivo. Circulation 1996;94(5): 932–8.

[45] Hatsukami TS, Ross R, Polissar NL, et al. Visualization of fibrous cap thickness and rupture in human atherosclerotic carotid plaque in vivo with highresolution magnetic resonance imaging. Circulation 2000;102(9):959–64.

[46] de Boer OJ, van der Wal AC, Teeling P, et al. Leucocyte recruitment in rupture prone regions of lipid-rich plaques: a prominent role for neovascularization? Cardiovasc Res 1999;41(2):443–9.

[47] Weiss CR, Arai AE, Bui MN, et al. Arterial wall MRI characteristics are associated with elevated serum markers of inflammation in humans. J Magn Reson Imaging 2001;14(6):698–704.

[48] Ruehm SG, Corot C, Vogt P, et al. Magnetic resonance imaging of atherosclerotic plaque with ultrasmall superparamagnetic particles of iron oxide in hyperlipidemic rabbits. Circulation 2001;103(3): 415–22.

[49] Yu X, Song SK, Chen J, et al. High-resolution MRI characterization of human thrombus using a novel fibrin-targeted paramagnetic nanoparticle contrast agent. Magn Reson Med 2000;44(6):867–72.

[50] Thackray BD, Burns DH, Ferguson MS, et al. A new method for studying plaque morphology. Am J Card Imaging 1995;9(3):149–56.

[51] Kang X, Polissar NL, Han C, et al. Analysis of the measurement precision of arterial lumen and wall areas using high-resolution MRI. Magn Reson Med 2000;44(6):968–72.

[52] Mitsumori LM, Hatsukami TS, Ferguson MS, et al. In vivo accuracy of multisequence MR imaging for identifying unstable fibrous caps in advanced human carotid plaques. J Magn Reson Imaging 2003;17(4): 410–20.

[53] Yuan C, Zhang SX, Polissar NL, et al. Identification of fibrous cap rupture with magnetic resonance imaging is highly associated with recent transient ischemic attack or stroke. Circulation 2002;105(2): 181–5.

[54] Shinnar M, Fallon JT, Wehrli S, et al. The diagnostic accuracy of ex vivo MRI for human atherosclerotic plaque characterization. Arterioscler Thromb Vasc Biol 1999;19(11):2756–61.

[55] Cai JM, Hatsukami TS, Ferguson MS, et al. Classification of human carotid atherosclerotic lesions with in vivo multicontrast magnetic resonance imaging. Circulation 2002;106(11):1368–73.

[56] Jaffer FA, O'Donnell CJ, Larson MG, et al. Age and sex distribution of subclinical aortic atherosclerosis: a magnetic resonance imaging examination of the Framingham Heart Study. Arterioscler Thromb Vasc Biol 2002;22(5):849–54.

[57] Corti R, Fayad ZA, Fuster V, et al. Effects of lipid-lowering by simvastatin on human atherosclerotic lesions: a longitudinal study by high-resolution, non-invasive magnetic resonance imaging. Circulation 2001;104(3):249–52.

[58] Shunk KA, Lima JA, Heldman AW, et al. Transesophageal magnetic resonance imaging. Magn Reson Med 1999;41(4):722–6.

[59] Shunk KA, Garot J, Atalar E, et al. Transesophageal magnetic resonance imaging of the aortic arch and descending thoracic aorta in patients with aortic atherosclerosis. J Am Coll Cardiol 2001;37(8):2031–5.

[60] Lima JA, Desai MY, Steen H, et al. Statin induced cholesterol lowering and plaque regression after 6 months of mri monitored therapy. Circulation 2004;10:2336–41.

[61] Manning WJ, Stuber M, Danias PG, et al. Coronary magnetic resonance imaging: current status. Curr Probl Cardiol 2002;27(7):275–333.

[62] Fischer SE, Wickline SA, Lorenz CH. Novel real-time R-wave detection algorithm based on the vector-cardiogram for accurate gated magnetic resonance acquisitions. Magn Reson Med 1999;42(2): 361–70.

[63] Stuber M, Botnar RM, Danias PG, et al. Submilli-meter three-dimensional coronary MR angiography with real-time navigator correction: comparison of navigator locations. Radiology 1999;212(2): 579–87.

[64] Hazirolan T, Gupta SN, Mohamed MA, et al. Reproducibility of black-blood coronary vessel wall MR imaging. J Cardiovasc Magn Reson, in press.

[65] Botnar RM, Kim WY, Bornert P, et al. 3D coronary vessel wall imaging utilizing a local inversion technique with spiral image acquisition. Magn Reson Med 2001;46(5):848–54.

[66] Ladd ME, Debatin JF. Interventional and intravascular MR angiography. Herz 2000;25(4):440–51.

[67] Hofmann LV, Liddell RP, Arepally A, et al. In vivo intravascular MR imaging: transvenous technique for arterial wall imaging. J Vasc Interv Radiol 2003;14(10):1317–27.

[68] Yang X, Atalar E. Intravascular MR imaging-guided balloon angioplasty with an MR imaging guide wire: feasibility study in rabbits. Radiology 2000;217(2): 501–6.

[69] Dion YM, Ben El Kadi H, Boudoux C, et al. Endovascular procedures under near-real-time magnetic resonance imaging guidance: an experimental feasibility study. J Vasc Surg 2000;32(5):1006–14.

[70] Spuentrup E, Ruebben A, Schaeffter T, et al. Magnetic resonance–guided coronary artery stent placement in a swine model. Circulation 2002;105(7): 874–9.

[71] Yang X, Atalar E, Li D, et al. Magnetic resonance imaging permits in vivo monitoring of catheter-based vascular gene delivery. Circulation 2001; 104(14):1588–90.

ELSEVIER
SAUNDERS

Magn Reson Imaging Clin N Am
13 (2005) 181–188

MAGNETIC
RESONANCE
IMAGING CLINICS
of North America

Emerging Functional MR Angiographic Techniques

Honglei Zhang, MD[a], Julianna M. Czum, MD[a],
Martin R. Prince, MD, PhD[a,b,*]

[a]*Weill Medical College of Cornell University, 1300 York Avenue, New York, NY 10021, USA*
[b]*Columbia College of Physicians and Surgeons, 630 West 168th Street, New York, NY 10032, USA*

With recent advances in hardware and software, MR angiography can now demonstrate significant stenoses in most anatomic territories with sensitivities and specificities in the range of 90%. Most technology-assessment studies compare the accuracy of MR angiography with that of conventional arteriography, because both allow assessment of luminal dimensions, such as the percentage of diameter stenosis or cross-sectional area stenosis. Knowledge of the functional significance of a visualized stenosis often is more important than the percentage of the area affected, however.

With conventional angiography, the standard procedure entails measurement of the trans-stenotic pressure gradient before angioplasty or stent placement. If a pressure gradient exists across a stenosis, dilating the lumen to eliminate or decrease the stenosis will result in greater blood flow to the end organ. In the absence of a trans-stenotic pressure gradient, however, revascularization techniques will not augment blood flow but still pose the risk of procedure-related complications. Thus, a newer goal of MR angiography techniques is to determine noninvasively the trans-stenotic pressure gradient for discriminating between hemodynamically significant and nonsignificant lesions.

Collateral vessels

In the presence of a hemodynamically significant stenosis, end-organ ischemia stimulates vasodilatation of adjacent small-caliber arteries, which serve as collateral pathways. These collaterals may ameliorate the effect of occlusive disease at rest but may not provide sufficient blood flow for normal functioning, because insufficient flow reserve remains available for recruitment. Collaterals are relatively easy to distinguish from named arteries because they increase in length as well as in diameter, resulting in tortuosity (Fig. 1). Profoundly tortuous arteries are referred to as "corkscrew" collaterals because of their characteristic appearance.

Direct visualization of collateral vessels by MR angiography has been reported to be a reliable indicator of hemodynamic significance in patients with prior repair of coarctation of the aorta [1]. Failure to visualize collaterals on MR angiography does not imply the absence of a trans-stenotic pressure gradient, because, depending on the achievable spatial resolution, these vessels may be too small to resolve adequately on MR angiography. One challenge in the depiction of collaterals with MR angiography is to improve spatial resolution while minimizing detrimental effects on the signal-to-noise ratio (S/N).

Flow measurement with phase-contrast sequences

Two-dimensional (2-D) measurement of the cine phase-contrast (PC) flow volume can be a reliable technique for noninvasively measuring velocity and flow in the blood vessels at the voxel level. The PC technique is based on the principle that magnetic field gradients introduce phase shifts in the MR signal arising from the flowing spins that are proportional to their velocity, enabling the construction of velocity maps from which the

---

* Corresponding author. 416 East 55th Street, New York, NY 10022.
E-mail address: map2008@med.cornell.edu (M.R. Prince).

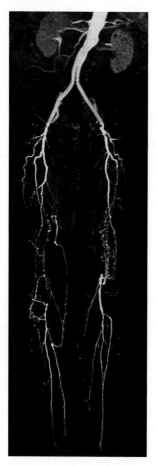

Fig. 1. A 65-year-old man with claudication. 3-D bolus-chase MR angiography shows occlusion of bilateral superficial femoral arteries and formation of collateral arteries.

volume of flow can be calculated simply by integrating the velocity measurements over the vessel cross-section [2]. 2-D cine PC performed after gadolinium-enhanced MR angiography has a higher S/N than noncontrast imaging [3]. Using cardiac gating and breath-holding, cine PC can demonstrate flow variations between systole and diastole with high spatial and temporal resolution [4].

PC flow measurement results are most accurate if the imaging plane is perpendicular to the long axis of the vessel of interest and flow encoding is set to interrogate through-plane flow. Motion-related errors caused by cardiac motion and arterial pulsatility can occur in the torso, especially in the thorax (eg, falsely elevated ascending aortic peak flow during systole). Pulse sequences have been designed to correct for this error by prescribing an imaging plane that is synchronized with cardiac motion.

At rest, patients have high-resistance triphasic flow in their peripheral arteries, consisting of peak forward flow during systole with transient reversal and then a plateau substantially below the peak forward flow. During exercise, muscle ischemia stimulates vasodilatation and decreased capillary resistance, which increases blood flow to the peripheral muscles and create a flatter waveform indicating low-resistance flow. When there is a hemodynamically significant stenosis or occlusion in a peripheral artery, the waveform will tend to be high resistance (triphasic wave form) proximal to the lesion and low resistance distal to the lesion (biphasic or monophasic waveform) (Fig. 2). A transition from high-resistance to low-resistance flow across a stenosis is evidence of hemodynamic significance. Cine PC can be exploited to measure the pulsatile, high-resistance triphasic blood flow in normal lower extremity arteries as well as the low-resistance flow that occurs distal to hemodynamically significant occlusive disease.

Flow-volume data obtained by integrating velocity–time curves over a cross-sectional arterial region of interest on PC images show high accuracy and excellent correlation with direct flow measurements in animal models and with indirect techniques such as clearance of para-aminohippurate and ^{133}Xenon washout measurements [5–7]. On PC flow curves, significant renal arterial stenosis results in delayed or absent early systolic peak with reduction in renal capillary resistance [8]. Renal flow can be indexed to the total volume of renal parenchyma: a renal flow index less than 1.5 mL/min/cm^3 predicts successful outcome of revascularization [9].

Combining cine PC data with MR angiography reduces interobserver variability on stenosis grading [8]. In the setting of a metallic renal artery stent, intraluminal flow may be obscured by susceptibility artifact, but flow measurement distal to the stent can assess in-stent stenosis [10]. Cine PC renal blood flow measurements obtained before and after pharmacologic intervention provide more physiologic data. For example, an angiotensin-converting enzyme (ACE) inhibitor markedly reduces flow to a kidney being supplied by a renal artery with a hemodynamically significant stenosis [11]. Different studies have showed controversial results in evaluating the significances of ACE inhibitor, however [12]. Further experiments are needed to clarify its usefulness and accuracy.

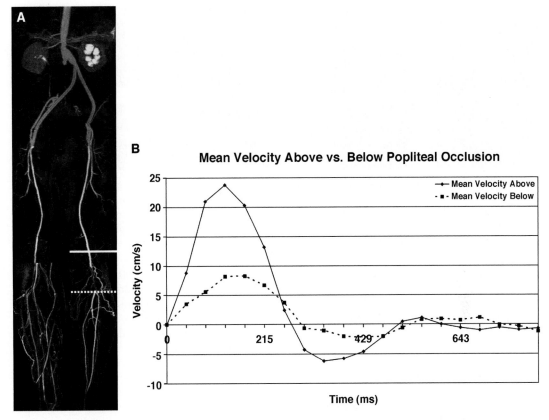

Fig. 2. A 56-year-old man with left calf pain at rest. (*A*) 3-D bolus-chase MR angiography shows left popliteal artery occlusion. (*B*) 2-D cine phase-contrast flow velocity measurements above and below popliteal occlusion show high-resistance, triphasic arterial flow proximal to the lesion and low-resistance flow distal to the lesion.

Ultrafast flow measurement

Ultrafast PC flow measurements are possible using echo planer imaging (EPI) and Fastcard PC (GE Medical Systems, Waukesha, Wisconsin). Multishot EPI PC imaging permits highly accurate flow measurement in pulsatile vessels during a breath-hold [13,14]. Particle-path visualization for time-resolved three-directional data sets in continuous slices covering the entire volume have been proposed to acquire time-resolved three-dimensional (3-D) velocity mapping of the flow in thoracic aorta [15].

Spin dephasing on three-dimensional phase contrast

On 3-D PC MR angiography, flow is encoded in all three axes. Flowing blood appears bright, with signal intensity directly related to flow velocity, and stationery tissues appear dark. With mild stenoses, laminar flow accelerates, creating a blooming effect that makes stenoses appear less severe. Through hemodynamically significant stenosis (>70% luminal narrowing, with a trans-stenotic pressure gradient), however, flow also accelerates but becomes disorganized and turbulent [16]. Flow jets created by pressure gradients also destroy MR phase coherence, causing loss of MR signal. This dephasing is especially prominent on 3-D PC MR angiography because of the relatively long echo times and proton motion during application of flow-encoding gradients [17].

Thus, with 3-D PC imaging, the underestimation of mild stenoses and overestimation of severe stenoses accentuates differences between unimportant mild stenoses and hemodynamically significant stenoses (Fig. 3). One in vitro study shows that the degree of this spin dephasing is directly correlated with the trans-stenotic pressure gradient [16]. The severity of stenosis on digital subtraction angiography, considered the reference standard, shows better correlation with severity

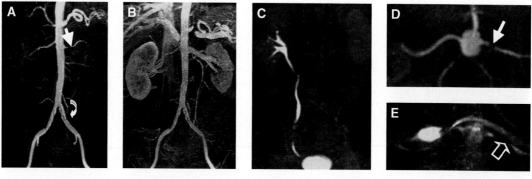

Fig. 3. Severe left renal artery stenosis (*arrow*) is better shown on arterial phase of 3-D gadolinium-enhanced MR angiography (*A, D*) with left kidney shrinkage, diminished cortical medullary differentiation in the venous phase (*B*), and asymmetrical gadolinium excretion on equilibrium phase (*C*). On 3-D PC (*E*), there is dephasing (*open arrow*) at the site of stenosis, indicating it is hemodynamically significant. Also noted is left common iliac artery dissection (*curved arrow*), which is useful for planning the approach to percutaneous angioplasty.

of spin dephasing on 3-D PC than with the length of dephasing [18].

3-D PC imaging is widely used in renal and carotid MR angiography [19–21]. Combining 3-D gadolinium MR angiography information with 3-D PC MR angiography offers more accurate grading of arterial stenosis by improving the specificity of MR angiography, because the number of false-positive interpretations of significant stenosis decreases with gadolinium-enhanced 3-D MR angiography.

Time-resolved MR angiography

Many techniques have been developed for obtaining functional information by temporally resolving the flow of contrast from arteries to veins. These methods include 2-D projection MR angiography, 3-D time-resolved imaging of contrast kinetics, fast 3-D spoiled gradient echo, vastly undersampled isotropic projection reconstruction (VIPR), periodically rotated overlapping parallel lines with enhanced reconstruction,

four-dimensional spiral MR angiography with sliding window reconstruction, and parallel imaging [22–30]. These techniques can now reconstruct 3-D data with temporal resolution faster than one frame per second and 2-D data at several frames per second. Time-resolved MR angiography is especially useful in vascular territories where the path of blood flow is uncertain and cannot be determined from static images of the vasculature (eg, in cases of congenital heart disease or peripheral arterial occlusive disease) or in cases of overlapping vessels (eg, in the circle of Willis and portal venous system) (Fig. 4) [31]. For example, a time-resolved 3-D imaging technique for an extended field-of-view performed during continuous table motion to obtain both functional (hemodynamic) and morphologic information can be performed by capturing the leading edge of the bolus as it travels down peripheral arteries [32,33].

Time-resolved MR angiography is also possible without contrast by taking advantage of ECG gating to acquire multiple images over the cardiac cycle to show how flow varies in systole and

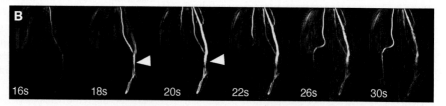

Fig. 4. A 59-year-old man with congestive heart failure after Fogarty balloon thrombectomy of a left femoral-popliteal bypass graft. (*A*) 3-D gadolinium-enhanced MR angiography is confusing because of venous contamination by left popliteal vein (*arrow*). (*B*) Time-resolved 2-D projection MR angiography, at 2 s/frame, shows an arterio-venous fistula (*arrowhead*) causing increased flow to the left leg. After the fistula was ligated, the congestive heart failure resolved.

diastole. A technique known as 'global coherent free precession' excites spins in the plane perpendicular to the artery and then acquires a projection image in the plane of the artery to illustrate flow pulsation over the cardiac cycle [34].

Functional evaluation of selected vascular pathology

Aortic coarctation and dissection

The morphologic severity of coarctation of the aorta may be difficult to evaluate, especially in the postrepair state. The physiologic severity of aorta coarctation can be assessed with cine PC MR imaging. Cine PC imaging is used to estimate flow volume at two locations in the aorta: one just distal to the coarctation site and the other at the level of the diaphragm. Normally, aortic flow decreases along its length. In cases of coarctation of the aorta, however, the more distal aortic flow at the level of the diaphragm is greater than the more proximal flow in the area just distal to the coarctation. This occurrence results from collateral filling of the descending aorta by the reversal of flow within the intercostal arteries, which represent a collateral pathway for arterial flow. The flow difference between the proximal and distal descending aorta can be quantified and represents the flow contributions of the collateral vessel. The presence of collateral filling accurately indicates the presence of a hemodynamically significant coarctation. This type of flow measurement can be helpful in cases where dilated collaterals may not be adequately demonstrated because of limited spatial resolution using spin echo imaging or 3-D contrast-enhanced MR angiography [35,36]. Determination of the peak velocity and flow volume also can be used to estimate the pressure gradient within the coarctation. A pressure gradient of more than 20 mm Hg as measured during cardiac catheterization is considered an indication for intervention [37].

In aortic dissection, as the overall aortic diameter increases, the ratio of the cross-sectional area of the false lumen to the true lumen increases, and the peak average velocity in the true lumen during systole decreases on cine PC imaging, a feature that can help determine prognosis and operability [38].

Renal artery stenosis

Loss of corticomedullary differentiation, poststenotic renal artery dilatation, asymmetry of kidney length, parenchymal thinning, and pattern of contrast excretion may help to diagnose renal artery stenosis [39]. Flow measurement with 2-D cine PC or 3-D PC imaging to detect spin dephasing is now a routine component of renal artery MR angiography in some institutions. Measurements of renal artery flow can be combined with additional pulse sequences (such as T1 measurements of flowing blood) to measure the gadolinium concentration in the renal artery (input) and renal vein (output), permitting exact calculation of the gadolinium clearance rate for each kidney and assessment of renal function [40]. Other functional techniques, including diffusion-weighted imaging, perfusion imaging, and the blood oxygen level–dependent (BOLD) effect, can be used to evaluate renal function and further determine the severity and hemodynamic significance of renal artery or mesenteric artery stenosis [41–44].

When evaluating renal arteries, the contrast arrival time in the renal cortex is similar for normal and ischemic kidneys, whereas the cortical transit time is much longer in kidneys with renal vascular disease and decreased function than in normal kidneys (40 seconds versus 15 seconds, respectively) [45]. Thus, in ischemic kidneys, the medullary enhancement rate is delayed and decreased. Low-dose gadolinium (2 mL) has been used to evaluate contrast enhancement of the renal cortex and medulla during MR renography [46].

Peripheral arterial occlusive disease

Often a borderline stenosis is not flow limiting at higher flow rates (eg, during exercise). During conventional angiography, a vasodilator such as priscoline can be used to increase flow to unmask a flow-limiting lesion. With MR angiography, flow to an extremity can be increased by inflating a blood pressure cuff to suprasystolic pressure (~200 mm Hg) for 3 minutes to induce transient ischemia. Upon cuff deflation, the time needed for the BOLD effect in calf muscles to return to normal can be measured. The BOLD effect is delayed in the presence of significant occlusive disease [47].

Phantom studies demonstrate that highly pulsatile flow, as in the limbs, needs ECG synchronization for flow measurement, increasing the duration of the PC scan. Fortunately, with cine PC, the blood flow volume can be examined in several vessels simultaneously in the same plane with a large field of view. A recent study in 50 healthy volunteers showed the mean blood flow was 353 mL/min in the femoral artery and 61.9 mL/min in the popliteal artery [48]. Femoral blood flow was related to age and gender, whereas popliteal blood flow was more related to calf muscle volume, after adjusting for age and gender. Another study showed that blood flow volume at rest was similar in volunteers and in patients. After exercise, however, patients with abnormal ankle–brachial indexes had diminished lower extremity arterial flow augmentation (a 2.6-fold increase in flow) compared with normal volunteers (a 4.8-fold increase in flow), indicating MR measurement of blood flow volume may aid in evaluating peripheral vascular disease [49].

In patients with occlusive peripheral arterial disease, the blood flow in the leg with occlusion or severe stenosis can be slower or faster than in the contralateral normal leg, because of the smaller cross-sectional diameter of collateral vessels or distal ischemia, which stimulates vasodilatation distal to occlusions [50]. Thus, time-resolved MR angiography must be interpreted with caution.

Pulmonary embolism

Pulmonary arteriography is not the preferred modality to diagnose pulmonary embolism because of its risk profile. In about 4% of patients with pulmonary embolism, acute pulmonary hypertension develops, causing diminished pulmonary flow and right ventricular dysfunction. MR angiography can demonstrate pulmonary arterial filling defects consistent with emboli with high accuracy [51,52]. Cross-sectional cine cardiac MR allows precise calculation of stroke volume, cardiac output, and ejection fraction to evaluate right heart function. Cine PC measurements of flow through the aorta and central pulmonary arteries enable calculation of the magnitude of right-to-left shunting in the setting of pulmonary hypertension [53,54]. In addition to demonstrating pulmonary emboli and their potential cardiac effects, MR imaging also can demonstrate deep vein thrombosis [55,56].

Portal venous system abnormality

Portal vein thrombosis is an important indication for MR angiography of the portal venous system. Cavernous transformation indicating chronic portal vein occlusion can be demonstrated easily by MR portography (Fig. 5). MR portography with PC flow measurement can provide a functional evaluation of portal hypertension and surgical portosystemic shunts. Contrast-enhanced MR angiography is promising as a noninvasive means to determine the resectability of

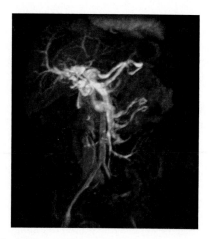

Fig. 5. A 21-year-old woman with lupus and abdominal pain. 3-D MR portography shows cavernous transformation of the portal vein.

pancreaticobiliary tumors involving the portal venous system. MR PC flow measurement is a simple and rapid technique for the assessment of portal venous patency, flow direction, and flow velocity. Pharmacologic stimulation of portal flow with nicardipine hydrochloride is useful for the evaluation of liver function [57]. Using MR techniques to measure flow in the azygous and hemiazygous veins may estimate the amount of portal flow being shunted from the liver in patients with cirrhosis [58–60].

Summary

As the accuracy of MR angiography approaches that of conventional digital subtraction angiography, further refinements of vascular analysis will focus on providing functional information about the normal and pathologic vasculature. In particular, PC flow measurement, time-resolved contrast-enhanced MR angiography, and detection of turbulent flow jets help to establish the functional significance of stenoses.

References

[1] Araoz PA, Reddy GP, Tarnoff H, et al. MR findings of collateral circulation are more accurate measures of hemodynamic significance than arm-leg blood pressure gradient after repair of coarctation of the aorta. J Magn Reson Imaging 2003;17:177–83.
[2] Dumoulin CL, Hart HRJ. Magnetic resonance angiography in the head and neck. Acta Radiol Suppl 1986;369:17–20.
[3] Prince MR, Grist TM, Debatin JF. 3D contrast MR angiography. Heidelberg (Germany): Springer-Verlag; 2003.

[4] Schoenberg SO, Essig M, Bock M, et al. Comprehensive MR evaluation of renovascular disease in five breath holds. J Magn Reson Imaging 1999;10:347–56.

[5] Wolf RL, King BF, Torres VE, et al. Measurement of normal renal artery blood flow: cine phase-contrast MR imaging vs clearance of p-aminohippurate. AJR Am J Roentgenol 1993;161:995–1002.

[6] Schoenberg SO, Knopp MV, Bock M, et al. Renal artery stenosis: grading of hemodynamic changes with cine phase-contrast MR blood flow measurements. Radiology 1997;203:45–53.

[7] de Haan MW, van Engelshoven JM, Houben AJ, et al. Phase-contrast magnetic resonance flow quantification in renal arteries: comparison with ^{133}Xenon washout measurements. Hypertension 2003;41:114–8.

[8] Schoenberg SO, Knopp MV, Londy F, et al. Morphologic and functional magnetic resonance imaging of renal artery stenosis: a multireader tricenter study. J Am Soc Nephrol 2002;13:158–69.

[9] Binkert CA, Debatin JF, Schneider E, et al. Can MR measurement of renal artery flow and renal volume predict the outcome of percutaneous transluminal renal angioplasty. Cardiovasc Intervent Radiol 2001;24:233–9.

[10] Shetty AN, Bis KG, Kirsch M, et al. Contrast-enhanced breath-hold three-dimensional magnetic resonance angiography in the evaluation of renal arteries: optimization of technique and pitfalls. J Magn Reson Imaging 2000;12:912–23.

[11] Soulez G, Oliva VL, Turpin S, et al. Imaging of renovascular hypertension: respective values of renal scintigraphy, renal Doppler US, and MR angiography. Radiographics 2000;20:1355–68.

[12] Lee VS, Rofsky NM, Ton AT, et al. Angiotensin-converting enzyme inhibitor-enhanced phase-contrast MR imaging to measure renal artery velocity waveforms in patients with suspected renovascular hypertension. AJR Am J Roentgenol 2000;174:499–508.

[13] Debatin JF, Davis CP, Felblinger J, et al. Evaluation of ultrafast phase-contrast imaging in the thoracic aorta. MAGMA 1995;3:59–66.

[14] Debatin JF, Leung DA, Wildermuth S, et al. Flow quantitation with echo-planar phase-contrast velocity mapping: in vitro and in vivo evaluation. J Magn Reson Imaging 1995;5:656–62.

[15] Bogren HG, Buonocore MH. 4D magnetic resonance velocity mapping of blood flow patterns in the aorta in young vs. elderly normal subjects. J Magn Reson Imaging 1999;10:861–9.

[16] Mustert BR, Williams DM, Prince MR. In vitro model of arterial stenosis: correlation of MR signal dephasing and trans-stenotic pressure gradients. Magn Reson Imaging 1998;16:301–10.

[17] Oshinski JN, Ku DN, Pettigrew RI. Turbulent fluctuation velocity: the most significant determinant of signal loss in stenotic vessels. Magn Reson Med 1995;33:193–9.

[18] Westenberg JJ, van der Geest RJ, Wasser MN, et al. Stenosis quantification from post-stenotic signal loss in phase-contrast MRA datasets of flow phantoms and renal arteries. Int J Card Imaging 1999;15:483–93.

[19] Hood MN, Ho VB, Corse WR. Three-dimensional phase-contrast magnetic resonance angiography: a useful clinical adjunct to gadolinium-enhanced three-dimensional renal magnetic resonance angiography. Mil Med 2002;167:343–9.

[20] Miller S, Schick F, Duda SH, et al. Gd-enhanced 3D phase-contrast MR angiography and dynamic perfusion imaging in the diagnosis of renal artery stenosis. Magn Reson Imaging 1998;16:1005–12.

[21] Benjamin MS, Gillams AR, Carter AP. Carotid MRA–what advantages do the turbo field-echo and 3D phase-contrast sequences offer? Neuroradiology 1997;39:469–73.

[22] Wang Y, Johnston DL, Breen JF, et al. Dynamic MR digital subtraction angiography using contrast enhancement, fast data acquisition, and complex subtraction. Magn Reson Med 1996;36:551–6.

[23] Du J, Carroll TJ, Wagner HJ, et al. Time-resolved, undersampled projection reconstruction imaging for high-resolution CE-MRA of the distal runoff vessels. Magn Reson Med 2002;48:516–22.

[24] Swan JS, Carroll TJ, Kennell TW, et al. Time-resolved three-dimensional contrast-enhanced MR angiography of the peripheral vessels. Radiology 2002;225:43–52.

[25] Mascalchi M, Cosottini M, Ferrito G, et al. Contrast-enhanced time-resolved MR angiography of spinal vascular malformations. J Comput Assist Tomogr 1999;23:341–5.

[26] Du J, Fain SB, Gu T, et al. Noise reduction in MR angiography with nonlinear anisotropic filtering. J Magn Reson Imaging 2004;19:632–9.

[27] Pipe JG. Motion correction with PROPELLER MRI: application to head motion and free-breathing cardiac imaging. Magn Reson Med 1999;42:963–9.

[28] Zhu H, Buck DG, Zhang Z, et al. High temporal and spatial resolution 4D MRA using spiral data sampling and sliding window reconstruction. Magn Reson Med 2004;52:14–8.

[29] Quick HH, Vogt FM, Maderwald S, et al. High spatial resolution whole-body MR angiography featuring parallel imaging: initial experience. Rofo 2004;176:163–9.

[30] Wilson GJ, Hoogeveen RM, Willinek WA, et al. Parallel imaging in MR angiography. Top Magn Reson Imaging 2004;15:169–85.

[31] Finn JP, Baskaran V, Carr JC, et al. Thorax: low-dose contrast-enhanced three-dimensional MR angiography with subsecond temporal resolution–initial results. Radiology 2002;224:896–904.

[32] Aksit P, Ho VB, Hood MN, et al. Single-injection, semi-automated multi-station bolus timing for optimization of 3D peripheral MR angiography. In: Program of the twelfth scientific meeting and exhibition

of the International Society for Magnetic Resonance in Medicine. Berkeley (CA): ISMRM; 2004. p. 228.

[33] Madhuranthakam AJ, Kruger DG, Riederer SJ, et al. Time-resolved 3D contrast-enhanced MRA of an extended FOV using continuous table motion. Magn Reson Med 2004;51:568–76.

[34] Rehwald WG, Chen EL, Kim RJ, et al. Noninvasive cineangiography by magnetic resonance global coherent free precession. Nat Med 2004;10:545–9.

[35] Steffens JC, Bourne MW, Sakuma H, et al. Quantification of collateral blood flow in coarctation of the aorta by velocity encoded cine magnetic resonance imaging. Circulation 1994;90:937–43.

[36] Holmqvist C, Stahlberg F, Hanseus K, et al. Collateral flow in coarctation of the aorta with magnetic resonance velocity mapping: correlation to morphological imaging of collateral vessels. J Magn Reson Imaging 2002;15:39–46.

[37] Campbell M. Natural history of coarctation of the aorta. Br Heart J 1970;32:633–40.

[38] Inoue T, Watanabe S, Masuda Y, et al. Evaluation of blood flow patterns of true and false lumens in dissecting aneurysms using MR phase-contrast techniques. Clin Imaging 1996;20:262–8.

[39] Zhang HL, Schoenberg SO, Resnick LM, et al. Diagnosis of renal artery stenosis: combining gadolinium-enhanced three-dimensional magnetic resonance angiography with functional magnetic resonance pulse sequences. Am J Hypertens 2003; 16:1079–82.

[40] Niendorf ER, Grist TM, Lee FT, et al. Rapid in vivo measurement of single-kidney extraction fraction and glomerular filtration rate with MR imaging. Radiology 1998;206:791–8.

[41] Li KC, Dalman RL, Wright GA. In vivo flow-independent T2 measurements of superior mesenteric vein blood in diagnosis of chronic mesenteric ischemia: a preliminary evaluation. Acad Radiol 1999;6:530–4.

[42] Chow LC, Chan FP, Li KC. A comprehensive approach to MR imaging of mesenteric ischemia. Abdom Imaging 2002;27:507–16.

[43] Juillard L, Lerman LO, Kruger DG, et al. Blood oxygen level-dependent measurement of acute intrarenal ischemia. Kidney Int 2004;65:944–50.

[44] Ries M, Basseau F, Tyndal B, et al. Renal diffusion and BOLD MRI in experimental diabetic nephropathy. Blood oxygen level-dependent. J Magn Reson Imaging 2003;17:104–13.

[45] Ros PR, Gauger J, Stoupis C, et al. Diagnosis of renal artery stenosis: feasibility of combining MR angiography, MR renography, and gadopentetate-based measurements of glomerular filtration rate. AJR Am J Roentgenol 1995;165:1447–51.

[46] Lee VS, Rusnek H, Johnson G, et al. MR renography with low-dose gadopentetate dimeglumine: feasibility. Radiology 2001;221:371–9.

[47] Lebon V, Brillault-Salvat C, Bloch G, et al. Evidence of muscle BOLD effect revealed by simultaneous interleaved gradient-echo NMRI and myoglobin NMRS during leg ischemia. Magn Reson Med 1998;40:551–8.

[48] Klein WM, Bartels LW, Bax L, et al. Magnetic resonance imaging measurement of blood volume flow in peripheral arteries in healthy subjects. J Vasc Surg 2003;38:1060–6.

[49] Pena CS, McCauley TR, Price TB, et al. Quantitative blood flow measurements with cine phase-contrast MR imaging of subjects at rest and after exercise to assess peripheral vascular disease. AJR Am J Roentgenol 1996;167:153–7.

[50] Prince MR, Chabra SG, Watts R, et al. Contrast material travel times in patients undergoing peripheral MR angiography. Radiology 2002;224: 55–61.

[51] Kruger S, Haage P, Hoffmann R, et al. Diagnosis of pulmonary arterial hypertension and pulmonary embolism with magnetic resonance angiography. Chest 2001;120:1556–61.

[52] Oudkerk M, van Beek EJ, Wielopolski P, et al. Comparison of contrast-enhanced magnetic resonance angiography and conventional pulmonary angiography for the diagnosis of pulmonary embolism: a prospective study. Lancet 2002;359:1643–7.

[53] Prince MR, Alderson PO, Sostman HD. Chronic pulmonary embolism: combining MR angiography with functional assessment. Radiology 2004;232: 325–6.

[54] Kreitner KF, Ley S, Kauczor HU, et al. Chronic thromboembolic pulmonary hypertension: pre- and postoperative assessment with breath-hold MR imaging techniques. Radiology 2004;232: 535–43.

[55] Sostman HD. MRA for diagnosis of venous thromboembolism. Q J Nucl Med 2001;45:311–23.

[56] Stern JB, Abehsera M, Grenet D, et al. Detection of pelvic vein thrombosis by magnetic resonance angiography in patients with acute pulmonary embolism and normal lower limb compression ultrasonography. Chest 2002;122:115–21.

[57] Nakano S, Katoh T, Ohki M, et al. Pharmacologically stimulated portal flow measurement by magnetic resonance imaging for assessment of liver function. Radiat Med 1999;17:21–6.

[58] Wu MT, Pan HB, Chen C, et al. Azygos blood flow in cirrhosis: measurement with MR imaging and correlation with variceal hemorrhage. Radiology 1996; 198:457–62.

[59] Ng WH, Chan YL, Sung JY, et al. Comparison of breath-hold 2D phase-contrast with non breath-hold cine phase-contrast MRA in the assessment of azygos venous blood flow in portal hypertension. MAGMA 2004;16:211–7.

[60] Debatin JF, Zahner B, Meyenberger C, et al. Azygos blood flow: phase contrast quantitation in volunteers and patients with portal hypertension pre- and postintrahepatic shunt placement. Hepatology 1996;24:1109–15.

ELSEVIER
SAUNDERS

Magn Reson Imaging Clin N Am
13 (2005) 189–203

MAGNETIC
RESONANCE
IMAGING CLINICS
of North America

Contrast Agents: Innovations and Potential Applications for Body MR Angiography

Maureen N. Hood, MS, RN, RT-R, MR*, Vincent B. Ho, MD

Department of Radiology and Radiological Sciences, Uniformed Services University of the Health Sciences,
4301 Jones Bridge Road, Bethesda, MD 20814-4799, USA

In 1985, Wedeen et al [1,2] described the ability of MR imaging to illustrate blood vessels by using flow-dependent techniques, methods now well known as time-of-flight MR angiography. It was not until the 1990s, however, with numerous innovations for the more reliable and robust method of contrast-enhanced (CE) MR angiography, that the use of MR imaging has become routine clinically for vascular diagnosis. Today a variety of gadolinium (Gd)-chelate contrast agents are commercially available in the United States for neurologic and body imaging applications, although none is approved yet by the Food and Drug Administration specifically for MR angiography. Although off-label, the use of contrast media for MR angiography [3,4] has been shown to be reliable, safe, and accurate in clinical practice [5–11] and in many centers has replaced more invasive x-ray catheter angiography as a primary standard for vascular diagnosis [12].

In its current implementation, CE MR angiography typically is performed using one of the commercially available extracellular Gd-chelate contrast agents with a three-dimensional (3D) fast spoiled gradient echo pulse sequence timed for contrast bolus filling of the target vasculature (Fig. 1). Vascular illustration on CE MR angiography is provided by the T1 shortening effects of Gd on blood. The preferential timing of 3D MR angiography data acquisition can be used to illustrate selectively the various arterial or venous phases of the contrast bolus. Arterial illustration is optimal during peak arterial enhancement, and venous illustration is optimal later during venous filling. Timing often can be difficult in patients with underlying cardiovascular diseases because their circulatory times (and contrast arrival times) may be variable. More recently, time-resolved imaging has afforded continuous dynamic viewing of arterial and venous bolus progression, which may be crucial for proper recognition of certain lesions [13]. The benefit of time-resolved MR angiography is the fact that dynamic imaging can be performed without the concerns of ionizing radiation exposure that are associated with x-ray-based studies, such as CT angiography and conventional x-ray angiography. Paralleling technologic improvements in MR angiography, numerous innovations in contrast agent development have occurred. These new investigational agents are in various phases of clinical development, but offer a variety of new opportunities for MR angiography. This article reviews some promising contrast agents and potential benefits for vascular imaging.

Contrast agents

As with other radiologic applications, a contrast agent not only must be safe, but also efficacious and cost-effective [14]. The key to the efficacy of an MR contrast agent is its ability to generate contrast-to-noise ratio (CNR), which, in the case of vascular imaging, is its ability to generate vessel-to-background CNR. One must not lose sight of the importance of tissue perfusion

The opinions or assertions contained herein are the private views of the authors and are not to be construed as official or reflecting the views of the Uniformed Services University of the Health Sciences or the Department of Defense.

* Corresponding author.
E-mail address: mhood@usuhs.mil (M.N. Hood).

1064-9689/05/$ - see front matter. Published by Elsevier Inc.
doi:10.1016/j.mric.2004.12.011

mri.theclinics.com

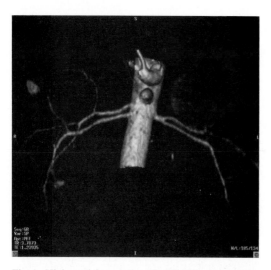

Fig. 1. High spatial resolution 3D CE MR angiography using 30 mL of Gd-DTPA. Arterial phase 3D CE MR angiography was optimized using MR fluoroscopic triggering and parallel imaging. The resulting volume-rendered view shows the accessory right renal artery and early bifurcation of the left renal artery in this otherwise normal individual. (Courtesy of William R. Corse, MD, Department of Radiology, Doylestown Hospital, Doylestown, PA.)

or tissue morphology, however, which in patients with vascular diseases may provide potentially complementary information. The additional finding of diminished end-organ perfusion may be crucial for determination of a vascular lesion's hemodynamic significance. More recently, tissue-specific contrast agents have been contemplated. These contrast agents target specific morphologic aspects of cardiovascular pathology, such as thrombus or atherosclerotic plaque. When considering potential contrast agents for MR angiography, one not only must consider the improvements in vascular signal, but also the benefits for various tissue-to-background CNR. This consideration is particularly important for the development of MR contrast agents, which often may be eclipsed by improvements in MR technology and changes in clinical therapeutic paradigms, which may make certain contrast applications obsolete. The efficacy of a contrast agent is highly dependent on the MR technique. The complexity of many cardiovascular diseases provides additional opportunities for novel implementations of various contrast agents into clinical practice.

The presence of contrast agents can provide improved CNR via two main mechanisms: proton

density and molecular dipolar interactions of the ion complexes with water [15,16]. In general, contrast agents can affect T1 and T2, and these effects vary based on a variety of conditions, such as contrast dose, injection rates, vascular concentration, and field strength. CE MR angiography using conventional Gd-chelate contrast agents typically relies on the shortened T1 relaxation time of blood by the arrival of contrast media into the vascular bed [17].

The MR imaging pulse sequences used should be optimized for the specific contrast agent and its specific application. Paramagnetic contrast agents, such as the currently commercially available Gd-chelate contrast agents, are the most widely used contrast agents for CE MR angiography. Paramagnetic contrast agents have a relaxivity that predominately causes a shortened T1, or longitudinal relaxation effect [18]. The Gd ion has a high relaxivity owing to its magnetic dipolar interactions with water; however, its toxicity requires the Gd ion to be highly complexed to ensure elimination from the body [16,19]. Chelating the Gd ion makes it safer for humans, but may lower its potential relaxivity. Gd-chelate contrast agents must be designed carefully for patient safety, while maintaining the relaxivity benefits of the agent. Currently the extracellular Gd-chelates that tumble slowly have been showing a higher relaxivity than chelates that have a faster tumbling speed [19]. Size of the molecule also can be a factor in relaxivity of an agent. Rigid macromolecular paramagnetic complexes have a long $1/T1$ time and result in high relaxivity [15,19].

The relaxivity of a compound depends on the compound's magnetic moment, electron spin relaxation time, and molecular interaction [15]. Gd-chelate contrast agents shorten T1 relaxation of blood, resulting in bright vascular signal on T1-weighted pulse sequences. Bright or positive enhancing agents have unpaired electrons that can be 18,000 times stronger than the hydrogen nucleus [15]. At low concentrations, paramagnetic agents are positive enhancers; however, at high concentrations, paramagnetic agents can cause significant T2* shortening effects, which can overpower the T1 contributions such that an actual decrease in vascular signal may be seen. Clinically, this T2* effect is seen most commonly as a result of a fast contrast injection rate (eg, >3 mL/sec), urinary concentration of Gd in the renal collecting system and bladder, or concentration of Gd in the central veins during the arterial phase imaging of a left antecubital venous injection [20].

Negative enhancing contrast agents work in a slightly different manner. The strong paramagnetic elements produce a localized disturbance in the magnetic field homogeneity, causing rapid dephasing of spins [15]. This disturbance causes the T2 and T2* relaxation times to decrease, resulting in local signal loss or negative enhancement. This type of negative enhancement that relies on "outer sphere" or rapid dephasing effect generally is best used with gradient echo or T2-weighted sequences [15,16].

The development of contrast agents is tied closely to pulse sequence design, which has confounded further the Food and Drug Administration approval process for many contrast agents. This is particularly true as the technical developments in MR imaging have accelerated greatly in recent years with rapid improvements in gradient performance, pulse sequence design, parallel imaging, and fast receiver technologies, which not only have revolutionized the speed of image acquisition, but also have changed the paradigms for CE MR angiography in clinical practice.

Vascular imaging considerations

Contrast agents for cardiovascular applications can be divided into several broad categories (Table 1). The first category comprises extracellular contrast agents, or the traditional Gd-chelate contrast agents, most of which are commercially available. These agents also are called *first-pass* or *nonspecific* agents and are relatively smaller in size. They have relatively shorter intravascular duration secondary to quick extravascular distribution into adjacent background tissues and urinary excretion within minutes of intravenous administration.

The next class of contrast agents comprises blood pool agents, also called *intravascular* contrast agents [21]. Blood pool agents preferentially remain within the vasculature at a fairly constant enhancement level for minutes (eg, >30 minutes) to hours after injection. Blood pool contrast agents are characterized by very slow or negligible diffusion across the capillary bed, which is attributed to their size or permeability coefficient [5,15,22]. By remaining principally within the blood pool, these agents can prolong the window of opportunity for CE MR angiography. The prolonged imaging window allows for not only high spatial resolution CE MR angiography, but also for the ability to perform CE MR angiography over different vascular regions during the same examination or for the ability to evaluate vascular disease over lengthened periods.

The third category of potential cardiovascular contrast agents targets specific tissues or lesions. These targeted agents specifically localize to a particular marker that may be associated with cardiovascular pathology, such as a component within thrombi or an atherosclerotic plaque. These contrast agents by virtue of their selective binding to tissue components also can be considered molecular imaging compounds.

Most contrast agents fall into one of the aforementioned three categories; however, some newer contrast agents have more than one effect. These agents may be considered hybrids and fall partially between categories. Some newer

Table 1
Select potential vascular contrast agents

Extracellular agents			Blood pool agents			Targeted/ smart agents
Traditional	Weak protein interaction	1 M concentrated	Strong protein interaction	Superparamagnetic iron oxides	Other macromolecular	
Gadodiamide (Omniscan)	Gd-BOPTA (MultiHance)	Gadobutrol (Gadovist)	B-22956	AMI-7228 (Ferumoxytol)	Gadofluorine-8	EP-2104R
Gadoteridol (ProHance)			MnDPDP	Ferumoxide (Feridex)	Gadomeritol (Vistarem)	
Gadoversetamide (OptiMARK)			MP-2269	NC100150 (Clariscan)	Gd-DTPA-17,24 (Gadomer-17)	
Gd-DOTA (Dotarem)			MS-325	P717 P760	Gd-DTPA-PEG MnHA/PEG-APD	
Gd-DTPA (Magnevist)				SH U 555 C (Supravist)	NMS60	

Gd-chelate contrast agents have been found to have various protein binding properties and have exhibited properties of an extracellular agent and a blood pool agent. One of these Gd-chelate contrast agents, Gadobenate dimeglumine (Gd-BOPTA) (MultiHance) also has hepatobiliary uptake. Conversely, blood pool agents also can be injected rapidly to enable first-pass arterial phase MR angiography techniques. Based on a review of the published literature and communication with various pharmaceutical company representatives, Table 2 summarizes some promising MR contrast agents for future body MR angiography.

Extracellular agents

Five low-molecular-weight (<1000 Da), extracellular Gd-chelate contrast agents currently are approved in the United States for neurologic and general body applications (see Table 2). Extracellular agents are used primarily for their T1 shortening effects and have become widely used for routine clinical 3D CE MR angiography. Numerous studies have shown their diagnostic effectiveness [8–11], and use of extracellular agents has been endorsed by at least one professional society [12]. Extracellular Gd agents generally are cleared from the circulatory system within 15 to 30 minutes of their injection. The usefulness of extracellular agents for MR angiography is based primarily on their effects during their first pass through the circulatory system. This basis for use results in several imaging limitations [23,24]. First, the duration of T1 shortening effects limits the acquisition window available for imaging, which by default also restricts the achievable spatial resolution of CE MR angiography. Second, the achievable T1 shortening effects (and vascular CNR) are limited by safety concerns related to contrast injection rates, T2* concerns, and maximal deliverable dose concerns. Third, optimized vascular illustration requires that timing and duration of image acquisition are coordinated with the period of peak vascular concentration of the contrast agent within the targeted vascular bed.

As described throughout this issue, CE MR angiography using current commercially available Gd-chelate contrast agents not only is reliable and accurate, but also easy to perform on almost all MR scanners using standard equipment and software (see Fig. 1). The rapid clearance of extracellular contrast agents is not detrimental because it enables the use of additional doses of contrast media for multiple different injections, assuming each injection is relatively small (eg, 0.1 mmol/kg dose each). Faster acquisition schemes and improved timing have enabled diagnostic quality MR angiography using smaller Gd-chelate doses such that multiple CE MR angiography scans of different regions can be performed in the same examination. In addition, the ability to perform MR angiography using lower doses has enabled more imaginative use of contrast agents for multiple evaluations, such as inclusion of MR colonography or myocardial perfusion during the same examination [25]. Most extracellular agents have roughly 40% to 50% of their concentration diffuse into the interstitium during the first pass through the circulatory system, however [15,26]. With each contrast injection, there is an accompanying increase in background signal and an inherent limitation on the achievable CNR of each successive CE application. These agents also are excreted from the body (primarily through glomerular filtration) faster than other agents, resulting in urinary contamination of later images.

A newer extracellular agent is a 1 M Gd-chelate, gadobutrol (Gadovist), which is available in Europe but not in the United States. Gadobutrol has double the concentration of Gd compared with conventional extracellular contrast agents [27,28]. An investigation by Knopp et al [21] found the higher concentration and smaller volume to be useful for ultrafast, multiphase pulmonary imaging. Some investigators [29–31] have proposed that gadobutrol may be better suited for first-pass CE MR angiography because its smaller volume for the same dose of Gd produces a "tighter" bolus and less venous contamination (Figs. 2 and 3). This agent also may be theoretically beneficial for the delivery of higher concentrations of Gd in patients with poor venous access in whom faster injection rates may not be clinically feasible; this is particularly true in pediatric patients.

Extracellular contrast agents with weak protein interaction

Extracellular contrast agents with weak protein interaction retain many of the qualities of traditional extracellular contrast agents but have additional benefits. Gd-BOPTA is one such agent that interacts with serum proteins in vivo [32].

Gd-BOPTA, approved in the United States for neurologic imaging, has a small molecular size, but also exhibits a weak, reversible binding to serum proteins. The weak protein interaction results in its persistence within vessels as seen in macromolecules. Clinical evaluations comparing Gd-BOPTA with other traditional Gd-chelate contrast agents (eg, Gd-diethylenetriaminepenta-acetic acid [DTPA]) have shown Gd-BOPTA to have increased T1 relaxivity (signal enhancement) and a prolonged duration for vascular enhancement—qualities ideal for CE MR angiography (Fig. 4) [32–34].

Blood pool agents

Blood pool contrast agents differ from extracellular agents by having a prolonged intravascular enhancement time (generally >30 minutes to hours) [15,35]. Similar to extracellular contrast agents, most blood pool agents also can be imaged during their first pass, but their main advantage is prolonged intravascular duration, which allows for higher spatial resolution imaging during the steady-state or equilibrium phase [15]. This longer enhancement period provides the operator the option to perform multiple high spatial resolution vascular scans of various body regions without the need for additional injections of contrast agent or concerns related to timing, as when using traditional extracellular Gd-chelate contrast agents. Blood pool agents also may play an important functional role. The assessment of blood volume, perfusion abnormalities, or oncologic applications may be improved by blood pool agents because they distribute primarily in the intravascular space instead of rapidly diffusing across the capillary beds into the interstitial space [36].

The main limitation of blood pool agents is that arteries and veins are well illustrated during the steady state (Fig. 5) [37]. In regions where the arteries and veins are intimately situated, such as within the calf and feet, proper segmentation of arteries from veins may be difficult or almost impossible. With higher spatial resolution imaging and improved computer segmentation tools, however, proper segmentation may not be as problematic in the near future [37,38].

Blood pool agents present unique clinical opportunities. One clinical application for blood pool agents may be for the detection of an occult bleeding site, such as may be the case in a gastrointestinal bleed. Currently, detection of an occult bleeding site is performed scintigraphically using tagged red blood cells, and imaging can be performed intermittently up to 18 to 24 hours postinjection [39]. In this case, the vascular persistence of a blood pool agent and MR imaging would be beneficial for detection over time. Another potential application of blood pool agents is the assessment of postoperative bleeding or extravascular leaks, such as an endoleak (Fig. 6) [40].

Not all blood pool agents are similar. Each blood pool agent is made to take advantage of various structures and functions of the vascular components—blood cells, plasma proteins, water, and vessel walls [19,22]. Some blood pool agents may be smaller molecules that interact or bind with a blood component to form macromolecules (eg, MS-325), which because of their size are retained within the circulation or are designed in such a way as to have slow diffusion across the capillary membrane [22]. Some blood pool agents are inherently large molecules (eg, ultrasmall superparamagnetic iron oxide agents [USPIOs]), with slow or no diffusion from vessels. A main concern for blood pool agents is their biologic half-life because ultimately their elimination from the body is desired. Persistence of a diagnostic contrast agent generally is not wanted because of potential toxicities or possibly its interference with other therapies or other MR evaluations. Blood pool agents, similar to other contrast agents, must be designed carefully not only for efficacy, but also for human safety, and timely biologic elimination is crucial.

Strong protein interacting agents

Several agents are currently in development that can become macromolecules after being injected into the blood plasma owing to their interactions with serum proteins [22,41]. These paramagnetic macromolecules are complexed through reversible interactions with blood serum proteins, such as albumin [35,42–44]. These interactions allow the macromolecules to reside in the vascular circulation for a longer time and allow for the agent to be eliminated from the body through the kidneys, reducing the toxicity risk compared with other blood pool agents [16]. Diphenylcyclohexl phosphodiester-Gd-DTPA (MS-325 or gadofosveset) (see Fig. 5) [44,45], 4-pentylbicyclo [2.2.2] octan-1-carboxyl-di-L-aspartyllysine-DTPA (MP-2269) [42,46–48], gadocoletic acid (B-22956) [49], and manganese dipyridoxyldiphosphate (MnDPDP) [50] are examples of strong protein interacting

Table 2
Overview of various contrast agents with current or potential use in cardiovascular imaging

Generic (trade name)	Vascular properties	Potential main use or targeted use(s)	Stage of development
Gadolinium agents			
Gadopentate dimeglumine, Gd-DTPA (Magnevist)	Extracellular	CNS/body	Commercially available
Gadoteridol (ProHance)	Extracellular	CNS/body	Commercially available
Gadodiamide (Omniscan)	Extracellular	CNS/body	Commercially available
Gadoversetamide (Optimark)	Extracellular	CNS/body	Commercially available
Gadobenate Dimeglumine, Gd-BOPTA (MultiHance)	Extracellular with weak protein interaction	CNS	Commercially available
Gadobutrol, gadolinium-DO3A-butriol (Gadovist)	Mainly extracellular	MRA	Commercially available (not in US)
Gadoterate meglumine, Gd-DOTA (Dotarem/Artirem)	Extracellular	CNS/body	Commercially available (not in US)
Gadofosveset (MS-325)	Blood pool agent	MRA and other applications	In registration (body MRA), phase II (cardiac, oncology applications)
Gadocoletic Acid (B-22956)	Blood pool agent	Coronary MRA	Phase II
Gadomeritol, P792 (Vistarem)	Blood pool agent	MRA	Phase II
Fibrin-binding peptide Gd chelate (EP-2104R)	Fibrin-binding molecular imaging agent	Thrombus in the body	Phase I
4-pentylbicyclo [2.2.2] octan-1-carboxyl-di-L-aspartyllysine-DTPA (MP-2269)	Nonaromatic small molecule blood pool agent	MRA	Preclinical
CH3-DTPA-Gd (NMS60)	Oligomer-based, weighted, super-extracellular fluid	MRA	Preclinical
Gadofluorine-8 (Gadofluorine)	Lymph imaging or blood pool agent	Atherosclerotic plaque imaging	Preclinical
Gadolinium-DOTA-dextran (P717)	Slow-clearance blood pool agent	MRA	Preclinical
Gd-DTPA-17, 24 cascade polymer (Gadomer-17)	Blood pool agent, cascade polymer	MRA vascularis, myocardium	Preclinical
Gadolinium - DTPA polyethylene glycol (Gd-DTPA-PEG)	Blood pool agent	MRA	Preclinical
Tetraazacyclodo decanetetraacetic acid DOTA (P760)	Macromolecular blood pool agent	MRA	Preclinical
Iron agents			
AMI 7228 (Ferumoxytol)	Ultrasmall superparamagnetic iron oxide	MRA contrast agent	Phase II
SH U 555 C, Ferucarbotran (Supravist)	Ultrasmall superparamagnetic iron oxide, blood pool agent	MRA	Phase I
Ferumoxides (Feridex)	Superparamagnetic iron oxide	Atherosclerotic plaque imaging	Preclinical
Feruglose, NC100150 (Clariscan)	Ultrasmall superparamagnetic iron oxide, blood pool agent	Cardiovascular imaging	Discontinued
Manganese agents			
Manganese dipyridoxyldiphosphate (MnDPDP)	Intracellular agent with protein binding	Myocardial viability	Preclinical
Manganese substituted hydroxylapatite (MnHA/PEG-APD)	Particle-based blood pool agent	MRA	Preclinical

Agents are grouped by central moiety; most of these agents still are undergoing clinical trial testing.
Abbreviations: CNS, central nervous system; MRA, magnetic resonance angiography.

Approximate vascular imaging time	Molecular size	Plasma half-life	Relaxivity (L/mmol · S-1)
First pass	Small (938 Da)	<20 min	r1 = 3.4 @ 1T
First pass	Small (559 Da)	<20 min	r1 = 3.7 @ 1T
First pass	Small (574 Da)	<20 min	r1 = 3.9 @ 1T
First pass	Small	<20 min	
First pass (+ hepatobiliary phase in liver)	Small (1058 Da)	<20 min	r1 = 4.6 @ 1T
First pass	Small (605 Da)	1.5 h	r1 = 3.6 @ 20 MHz
First pass	Small (560 Da)	41 min	r1 = 2.9 @ 60 MHz
1 h	Small (957 Da)	>4 h	r1 = 30–50 @ 1T
First pass blood pool	Small (1059 Da)	Approximately 7 h	
	6.47 Da		r1 = 29 @ 60 MHz
Blood persistent	Small (67 kDa)	142 min (rabbit)	
	2158 Da		r1 = 8.3 @ 1.5 T
Approximately 90 min	5 nm	28 min	r1 = 17 @ 1.5 T
	52 kDa	>180 min	r1 = 9.4 @ 60 MHz
Vessel = 10 min, myocardium = 30 min	Intermediate (30 kDa)		r1 = 11 @ 1T
			r1 = 6.0 @ 1T
	Intermediate (5.93 kDa)	59 min	r1 = 23.3 @ 60 MHz
	30 nm	10–14 h	r1 = 25 @ 0.47 T
First pass, plus 42 min equilibrium phase MRA	62 nm	3.9–5.8 h and 2.4–3.9 h	r1 = 24 @ 0.47 T
120 min	20 nm		
			r1 = 2.3 @ 1T
Blood persistent	Small particle	50 min (rabbit)	

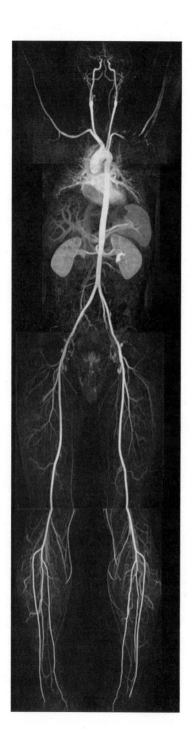

blood pool agents currently in human clinical trials. These agents have been found to be efficacious for first-pass imaging and steady-state imaging.

Macromolecular blood pool agents

Macromolecular blood pool agents are designed to remain primarily within the distribution of the blood vasculature because their size prevents normal diffusion across the capillary bed or through the glomerular endothelium [15]. Many macromolecular agents have been extracellular Gd agents that have been bound to albumin, dextran, or polylysine [36,51]. These agents are very large (43,000–94,000 Da) and have two to four times the relaxivity of extracellular agents [43,52,53].

The macromolecular agents currently in testing are designed primarily to have a Gd, manganese, or iron central moiety. Among the Gd-based agents are Gadomeritol (P792) [54,55], Gadomer-17 [56,57], NMS60 [58], Gd-DTPA-PEG [59], and Gadofluorine-8 [60,61]. An example of a macromolecular manganese agent is MnHA/PEG-APD [62], which is currently in early research. There are two main types of iron agents, superparamagnetic iron oxide agents (SPIOs) and USPIOs. SPIOs, such as monocrystalline iron oxide nanoparticles [63], are in early development. The USPIO agents have been receiving more attention as blood pool agents. SH U 555 C [64–67], AMI-7228 (Ferumoxytol) (see Fig. 6) [40,68], NC100 150 [69–72], P717 [41,73,74], and P760 [41,73–75] are among the USPIOs undergoing investigative studies that show potential for MR angiography. USPIOs have tended to have a high degree of T2* effect on first-pass imaging [13]. Further research into T2* effects with contrast agents undoubtedly will

Fig. 2. Whole-body 3D CE MR angiography using 1 M gadobutrol. Four stations were acquired using a bolus chase moving table acquisition technique synchronized with the arterial passage of a 20-mL dose of gadobutrol administered intravenously using a biphasic injection rate (1.3 mL/sec and 0.7 mL/sec) and a 30-mL saline flush injected at 0.7 mL/sec. Imaging was accelerated using multiple whole-body phased array coils and parallel imaging with an acceleration factor of 2. Note the good arterial signal and relative absence of venous contamination, especially in the calf, the last or terminal station of the bolus chase examination. (Courtesy of Bernd Tombach, MD, Department of Radiology, University of Muenster, Muenster, Germany.)

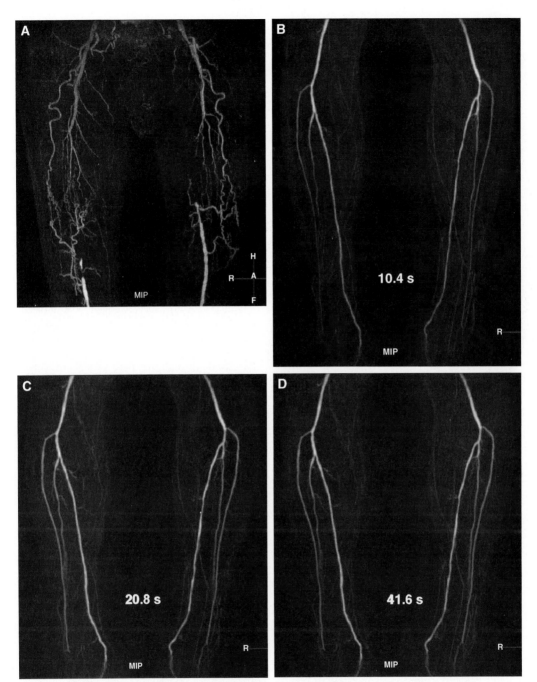

Fig. 3. (*A–E*) Time-resolved calf 3D CE MR angiography using a "keyhole" technique during an intravenous injection of 1 M of gadobutrol. In this patient with bilateral superficial femoral artery occlusion (*A,* coronal MIP from moving table 3D CE MR angiography), multiphase 3D CE MR angiography (*B–E,* select time points) of the calf was performed using a keyhole technique. The keyhole technique is an example of pulse sequence innovation whereby high temporal and high spatial resolution 3D data sets can be acquired by using a selective k-space sampling scheme that samples the central k-space data at a higher temporal rate. Individual 3D volumes for each central k-space time point are reconstructed using shared peripheral k-space data. This time-resolved method provides high spatial and high temporal resolution, enabling the excellent visualization of the arterial and venous enhancement of the calf vessels. (Courtesy of Bernd Tombach, MD, Department of Radiology, University of Muenster, Muenster, Germany.)

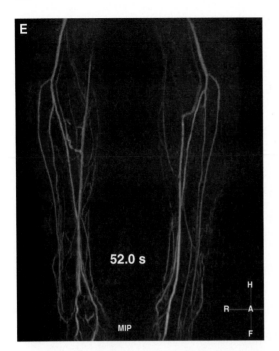

52.0 s

MIP

Fig. 3 (*continued*)

occur before USPIO agents become available for MR angiography.

Other contrast agents

Contrast agents that can be designed to target a particular tissue or pathologic entity could be valuable not only in MR angiography, but also for potentially therapeutic applications [19]. These agents could be designed to target the receptor sites on the cell surface or a tumor or other pathologic tissue. Safety reasons have mostly precluded cellular receptor binding because of metabolic equilibrium problems [19]. Cell surface targeting, labeled antibodies, receptor targeting, internalization, and direct imaging of gene expression are targeted agents in development. Targeted contrast agents may increase the specificity of MR imaging.

Gd-DTPA-labeled fibrinogen is a molecular agent in phase I clinical trials that is designed to target thrombus notably in the coronary arteries [76]. This agent is designed to take advantage of the local thrombosis that occurs in sites of

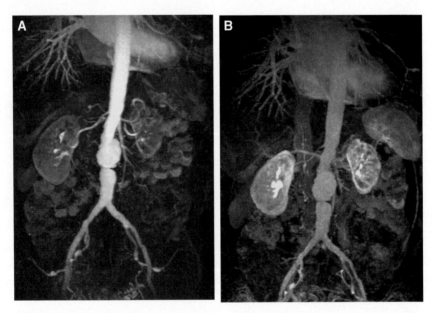

Fig. 4. (*A* and *B*) 3D CE MR angiography in a patient with an infrarenal abdominal aortic aneurysm using two different Gd-chelate contrast agents. One 3D CE MR angiography scan was performed with a 0.1-mmol/kg dose of Gd-BOPTA (*A*), and a second 3D CE MR angiography scan was performed with a 0.2-mmol/kg dose of Gd-DTPA (*B*). Although there are some differences in timing between acquisitions, the vascular signal using a single dose of the Gd-BOPTA is comparable to that using twice the dose of a traditional extracellular Gd-chelate contrast agent (Gd-DTPA). Gd-BOPTA has improved relaxivity, which is to some extent attributable to its weak protein interaction. As a result, relatively lower doses of Gd-BOPTA can be used to produce diagnostic 3D CE MR angiography. (Courtesy of Drs. Mathias Goyan and Stefan Ruehm, University Hospital Essen, Essen, Germany.)

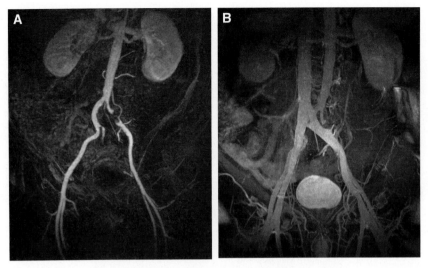

Fig. 5. Aortoiliac CE MR angiography using the blood pool agent MS-325 (gadofosveset). (*A*) Arterial phase CE MR angiography during the first pass of the contrast bolus illustrates the aortoiliac arteries. (*B*) Subsequent CE MR angiography during steady state depicts equally well the central abdominal veins and the aorta and its branches. (Courtesy of Dr. Mark Edelman and Epix Pharmaceuticals, Cambridge, MA.)

ruptured atherosclerotic plaque and the so-called white thrombi that forms in early acute coronary syndrome or acute in-stent thrombosis [76].

Two other groups of agents that can be used as targeted agents for thrombus imaging are the SPIOs and USPIOs. These agents can be used in quantifying monocytes that aggregate in atherosclerotic lesions [77,78]. It is theorized that the inflammatory process causes increased macrophage activity, and increase in proteases may contribute to the breakdown of the fibrous cap of the plaque [79,80]. SPIOs and USPIOs are contrast agents that can target monocyte recruitment into the atherosclerotic plaques, identifying plaque at risk for rupture and potential occlusion. This technique also could be used to assess the status of plaque burden in response to various therapies, such as statin medications [81]. The iron particles from these agents are absorbed by the atherosclerotic plaques via newly recruited monocytes [82,83]. The contrast injection is given 5 to 7 days before MR imaging, then high-resolution MR imaging of the vessels of interest is performed.

Smart contrast agents, as opposed to targeted contrast agents, depend on specific stimuli in the immediate environment for relaxivity [19]. Temperature or pH sensitivity, oxygen pressure response, enzyme response, and metal ion concentration dependency are a few examples of local environmental conditions that can be exploited to cause contrast enhancement [19].

Summary

The future of CE MR angiography is full of a wide variety of imaging options, from time-resolved CE MR angiography, to steady-state high-resolution imaging, to tissue-specific imaging. The growth in the complexity of contrast agent formulation for CE MR angiography and improvements in pulse sequence design are providing countless opportunities for improved applications of MR imaging and MR angiography for the evaluation of cardiovascular disease. In the 1990s, tremendous growth in the clinical use of MR angiography occurred, notably with the invention of CE MR angiography. It is hoped and expected that this growth will continue as these agents become commercially available for MR angiography.

Acknowledgments

The authors thank the following pharmaceutical vendors and representatives for their assistance in the compilation of the agents listed in this article: Advanced Magnetics, Inc.—Paula Jacobs; Berlex Laboratories—Fran Kashanian; Bracco—Miles

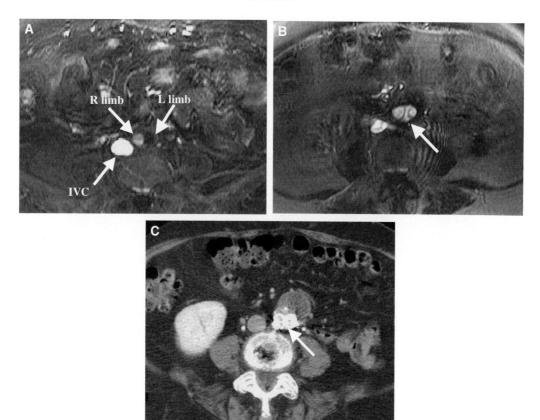

Fig. 6. An example of an endoleak in an 83-year-old woman. (*A*) At 8 minutes after injection of AMI-7228 (ferumoxytol), no signal is seen in the left lower limb graft, where it was buttressed by a cobalt alloy wall stent on axial MR angiography with fat suppression. IVC, inferior vena cava. (*B*) On arterial phase MR angiography at a slightly more proximal location, a tiny endoleak (*arrow*) is noted at the level of the graft bifurcation. (*C*) On arterial phase CT angiography, a metallic artifact caused by the graft obscures visualization of the endoleak area (*arrow*). (Courtesy of Hale Ersoy and Martin Prince, Department of Radiology, Weill Medical College of Cornell University.)

Kirchin; Epix Pharmaceuticals—Robert Weisskoff and Andrea Wiethoff; GE Healthcare—Tom Coogan; Tyco Healthcare—Peri Periasamy.

References

[1] Wedeen VJ, Rosen BR, Chesler D, Brady TJ. MR velocity imaging by phase display. J Comput Assist Tomogr 1985;9:530–6.

[2] Wedeen VJ, Meuli RA, Edelman RR, et al. Projective imaging of pulsatile flow with magnetic resonance. Science 1985;230:946–8.

[3] Runge VM. Safety of approved MR contrast media for intravenous injection. J Magn Reson Imaging 2000;12:205–13.

[4] Runge VM, Knopp MV. Off-label use and reimbursement of contrast media in MR. J Magn Reson Imaging 1999;10:489–95.

[5] Knopp MV, von Tengg-Kobligk H, Floemer F, Schoenber SO. Contrast agents for MRA: future directions. J Magn Reson Imaging 1999;10:314–6.

[6] Runge AM. Safety of magnetic resonance contrast media. Top Magn Reson Imaging 2001;12:309–14.

[7] Marti-Bonmati L, Vega T, Benito C, et al. Safety and efficacy of Omniscan (gadodiamide injection) at 0.1 mmol/kg for MRI in infants younger than 6 months of age: phase III open multicenter study. Invest Radiol 2000;35:141–7.

[8] Tan KT, van Beek EJ, Brown PW, van Delden OM, Tijssen J, Ramsay LE. Magnetic resonance angiography for the diagnosis of renal artery stenosis: a meta-analysis. Clin Radiol 2002;57: 617–24.

[9] Vasbinder GB, Nelemans PJ, Kessels AG, Kroon AA, de Leeuw PW, van Engelshoven JM. Diagnostic tests for renal artery stenosis in patients suspected of having renovascular hypertension: a meta-analysis. Ann Intern Med 2001;135:401–11.

[10] Nelemans PJ, Leiner T, de Vet HC, van Engelshoven JM. Peripheral arterial disease: meta-analysis of the diagnostic performance of MR angiography. Radiology 2000;217:105–14.

[11] Koelemay MJ, Lijmer JG, Stoker J, Legemate DA, Bossuyt PM. Magnetic resonance angiography for the evaluation of lower extremity arterial disease: a meta-analysis. JAMA 2001;285:1338–45.

[12] Yucel EK, Anderson CM, Edelman RR, et al. A scientific statement: magnetic resonance angiography: update on applications for extracranial arteries. Circulation 1999;100:2284–301.

[13] Knopp MV, Kirchin MA. Contrast agents for magnetic resonance angiography: current status and future perspectives. In: Schneider G, Prince MR, Meaney JF, Ho VB, editors. Magnetic resonance angiography: techniques, indications and practicalapplications. Milan (Italy): Springer-Verlag; 2004. p. 67–80.

[14] Runge VM. A review of contrast media research in 1999–2000. Invest Radiol 2001;36:123–30.

[15] Brasch RC. New directions in the development of MR imaging contrast media. Radiology 1992;183:1–11.

[16] Adzamil K, Spiller M, Koenig SH. Water-proton relaxation by a noncovalent albumin-binding gadolinium chelate: an NMRD study of a potential blood pool agent. Acad Radiol 2002;9:S11–6.

[17] Prince MR. Gadolinium-enhanced MR aortography. Radiology 1994;191:155–64.

[18] Runge VM. Contrast media—basic principles. The CMRS Vision 1998;December:17–23.

[19] Jacques V, Desreux JF. New classes of MRI contrast agents. Top Curr Chem 2002;221:123–64.

[20] Tirkes AT, Rosen MA, Siegelman ES. Gadolinium susceptibility artifact false positive stenosis isolated to the proximal common carotid artery in 3D dynamic contrast medium enhanced MR angiography of the thorax—a brief review of causes and prevention. Int J Cardiovasc Imaging 2003;19:151–5.

[21] Knopp MV, von Tengg-Kobligk H, Floemer F, Schoenberg SO. Contrast agents for MRA: future directions. J Magn Reson Imaging 1999;10:314–6.

[22] Schalla S, Higgins CB, Saeed M. Contrast agents for cardiovascular magnetic resonance imaging: current status and future directions. Drugs RD 2002;3:285–302.

[23] Svensson J, Petersson S, Stahlberg F, Larsson EM, Leander P, Olsson LE. Image artifacts due to a time-varying contrast medium concentration in 3D contrast-enhanced MRA. J Magn Reson Imaging 1999;10:919–28.

[24] Ho VB, Foo TKF, Czum JM, Marcos H, Choyke PL, Knopp MV. Contrast-enhanced magnetic resonance angiography: technical considerations for optimized clinical implementation. Top Magn Reson Imaging 2001;12:283–99.

[25] Goyen M, Goehde SC, Herborn CU, et al. MR-based full-body preventative cardiovascular and tumor imaging: technique and preliminary experience. Eur Radiol 2004;14:783–91.

[26] Weinmann HJ, Brasch RC, Press WR, Wesby GE. Characteristics of gadolinium-DTPA complex: a potential NMR contrast agent. AJR Am J Roentgenol 1984;142:619–24.

[27] Goyen M, Herborn CU, Florian MV, et al. Using a 1 M Gd-chelate (gadobutrol) for total-body three-dimensional MR angiography: preliminary experience. J Magn Reson Imaging 2003;17:565–71.

[28] Fink C, Bock M, Kiessling F, et al. Time-resolved contrast-enhanced three-dimensional pulmonary MR-angiography: 1.0 M gadobutrol vs. 0.5 M gadopentetate dimeglumine. J Magn Reson Imaging 2004;19:202–8.

[29] Leung DA, Hagspiel KD, Angle JF, Spinosa DJ, Matsumoto AH, Butty S. MR angiography of the renal arteries. Radiol Clin North Am 2002;40:847–65.

[30] Tombach B. Whole-body CE-MRA with Gadovist. Eur Radiol 2004;14(Suppl 5):M26–7.

[31] Tombach B. 1 M Gd-chelates for MRA—a 3 year experience in clinical routine [abstract]. Program of the 2004 Magnetic Resonance Angiography Workshop. London, Ontario, Canada, 2004. p. 84.

[32] Cavagna FM, Maggioni F, Castelli PM, et al. Gadolinium chelates with weak binding to serum proteins: a new class of high-efficiency, general purpose contrast agents for magnetic resonance imaging. Invest Radiol 1997;32:780–96.

[33] Knopp MV, Giesel FL, von Tengg-Kobligk H, et al. Contrast-enhanced MR angiography of the run-off vasculature: intraindividual comparison of gadobenate dimeglumine with gadpentetate dimeglumine. J Magn Reson Imaging 2003;17:694–702.

[34] Knopp MV, Schoenberg SO, Rehm C, et al. Assessment of gadobenate dimeglumine for magnetic resonance angiography: phase I studies. Invest Radiol 2002;37:706–15.

[35] Saeed M, Wendland MF, Higgins CB. Blood pool MR contrast agents for cardiovascular imaging. J Magn Reson Imaging 2000;12:890–8.

[36] Schmiedl U, Brasch RC, Ogan MD, Mosely ME. Albumin labeled with Gd-DTPA: an intravascular contrast-enhancing agent for magnetic resonance blood pool and perfusion imaging. Acta Radiol 1990;S374:99–102.

[37] van Bemmel CM, Wink O, Verdonck B, Viergever MA, Niessen WJ. Blood pool contrast-enhanced MRA: improved arterial visualization in the steady state. IEEE Trans Med Imaging 2003;22:645–52.

[38] van Bemmel CM, Spreeuwers LJ, Viergever MA, Niessen WJ. Level-set-based artery-vein separation in blood pool agent CE-MR angiograms. IEEE Trans Med Imaging 2003;22:1224–34.

[39] Gupta H, Weissleder R, Bogdanov AA Jr, Brady TJ. Experimental gastrointestinal hemorrhage: detection with contrast-enhanced MR imaging and scintigraphy. Radiology 1995;196:239–44.

[40] Ersoy H, Jacobs P, Kent CK, Prince MR. Blood pool MR angiography of aortic stent-graft endoleak. AJR Am J Roentgenol 2004;182:1181–6.

[41] Weinmann HJ, Bauer H, Ebert W, et al. Comparative studies on the efficacy of MRI contrast agents in MRA. Acad Radiol 2002;9:S135–6.

[42] Wallace RA, Haar JP, Miller DB, et al. Synthesis and preliminary evaluation of MP-2269: a novel, nonaromatic small-molecule blood-pool MR contrast agent. Magn Reson Med 1998;40:733–9.

[43] Vexler VS, Clement O, Schmitt-Willich H, Brasch RC. Effect of varying the molecular weight of the MR contrast agent Gd-DTPA-polylysine on blood pharmacokinetics and enhancement patterns. J Magn Reson Imaging 1994;4:381–8.

[44] Parmelee DJ, Walovitch RC, Ouellet HS, Lauffer RB. Preclinical evaluation of the pharmacokinetics, biodistribution, and elimination of MS-325, a blood pool agent for magnetic resonance imaging. Invest Radiol 1997;32:741–7.

[45] Stuber M, Botnar RM, Danias PG, et al. Contrast agent-enhanced, free-breathing three-dimensional coronary magnetic resonance angiography. J Magn Reson Imaging 1999;10:790–9.

[46] Ni Y, Adzamli K, Miao Y, et al. MRI contrast enhancement of necrosis by MP-2269 and gadophrin-2 in a rat model of liver infarction. Invest Radiol 2001;36:97–103.

[47] Flacke S, Allen JS, Chia JM, et al. Characterization of viable and nonviable myocardium at MR imaging: comparison of gadolinium-based extracellular and blood pool contrast materials versus manganese-based contrast materials in a rat myocardial infarction model. Radiology 2003;226:731–8.

[48] Adzamli K, Toth E, Periasamy MP, Koenig SH, Merbach AE, Adams MD. H-NMRD and O-NMR assessment of water exchange and rotational dynamics of two potential MRI agents: MP-1177 (an extracellular agent) and MP-2269 (a blood pool agent). MAGMA 1999;8:163–71.

[49] Paetsch I, Huber M, Bornstedt A, et al. Improved three-dimensional free-breathing coronary magnetic resonance angiography using gadocoletic acid (B-22956) for intravascular contrast enhancement. J Magn Reson Imaging 2004;20:288–93.

[50] Bremerich J, Saeed M, Arheden H, Higgins CB, Wendland MF. Normal and infracted myocardium: differentiation with cellular uptake of manganese at MR imaging in a rat model. Radiology 2000;216: 524–30.

[51] Kroft LJM, de Roos A. Blood pool contrast agents for cardiovascular MR imaging. J Magn Reson Imaging 1999;10:395–403.

[52] Loubeyre P, Ahao S, Canet E, Benderbous HAS, Revel D. Ultrasmall superparamagnetic iron oxide particles (AMI 227) as a blood pool contrast agent for MR angiography: experimental study in rabbits. J Magn Reson Imaging 1997;7:958–62.

[53] Schwitter J, Saeed M, Wendland MF, et al. Influence of severity of myocardial injury on distribution of macromolecules: extravascular versus intravascular gadolinium-based magnetic resonance contrast agents. J Am Coll Cardiol 1997;30:1086–94.

[54] Ruehm SG, Christina H, Violas X, Corot C, Debatin JF. MR angiography with a new rapid-clearance blood pool agent: initial experience in rabbits. Magn Reson Med 2002;48:844–51.

[55] Dirksen MS, Kaandorp TAM, Lamb HJ, Doornbos J, Corot C, de Roos A. Three-dimensional navigator coronary MRA with the aid of a blood pool agent in pigs: improved image quality with inclusion of the contrast agent first-pass. J Magn Reson Imaging 2003;18:502–6.

[56] Gerber BL, Bluemke DA, Chin BB, et al. Single-vessel coronary artery stenosis: myocardial perfusion imaging with gadomere-17 first-pass MR imaging in a swine model of comparison with gadopentetate dimeglumine. Radiology 2002;225:104–12.

[57] Clarke SE, Weinmann HJ, Lucas AR, Rutt BK. Comparison of two blood pool contrast agents for 0.5-T MR angiography: experimental study in rabbits. Radiology 2000;214:787–94.

[58] Bammer R, de Crespigny AJ, Howard D, et al. A comparative evaluation of CH3-DTPA-Gd (NMS60) for contrast enhanced magnetic resonance angiography. Magn Reson Imaging 2004;22:619–24.

[59] Li KC, Pelc LR, Napel SA, et al. MRI of pulmonary embolism using Gd-DTPA-polyethylene glycol polymer enhanced 3D fast gradient echo technique in a canine model. Magn Reson Imaging 1997;15: 543–50.

[60] Misselwitz B, Platzek J, Weinmann HJ. Early MR lymphography with gadofluorine M in rabbits. Radiology 2004;231:682–8.

[61] Barkhausen J, Ebert W, Heyer C, Debatin JF, Weinmann HJ. Detection of atherosclerotic plaque with gadofluorine-enhanced magnetic resonance imaging. Circulation 2003;108:605–9.

[62] Adzamli K, Dorshow RB, Hynes MR, Nosco DL, Adams MD. Characterization of polyethylenglycol-stabilized, manganese-substituted hydroxylaptite (MnHA-PEG): a potential MR blood pool agent. Acta Radiol 1997;412(Suppl):73–8.

[63] Krause MHJ, Kwong KK, Gragoudas ES, Young LHY. MRI of blood volume with superparamagnetic iron in choroidal melanoma treated with thermotherapy. Magn Reson Imaging 2004;22: 779–87.

[64] Tombach B, Reimer P, Mahler M, Ebert W, Pering C, Heindel W. First-pass and equilibrium phase MRA following intravenous bolus injection of SH U 555 C: phase I clinical trial in elderly volunteers with risk factors for arterial vascular disease. Acad Radiol 2002;9:S425–7.

[65] Wacker FK, Reither K, Ebert W, Wendt M, Lewin JS, Wolf KJ. MR image-guided endovascular procedures with the ultrasmall superparamagnetic iron oxide SH U 555 C as an intravascular contrast agent: study in pigs. Radiology 2003;26:459–64.

[66] Reimer P, Bremer C, Allkemper T, et al. Myocardial perfusion and MR angiography of chest with SH U 555 C: results of placebo-controlled clinical phase I study. Radiology 2004;231:474–81.

[67] Reimer P, Allkemper T, Matuszewski L, Balzer T. Contrast-enhanced 3D-MRA of the upper abdomen with a bolus-injectable SPIO (SH U 555 A). J Magn Reson Imaging 1999;10:65–71.

[68] Le Duc G, Vader Elst L, Colet JM, et al. Ultrasmall particulate iron oxide as contrast agents for magnetic resonance spectroscopy: a dose effect study. J Magn Reson Imaging 2001;13:619–26.

[69] Klein C, Schalla S, Schnackenberg B, et al. Improvement of image quality of non-invasive coronary artery imaging with magnetic resonance by the use of the intravascular contrast agent Clariscan (NC100150 injection) in patients with coronary artery disease. J Magn Reson Imaging 2003;17:656–62.

[70] Taylor AM, Panting JR, Keegan J, et al. Safety and preliminary findings with the intravascular contrast agent NC100150 injection for MR coronary angiography. J Magn Reson Imaging 1999;9:220–7.

[71] Schoenberg SO, Aumann S, Just A, et al. Quantification of renal perfusion abnormalities using an intravascular contrast agent (part 2): results in animals and humans with renal artery stenosis. Magn Reson Med 2003;49:288–98.

[72] Larsson EM, Sunden P, Olsson CG, et al. MR venography using an intravascular contrast agent: results from a multicenter phase 2 study of dosage. AJR Am J Roentgenol 2003;180:227–32.

[73] Corot C, Violas X, Robert P, Port M. Pharmacokinetics of three gadolinium chelates with different molecular sizes shortly after intravenous injection in rabbits: relevance to MR angiography. Invest Radiol 2000;35:213–8.

[74] Corot C, Violas X, Robert P, Port M. Arterial concentration profiles of two blood pool agents and Gd-DOTA after intravenous injection in rabbits. Acad Radiol 2002;9:S137–9.

[75] Port M, Corot C, Raynal I, et al. P760: a new gadolinium complex characterized by a low rate of interstitial diffusion. Acad Radiol 2002;9:S17–9.

[76] Botnar RM, Buecker A, Wiethoff AJ, et al. In vivo magnetic resonance imaging of coronary thrombosis using a fibrin-binding molecular magnetic resonance contrast agent. Circulation 2004;110:1463–6.

[77] Litovsky S, Modjid M, Zarrabi A, Casscells SW, Willerson JT, Naghavi M. Superparamagentic iron oxide-based method for quantifying recruitment of monocytes to mouse atherosclerotic lesions in vivo: enhancement by tissue necrosis factor-α, interleukin-1 β, and interferon-γ. Circulation 2003; 107:1545–9.

[78] Johansson LO, Bjornerud A, Ahlstrom HK, Ladd DL, Fuji DK. A targeted contrast agent for magnetic resonance imaging of thrombus: implications of spatial resolution. J Magn Reson Imaging 2001; 13:615–8.

[79] Shah PK, Falk E, Badimon JJ, et al. Human monocyte-derived macrophages induce collagen breakdown in fibrous caps of atherosclerotic plaques: potential role of matrix-degrading metalloproteinases and implications for plaque rupture. Circulation 1995;92:1565–9.

[80] Carr SC, Farb A, Pearce WH, Virmani R, Yao JS. Activated inflammatory cells are associated with plaque rupture in carotid artery stenosis. Surgery 1997; 122:757–63.

[81] Zhao XQ, Yuan C, Hatsukami TS, et al. Effects of prolonged intensive lipid-lowering therapy on the characteristics of carotid atherosclerotic plaques in vivo by MRI. Arterioscler Thromb Vasc Biol 2001; 21:1623–9.

[82] Kim CJ, Khoo JC, Gillotte-Taylor K, et al. Polymerase chain reaction-based method for qualifying recruitment of monocytes to mouse atherosclerotic lesions in vivo: enhancement by tumor necrosis factor-α and interleukin-1β. Arterioscler Thromb Vasc Biol 2000;20:1979–82.

[83] Rosenfeld ME. Leukocyte recruitment into developing atherosclerotic lesions: the complex interaction between multiple molecules keeps getting more complex. Arterioscler Thromb Vasc Biol 2002;22:361–3.

ELSEVIER
SAUNDERS

Magn Reson Imaging Clin N Am
13 (2005) 205–209

**MAGNETIC
RESONANCE
IMAGING CLINICS**
of North America

Index

Note: Page numbers of article titles are in **boldface** type.

A

Abdominal aorta, contrast-enhanced MR
angiography of, 65–69
three-dimensional, 69
dissection of, 81
MR angiography of, **65–89**
selected conditions of, MR angiography in,
79–85

Abdominal aortic aneurysm(s), incidence of, 79
MR angiography in, 79–81

Aneurysm(s), abdominal aortic, incidence of, 79
MA angiography in, 79–81
aortic, cine MR imaging of, 49–50, 51
MR imaging of, 56
coronary, in child, MR angiography in, 169
of thoracic aorta, MR imaging of, 59–60
thoracoabdominal, 81

Angiograms, magnetic resonance, interpretation
of, 29–30

Angiography, magnetic resonance. See *Magnetic
resonance angiography.*

Aorta, abdominal. See *Abdominal aorta.*
atherosclerosis of, MR imaging of, 174–175
coarctation of. See *Coarctation of aorta.*
dissection of. See *Aortic dissection.*
MR imaging of, transesophageal MR imaging
for, 175, 176
thoracic. See *Thoracic aorta.*
thoracoabdominal, MR imaging of, 60–61

Aortic aneurysm, cine MR imaging of, 49–50, 51
MR imaging in, 56

Aortic arch, anatomy of, 56–57
MR imaging of, 57

Aortic dissection, 80–81
abdominal aorta, 81
definition of, 81
in cystic medial necrosis, 54, 56
into iliac arteries, MR angiography in, 67–68
thoracoabdominal, MR angiography in, 80–81
with chest pain, MR aortography in, 41–42

Aortic root, MR imaging of, 52–54

Arterial occlusive disease, peripheral,
MR angiography in, 185–186

Artery(ies), carotid, atherosclerosis of,
MR imaging of, 173–174
coronary, imaging of, 17–19
MR angiography of, 52
MR imaging of, 54, 175–177
peripheral, MR angiography of, **91–111**
renal. See *Renal artery(ies).*
stenosis of, contrast-enhanced MR
angiography in, 106

Atherosclerosis, aortic, MR imaging of, 174–175
carotid, MR imaging of, 173–174
coronary, MR imaging of, 175–177
diffuse, 3-D contrast-enhanced
MR angiography in, 70, 71, 77
flow-limiting stenosis of, 171
incidence of, 171
intravascular MR imaging in, 177
MR imaging in, **171–180**
future of, 177–178
technical considerations for, 172
of lower extremity, axillary bifemoral bypass
graft in, 156
clinical presentations of, 153–154
diagnostic tools in, 154–157
future advances in, 158–159
hybrid contrast-enhanced MR angiography
in, 155
report on, 157–158
plaque in, morphology of, MR imaging to
assess, 172–173
MR imaging to characterize, 173
predisposing factors for, 91

Atherosclerotic renal artery stenosis, bilateral,
MR angiography in, 138–139
MR angiography in, 137–138, 141

C

Cardiac MR angiography, 17–19

1064-9689/05/$ - see front matter © 2005 Elsevier Inc. All rights reserved.
doi:10.1016/S1064-9689(05)00014-0

mri.theclinics.com

Carotid artery, atherosclerosis of, MR imaging of, 173–174

Celiac artery stenosis, with atherosclerosis, 82

Chest, veins of, thrombo-occlusive disease of, 119–120

Child(ren), coronary aneurysms in,
MR angiography in, 169
infants and, contrast-enhanced
MR angiography in, **161–170**

Circulation, infrapopliteal, venous enhancement in, MR imaging and, 98–99

Coarctation of aorta, 57, 58
functional MR angiography in, 185
time-resolved contrast-enhanced MR angiography in, 163, 164, 165–167

Collateral vessels, direct visualization of, by MR angiography, 181

Computed tomography, advantages of MR angiography over, 41

Congestive heart failure, MR angiography in, 184

Contrast agents, 189–191
blood pool, clinical opportunities with, 193
limitation of, 193
strong protein interacting, 193–196
extracellular, 192–193
with weak protein interaction, 192–193
first-pass, 191
for cardiovascular applications, 194–195
categories of, 191–192
for MR angiography, 105
innovations in, and applications for body MR angiography, **189–203**
intravascular, 191
macromolecular blood pool, 196–198

Contrast-enhanced MR angiography, 2, 95
and time-of-flight MR angiography, compared, 97
examination using, 3–5
hybrid, in atherosclerotic disease of lower extremity, 155
in arterial stenosis, 106
in infants and children, **161–170**
clinical applications of, 167–169
technical considerations in, 162
moving table, enhancements to, 99–107
of peripheral arteries, 96–98
of abdominal aorta, 65–69
of peripheral vasculature, 95
single-scan location studies in, 3, 4

three-dimensional, 45–49
contrast considerations for, 71–72
for periprocedural evaluation, 86
for renal transplant evaluation, 85, 86
image processing and interpretation for, 77
in presurgical roadmapping, 86
k-space acquisition schemes for, 76–77
of abdominal aorta, 69
of endovascular abdominal aortic aneurysm repair and graft surveillance, 86
patient positioning for, 69
phase-contrast imaging, 78–79
postcontrast gradient echo imaging, 77–78
pulse sequence selection and scan prescription for, 69–71
steady-state free precession, 78
timing options for, 72–76
three station moving table, 92
time-resolved, in coarctation of aorta, 163, 164, 165–167
two-dimensional, 100

Contrast-enhanced MR venography, three-dimensional, 119–122

Coronary aneurysms, in child, MR angiography in, 169

Coronary artery(ies), atherosclerosis of, MR imaging of, 175–177
imaging of, 17–19
MR angiography of, 52
MR imaging of, 54

Cystic medial necrosis, aortic dissection in, 54, 56

D

Diaphragm, descending thoracic aorta and, 60–61

Dynamic two-dimensional thick-slice projection, 5–6

E

Echo planer imaging, ultrafast flow measurements using, 183

Endoscopy, virtual vascular, and MR angiography, 27–28, 30

F

Fibrinogen, Gd-DTPA-labeled, 198–199

Fibromuscular dysplasia, MR angiography in, 82–84, 139–140

G

Gadobutrol, 194, 196, 197

Gadofosveset, 194, 199

Gadolinium, -chelate contrast agents, 189, 190

H

Heart failure, congestive, MR angiography in, 184

Hemodialysis shunts, MR angiography of, 146

Hepatic artery, replaced, MR angiography of, 83

Heterotaxy, MR angiography in, 166

Hypertension, 3-D contrast-enhanced
MR angiography in, 74–75
MR angiography in, 140, 142

I

In-flow MR angiography, 48–51

Infants, and children, contrast-enhanced
MR angiography in, **161–170**

Infrapopliteal circulation, venous enhancement
in, MR imaging and, 98–99

K

Kidneys, anatomy of, MR angiography and, 133
disease of. See *Renal disease.*

Kppel-Trenauny syndrome, MR venography in,
125

L

Leriche syndrome, MR angiography in, 66

Liver, transplantation of, MR imaging evaluation
for, 168

Lower extremity(ies), atherosclerotic disease of.
See *Atherosclerosis, of lower extremity.*
MR venography of, 122–125

M

Magnetic resonance angiograms, interpretation
of, 29–30

Magnetic resonance angiography, abdominal,
basic considerations for, 65–69
adjunctive techniques with, 49–52
advantages over computed tomography, 41
aortoiliac and femoropopliteal, 100, 106
black blood, 51–52, 79
bright blood, 49–51, 77–79

cardiac, 17–19
cine, of aortic aneurysm, 49–50, 51
contrast agents for, 105
contrast-enhanced. See *Contrast-enhanced
MR angiography.*
data processing and presentation in, 24–29
filters and zero-filling in, 24–25
functional, emerging techniques of, **181–188**
in aortic dissection, 185
in coarctation of aorta, 185
in-flow, 48–51
in renal disease. See *Renal disease.*
in vascular interventional planning, **153–160**
incidental findings in, 36–37
infrapopliteal, 100, 106
interpretation of, **23–40**
maximum intensity projection in, 26–27, 29
multiplanar reformation in, 26
multiple-scanning location, 11–15
multiple-station image stitching in, 29
multistation multi-injection, of peripheral
arteries, 95–96
of abdominal aorta, **65–89**
of coronary arteries, 52
of peripheral arteries, **91–111**
methodologies of, 94–98
relevant anatomy for, 91–93
scope of, 93–94
of thoracic aorta, 43–45, 52–57
parallel imaging in, 102
phase-contrast. See *Phase-contrast
MR angiography.*
physics of, **1–22**
pitfalls of, and artifacts on, 30–36
postprocessing in, 105–107
projection recontruction and, 9–10
receiver coils for, 105
"segmented" k-space approach for, 101
"shoot 'n' scoot" approach for, 101, 102
signal intensity and, 1, 2
single-station, of peripheral vasculature, 95,
96, 98
steady state free precession, 41–42
subsecond contrast-enhanced, 41–42
subtraction technique in, 25–26
surface rendering in, 27
technique of, 23–24
three-dimensional time-resolved acquisition
imaging of contrast kinetics, 101
three-dimentional reconstruction techniques
in, 26–29
time-of-flight, 1, 48–51, 94–95
and contrast-enhanced, compared, 97

Magnetic resonance angiography (*continued*)
  time-resolved. See *Time-resolved*
    MR angiography.
  tourniquets to slow circulation during,
    102–104
  universal, of peripheral arteries, 94
  universal goal of, 108
  vascular segmentation in, 29
  virtual vascular endoscopy and, 27–28, 30
  volume rendering in, 27

Magnetic resonance aortography, in aortic
  dissection with chest pain, 41–42

Magnetic resonance imaging, in atherosclerosis,
  171–180

Magnetic resonance renography, in renal disease,
  136

Magnetic resonance venography. See *Venography,*
  MR.

Marfan's syndrome, MR angiography in, 54, 55

Mesenteric ischemia, MR angiography in, 65, 66,
  82, 84–85

P

Peripheral arteries, MR angiography of, **91–111**

Phase-contrast MR angiography, 15–16, 95
  flow measurement with, 181–183
  three-dimensional, spin dephasing on, 183–184

Phase-contrast MR venography, 115

Portal venous system, abnormality of, MR
  angiography in, 186

Pulmonary embolism, MR angiography in, 186

Pulmonary venous return, repair of, subsecond
  MR angiography following, 162

R

Renal artery(ies), atherosclerotic stenosis of,
    bilateral, MR angiography in, 138–139
      MR angiography in, 137–138, 141
  dissection of, MR angiography in, 141–143
  stenosis of, functional MR angiography in, 185
    MR angiography in, 81–82
  supernumerary, MR angiography in, 84

Renal disease, MR angiography in, **131–151**
  applications of, 136–146
  flow measurements for, 134–135
  perfusion measurements for, 135–136
  renal anatomy and, 133

technical considerations in, 132–133
  techniques of, 132–136
  MR renography in, 136

Renal transplant(s), evaluation of, 3-D
  contrast-enhanced MR angiography for, 85, 86
    MR angiography for, 144–146
  surveillance of, MR angiography in, 85, 86

Renal vein, thrombosis of, MR angiography in,
  144

"Ringing artifact", 3-D contrast-enhanced
  MR angiography in, 76

S

Scimitar syndrome, MR angiography in, 165

Sinotubular junction, MR imaging of, 54, 55

Sinuses of Valsalva, MR imaging of, 52, 53

SPIOs, 199

Splenomegaly, MR angiography in, 169

Steady state free precession MR angiography,
  41–42

Subsecond contrast-enhanced angiography, 41–42

T

Takayasu arteritis, renal artery stenosis in, 140,
  143

Thoracic aorta, aneurysm of, MR imaging of,
    59–60
  ascending, MR imaging of, 54–56
  descending, diaphragm and, 60–61
    MR imaging of, 59–60
  MR angiography of, clinical considerations
    for, 43–45
  posttraumatic pseudoaneurysms of, 58, 59
  selected studies of, MR angiography of, 52–57

Thoracoabdominal aneurysms, 81

Thoracoabdominal aorta, MR imaging of, 60–61

Thoracoabdominal aortic dissection,
  MR angiography in, 80–81

Thromboembolic disease, venous, 113

Thrombo-occlusive disease, of veins of chest,
  119–120

Thrombosis, deep vein, MR venography in, 116,
  118, 123

Thrombus, direct imaging of, MR venography in,
  118–126

Time-of-flight effect, 1–2

Time-of-flight MR angiography, 1, 48–51,
94–95
and contrast-enhanced angiography,
compared, 97

Time-of-flight MR venography, 114–115

Time-resolved MR angiography, 5–6, 99–100,
184–185
contrast-enhanced, in coarctation of aorta,
163, 164, 165–167
fast three-dimensional imaging, 8–9
in infants and children, 162–167
of contrast kinetics, 6–8
parallel imaging, 10–11

Transesophageal MR imaging, for aortic
MR imaging, 175, 176

Transplants, renal. See *Renal transplant(s)*.

U

Upper extremity(ies), MR venography of,
119–122

USPIOs, 199

V

Vascular interventional planning, role
of MR angiography in, **153–160**

Vein(s), malformations of, MR venography in,
125–126
of chest, thrombo-occlusive disease of,
119–120
renal, thrombosis of, MR angiography in, 144

Vena cava, inferior, MR venography of, 122–125
superior, MR venography of, 119–122

Venography, MR, **113–129**
background of, 113
in direct thrombus imaging, 118–126
non-contrast-enhanced, 114
nonenhanced flow-independent sequences,
115–116
phase-contrast, 115
techniques for, 113
three-dimensional contrast-enhanced,
117–118
image analysis in, 118
pulse sequences in, 118
time-of-flight, 114–115

Venous thromboembolic disease, 113

Changing Your Address?

Make sure your subscription changes too! When you notify us of your new address, you can help make our job easier by including an exact copy of your Clinics label number with your old address (see illustration below.) This number identifies you to our computer system and will speed the processing of your address change. Please be sure this label number accompanies your old address and your corrected address—you can send an old Clinics label with your number on it or just copy it exactly and send it to the address listed below.

We appreciate your help in our attempt to give you continuous coverage. Thank you.

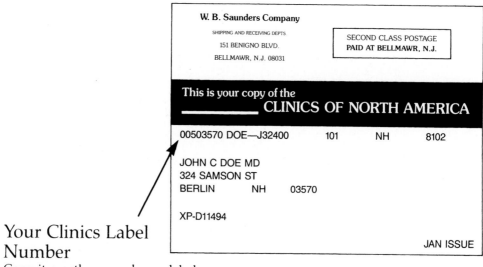

Your Clinics Label Number

Copy it exactly or send your label
along with your address to:
W.B. Saunders Company, Customer Service
Orlando, FL 32887-4800
Call Toll Free 1-800-654-2452

Please allow four to six weeks for delivery of new subscriptions and for processing address changes.

Practice, Current, Hardbound:
SATISFACTION GUARANTEED

❑ **Adolescent Medicine Clinics**
❑ Individual $95
❑ Institutions $133
❑ *In-training $48

❑ **Anesthesiology**
❑ Individual $175
❑ Institutions $270
❑ *In-training $88

❑ **Cardiology**
❑ Individual $170
❑ Institutions $266
❑ *In-training $85

❑ **Chest Medicine**
❑ Individual $185
❑ Institutions $285

❑ **Child and Adolescent Psychiatry**
❑ Individual $175
❑ Institutions $265
❑ *In-training $88

❑ **Critical Care**
❑ Individual $165
❑ Institutions $266
❑ *In-training $83

❑ **Dental**
❑ Individual $150
❑ Institutions $242

❑ **Emergency Medicine**
❑ Individual $170
❑ Institutions $263
❑ *In-training $85
❑ Send CME info

❑ **Facial Plastic Surgery**
❑ Individual $199
❑ Institutions $300

❑ **Foot and Ankle**
Individual $160
Institutions $232

❑ **Gastroenterology**
❑ Individual $190
❑ Institutions $276

❑ **Gastrointestinal Endoscopy**
❑ Individual $190
❑ Institutions $276

❑ **Hand**
❑ Individual $205
❑ Institutions $319

❑ **Heart Failure (NEW in 2005!)**
❑ Individual $99
❑ Institutions $149
❑ *In-training $49

❑ **Hematology/Oncology**
❑ Individual $210
❑ Institutions $315

❑ **Immunology & Allergy**
❑ Individual $165
❑ Institutions $266

❑ **Infectious Disease**
❑ Individual $165
❑ Institutions $272

❑ **Clinics in Liver Disease**
❑ Individual $165
❑ Institutions $234

❑ **Medical**
❑ Individual $140
❑ Institutions $244
❑ *In-training $70
❑ Send CME info

❑ **MRI**
❑ Individual $190
❑ Institutions $290
❑ *In-training $95
❑ Send CME info

❑ **Neuroimaging**
❑ Individual $190
❑ Institutions $290
❑ *In-training $95
❑ Send CME info

❑ **Neurologic**
❑ Individual $175
❑ Institutions $275

❑ **Obstetrics & Gynecology**
❑ Individual $175
❑ Institutions $288

❑ **Occupational and Environmental Medicine**
❑ Individual $120
❑ Institutions $166
❑ *In-training $60

❑ **Ophthalmology**
❑ Individual $190
❑ Institutions $325

❑ **Oral & Maxillofacial Surgery**
❑ Individual $180
❑ Institutions $280
❑ *In-training $90

❑ **Orthopedic**
❑ Individual $180
❑ Institutions $295
❑ *In-training $90

❑ **Otolaryngologic**
❑ Individual $199
❑ Institutions $350

❑ **Pediatric**
❑ Individual $135
❑ Institutions $246
❑ *In-training $68
❑ Send CME info

❑ **Perinatology**
❑ Individual $155
❑ Institutions $237
❑ *In-training $78
❑ Send CME info

❑ **Plastic Surgery**
❑ Individual $245
❑ Institutions $370

❑ **Podiatric Medicine & Surgery**
❑ Individual $170
❑ Institutions $266

❑ **Primary Care**
❑ Individual $135
❑ Institutions $223

❑ **Psychiatric**
❑ Individual $170
❑ Institutions $288

❑ **Radiologic**
❑ Individual $220
❑ Institutions $331
❑ *In-training $110
❑ Send CME info

❑ **Sports Medicine**
❑ Individual $180
❑ Institutions $277

❑ **Surgical**
❑ Individual $190
❑ Institutions $299
❑ *In-training $95

❑ **Thoracic Surgery (formerly Chest Surgery)**
❑ Individual $175
❑ Institutions $255
❑ *In-training $88

❑ **Urologic**
❑ Individual $195
❑ Institutions $307
❑ *In-training $98
❑ Send CME info

Order your subscription today. Simply complete and detach this card and drop it in the mail to receive the best clinical information in your field.